PENGUIN BOOKS

EVERYWOMAN

Derek Llewellyn-Jones OBE MD MAO FRCOG FRACOG is former Associate Professor of Obstetrics and Gynaecology at the University of Sydney. He is the author of numerous highly successful books including *Breastfeeding: How to Succeed* (1983), *Sexually Transmitted Diseases* (1990) and *Everywoman's Middle Years* (1992). He has also written medical textbooks including the standard work *Fundamentals of Obstetrics and Gynaecology.*

'The text is presented in elegant yet honest language, which neither irritates the informed reader, nor condescends to the lay reader; and this is no mean feat . . . Altogether a book which deserves to run into many editions, since it is undoubtedly a classic of its kind' – Claire Rayner

'A sensible, straightforward account of the way a woman's body works . . . in pregnancy and childbirth, at the menopause, in illness and after surgery' – Sheila Kitzinger

'Derek Llewellyn-Jones's brilliant gynaecological guide which contains the finest account of pregnancy and childbirth I have come across. Extending back to menstruation, forward to the menopause, *Everywoman* deals sensitively and thoroughly with every physical and psychological aspect of internal female development' – Jill Weldon, *Vogue*

By the same author

Fundamentals of Obstetrics and Gynaecology
Breast Feeding: How to Succeed
Sexually Transmitted Diseases
Everywoman's Middle Years

Everywoman

A Gynaecological Guide for Life

Derek Llewellyn-Jones

OBE, MD, MAO, FRCOG, FRACOG

New edition
fully revised and updated

PENGUIN BOOKS

PENGUIN BOOKS

Published by the Penguin Group
Penguin Books Ltd, 27 Wrights Lane, London W8 5TZ, England
Penguin Books USA Inc., 375 Hudson Street, New York, New York 10014, USA
Penguin Books Australia Ltd, Ringwood, Victoria, Australia
Penguin Books Canada Ltd, 10 Alcorn Avenue, Toronto, Ontario, Canada M4V 3B2
Penguin Books (NZ) Ltd, 182–190 Wairau Road, Auckland 10, New Zealand

Penguin Books Ltd, Registered Offices: Harmondsworth, Middlesex, England

First published by Faber and Faber 1971
Published in Faber Paperbacks 1972
Second edition 1978
Third edition 1982
Fourth edition 1986
Fifth edition 1989
Published in Penguin Books 1992
Sixth edition published in Penguin Books 1993
3 5 7 9 10 8 6 4 2

Printed in England by Clays Ltd, St Ives plc

National Library of Australia
Cataloguing-in Publication datta:

Llewellyn-Jones, Derek, 1923–
Everywoman: a gynaecological guide for life

6th ed.
includes index
ISBN 0 14 01705 3.

1. Gynaecology – Popular works.   2. Obstetrics – Popular works   3.
Women – Health and hygiene   4.Title

Contents

Illustrations

Illustrations by Susan Harniess and Lorraine Ellis

Tables

Preface

When *Everywoman* was published in 1971, I hoped that it would provide a helpful source of information for women who were interested in their bodies and in the changes which occur during each period of their lives. Judging from the gratifying sales of the book, my hope has been realized!

But because of changes in attitude to woman's role in society, and to her sexuality, and because medical science has made considerable advances in all fields of study, including obstetrics and gynaecology, a revised sixth edition is needed. In this edition I have made many alterations, including rewriting several of the chapters. I hope that the information is as up to date as possible.

It is my firm belief that modern woman is interested in her femininity and wants information which, all too often, she is not given when she consults a doctor. Although attitudes are changing, some doctors still behave in an authoritarian way (I'll tell the little woman as much as is good for her to know), rather than involving the woman in her own health care as an active participant.

Some readers have complained that I write 'he' when referring to a doctor, although about half of all medical students are women, and over 20 per cent of doctors are women. As it is clumsy to write 'he or she', I hope readers will take 'he' to include 'she'. This also applies to babies who have been called 'he' rather than 'it'. 'He' should be taken to include 'she'.

It also should be added that I neglected to state that in many places midwives conduct most of the antenatal care and when I write doctor, this term should be used to incorporate midwives. The same criticism applies to the care of a woman during the birthing process (Chapter 14). Often a midwife will be in charge, so that the word doctor should include midwife.

PREFACE

Once again I acknowledge the help I have received from interested readers, from Members of the Childbirth Education Association, the Australian Society of Obstetric Physiotherapists, the Nursing Mothers Association of Australia and from some of my colleagues, in preparing this new edition.

I am most grateful to Julia Sundin, childbirth educator and physio-therapist, for her considerable help in revising the section on 'Prepared Childbirth' (previously called Psychoprophylaxis) and the section on postnatal exercises.

DEREK LLEWELLYN-JONES

CHAPTER 1

A Woman is Different

A woman is obviously different from a man. The anatomical difference is clear but, as well, women have a different perception of many experiences, although how much this is due to prevailing cultural attitudes and how much to gender difference is not clear.

The anatomical differences are apparent at once, particularly in the development of a woman's breasts. Among Western communities, the breast has a unique sexual symbolism, and even if fashion diminishes its rotundity, the hemispherical mammary glands are a potent attraction for the male eye. In more primitive communities, where breasts are habitually exposed, they have little sexual connotation, being considered for what they are – a source of nourishment for the infant.

The more specific anatomical differences are of the genital organs. The male external genitals – the penis and the testicles – are absent in women, a fact which suggested to Freud that many of women's sexual problems related to an envy for the absent penis and a complex that the testicles had been castrated. Woman was therefore a mutilated male, and inferior to man. Freud was more than unfair to women, and considerably confused about women, possibly because of his own upbringing in a traditional Jewish middle-class family. He held that woman had a smaller intellectual capacity, a far greater vanity, a constitutional passivity, a weaker sexuality, and a greater disposition to neurosis. At the same time, he considered her enigmatic, her femininity a complicated process, her psychology involved. Studies over the past half-century have shown that Freud's view of woman as an inferior, mutilated male is incorrect, and his assessment of her inferiority and her instability is more an indictment of the cultural environment in which she is brought up, than of her inherited make-up. In other words, a woman behaves in a certain way because she is brought up to believe that society expects her to behave in that way. This does not imply that she is weaker or inferior to a man, even if both women and men are brought up by society to believe this. Indeed, longevity studies show that the female is stronger than the male, less likely to be aborted when in her mother's womb, more likely to be born alive, less likely to succumb to infection in the first years of life, and more likely to live beyond the age of 65.

Given the opportunity, a woman can succeed in most activities as well as a man, but in one activity she is unique. The human female is a mammal. She carries her infant in the womb until it is sufficiently well developed to survive, or at least to suck, she suckles it and cares for it. This process of internal development of the infant is only possible because the womb – or uterus – is in a protected position, enclosed by the strong bones of the female pelvis.

Although the uterus is central to the anatomical difference between male and female, the most obvious differences are those of the external genitalia, which will be described first. After that, the internal genital organs, the vagina, the uterus, the oviducts (Fallopian tubes) and the ovaries will be described, for if a woman has some idea of her anatomy, much of what follows in this book will be easily understood.

The external genitalia in the female

The anatomical name for the area of the external genitalia in the female is the *vulva*. It is made up of several structures which surround the entrance to the vagina, and each of which has its own separate function (Fig. 1/1). The *labia majora* (or the large lips of the vagina) are two large folds of skin which contain sweat glands and hair follicles embedded in fat. The size of the labia majora varies considerably. In infancy and in old age they are small, and the fat is not present; in the reproductive years, between puberty and the menopause, they are well filled with fatty tissue. In front (looked at from between the legs), they join together in the pad of fat which surmounts the pelvic bone, and which was called the mount of Venus (*mons veneris*) by the ancient anatomists, when they noted that it was most developed in the reproductive years. Both of the labia, and more particularly the mons veneris, are covered with hair, the quantity of which varies from woman to woman. The pubic hair on the abdominal side of the mons veneris terminates in a straight line, while in the male the hair stretches upwards in an inverted 'V' to reach the umbilicus (Fig. 1/2). The inner surfaces of the labia majora are free from hair, and are separated by

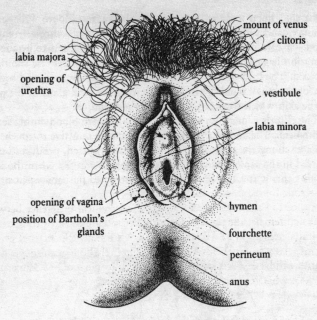

FIG. 1/1   The external genitals in a virgin.

a small groove from the thin labia minora, which guard the entrance to the vagina.

The *labia minora* (the small lips) are delicate folds of skin which contain little fatty tissue. They vary in size, and it was once believed that large labia minora were due to masturbation, which at that time was considered evil. It is now known that this is nonsense. In front, the labia minora split into two folds, one of which passes over and the other under the *clitoris*, and at the back they join to form the *fourchette*, which is always torn during childbirth. In the reproductive years, the labia minora are hidden by the enlarged labia majora, but in childhood and old age the labia minora appear more prominent because the labia majora are relatively small.

The *clitoris* is the exact female equivalent of the male penis. The fold of the labia minora which passes over it is equivalent to the male foreskin (prepuce). It is called the 'hood' and it covers and protects the sensitive end (or glans) of the clitoris. Some sexologists believe that an

3

'adherent' hood reduces a woman's ability to achieve full sexual pleasure, and have devised operations to 'free' the clitoris from the hood – a sort of circumcision of the clitoris. It is unlikely that the operation has anything more than a psychological effect and should be avoided. The fold of skin which passes under the clitoris is the equivalent of the small band of tissue which joins the pink glans of the penis to the skin which covers it. It is called the *frenulum*.

The clitoris is made up of tissue which fills with blood during sexual excitement. The end of the clitoris is often very sensitive to touch, but the area along the shaft of the clitoris, if stimulated, produces sexual arousal in the same way that a man is sexually aroused when the shaft of his penis is stimulated. In sexual intercourse, the movement of the

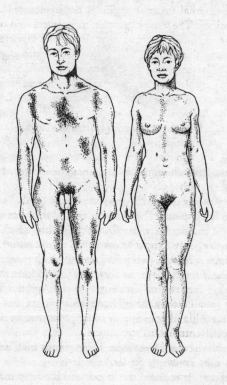

FIG. 1/2 The male and female from the front.

man's penis in the vagina indirectly stimulates the clitoris and can lead to the woman having an orgasm. Many women do not get an orgasm during sexual intercourse but have deeply satisfying orgasms if they masturbate their clitoral area with their own finger or hand, or if their sexual partner caresses the area with finger or tongue (see p. 60). The clitoris varies considerably in size, but is usually that of a green pea. As sexual excitement mounts, the clitoris increases in size. Once again this varies considerably between individuals.

The cleft below the clitoris and between the labia minora is called the *vestibule* (or entrance). Just below the clitoris is the external opening of that part of the urinary tract (the *urethra*) which connects the bladder to the outside world. In old women the urethral orifice may stretch and the lining of the lower part of the urethra may be exposed.

Below the external urethral orifice is the hymen, which surrounds the vaginal orifice. The hymen is a thin incomplete fold of membrane, which has one or more apertures in it. It varies considerably in shape and in elasticity, but is generally stretched or torn during the first attempt at sexual intercourse. The tearing is usually followed by a minute amount of bleeding. In many cultures the rupture of the hymen (also called the maidenhead), and the consequent bleed, is considered a sign that the girl was a virgin at the time of marriage, and the bed is inspected on the morning after the first night of the honeymoon for evidence of blood. Although an 'intact' hymen is considered a sign of virginity, it is not a reliable sign, as in some cases coitus fails to cause a tear, and in others the hymen may have been torn previously by exploring fingers, either of the girl herself or of her sexual partner. The stretching and tearing of the hymen at a first intercourse may be painful, particularly if the partners are apprehensive or ignorant of sexual matters. If the couple are well adjusted, the discomfort is minimal. Childbirth causes a much greater tearing of the hymen, and after delivery only a few tags remain. They are called *carunculae myrtiformes* (Fig. 1/3). Just outside the hymen, still within the vestibule but deep beneath the skin, are two collections of erectile tissues which fill with blood during sexual arousal. Deep in the backward part of the vestibule are two pea-sized glands which also secrete fluid during sexual arousal and moisten the entrance to the vagina, so that the penis may more readily enter it without discomfort. These glands occasionally become infected. They are known as *Bartholin's glands.*

The area of the vulva between the posterior fourchette and the anus, and the muscles which lie under the skin, form a pyramid-shaped

5

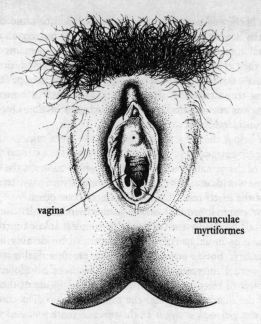

vagina

caruncula
myrtiformes

FIG. 1/3   The external genitals in a woman who has had a child.

wedge of tissue separating the vagina and the rectum. It is called the *perineum*, and of considerable importance in childbirth.

It is a matter of constant surprise to me that a large number of women have never looked at their own or any other woman's external genitals, and consequently are concerned that they may be abnormal. I should say, first, that the diagram on page 3 is idealized to some extent and that a considerable range of shapes and sizes of labia minora, the hymen and the hood of the clitoris are usual; so that if a woman looks at her external genitals with a mirror (and women should do this!) and finds that what she sees is not exactly like the diagram she should not be worried, as biological variations are very wide, particularly in the length and shapes of the labia minora.

This reluctance to look at one's own genitals is a feminine trait (after all men constantly look at and touch their external genitals) and has its origin in the attitudes that many mothers give their daughters about their genitals. These attitudes are that the external genitals are 'private', ugly, should never be touched or 'played with', have a smell, and are 'dirty'. Such indoctrination in childhood can have sad consequences to a woman's image of her own body and in her sexual response. Even the medical word for the external genitals of a woman is negatively loaded: it is the *pudendum* – which derives from the Latin word *pudere* 'to be ashamed'. A woman should not be ashamed of or disgusted by her external genitals and should look at them to become familiar with their unique shape.

The internal genital organs

The *vagina* is a muscular tube which stretches upwards and backwards from the vestibule to reach the uterus. As well as being muscular, it contains a well-developed network of veins which become distended in sexual arousal. Normally the walls of the vagina lie close together, the vagina being a potential cavity which is distended by intravaginal tampons used during mensturation, by the penis during sexual intercourse; and during childbirth, when it stretches very considerably to permit the baby to be born. The vagina is about 9cm (3¾in) long, and at the upper end the *cervix* (or neck) of the uterus projects into it (Fig. 1/4). The vagina lies between the bladder in front and the rectum (or back-passage) behind. At the sides it is surrounded and protected by the strong muscles of the floor of the pelvis. Unless the vagina has been damaged, injured or tightened at operation, or has not developed due to an absence of sex hormones, its size is adequate for sexual intercourse. A woman who menstruates has a normal-sized vagina, and 'difficulty' at intercourse is not due to her being 'small made'. This is a myth. The cause lies not in the vagina, but in a mental fear of sexual intercourse which leads the woman to tighten the muscles which support the vagina to such an extent that sexual intercourse is painful.

The vagina is a remarkable organ. Not only is it capable of great distension, but it keeps itself clean. The cells which form its walls are 30 cells deep, lying on each other like the bricks of a house wall. In the reproductive years, the top layer of cells is constantly being shed into the vagina, where the cells are acted upon by a small bacillus which normally lives there, to produce lactic acid. The lactic acid then kills any contaminating germs which may happen to get into the vagina. Because of this, 'cleansing' vaginal douches, so popular at one time in the USA, are unnecessary. In childhood, the wall of the vagina is thin, and the production of lactic acid does not take place. However, this

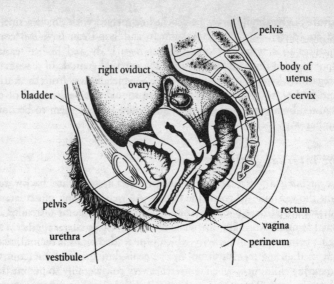

FIG. 1/4 The internal genital organs of the female.

is of little importance, because the vagina is not usually contaminated at this age. In old age, the lining becomes thin once again, and few cells are shed. Because of this, little or no lactic acid is formed, and contaminating germs may grow. This sometimes results in inflammation of the vagina.

The *uterus* is an even more remarkable organ than the vagina. Before pregnancy it is pear-shaped, averages 9cm (3¾in) in length, 6cm (2½in) in width at its widest point, and weighs 60g (2oz). In pregnancy, it enlarges to weigh 1000g (2¼lb), and is able to contain a baby measuring 40cm (17in) in length. It is able to undergo these changes because of the complex structure of its muscle and its exceptional response to the female sex hormones. The uterus is a hollow, muscular organ, which is located in the middle of the bony pelvis, lying between the bladder in front and the bowel behind (Fig. 1/4). It is pear-shaped, and its muscular front and back walls bulge into the cavity which is normally narrow and slitlike, until pregnancy occurs. Viewed from in front, the cavity is triangular, and is lined with a special tissue made up of glands in a network of cells. This tissue is called the endometrium, and it undergoes changes during each menstrual cycle. For descriptive purposes, the uterus is divided into an upper part, or *body*, and a lower portion, or *cervix uteri*. The word cervix means neck, so that the 'cervix uteri' means the neck of the womb. The cavity is narrow in the cervix, where it is called the cervical canal; widest in the body of the uterus; and then narrows again towards the cornu (or horn), where the cavity is continuous with the hollow of the Fallopian tube (Fig. 1/5). The cervix projects into the upper part of the vagina, and is a particular place where cancer sometimes develops. As it is readily accessible for examination, early changes in the cells indicating that cancer may be about to occur can be sought by special methods. This is discussed in more detail in Chapter 21. The lower part of the uterus and the upper part of the cervix are supported by a sling of special tissues, which stretch to the muscles of the pelvic wall in a fan-like manner. These supports may be stretched in childbirth, leading to a 'prolapse' later in life. With better obstetrics, and better education for childbirth, this complication is much less likely to occur today.

Normally the uterus lies bent forward at an angle of 90° to the vagina, resting on the bladder. As the bladder fills, it rotates backwards; as it empties, the uterus falls forward. In about 10 per cent of women

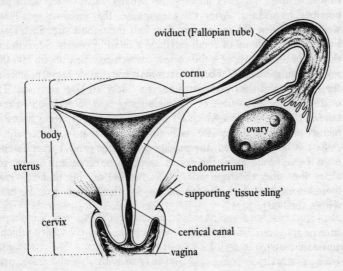

FIG. 1/5   The cavity of the uterus, and tubes.

the uterus lies bent backwards. This is called *retroversion*. In the past it was considered a serious condition, causing backache, sterility and many other complaints. There were many operations for its cure. Today it is known that unless the retroversion is due to infection or to a peculiar condition called endometriosis, it is unimportant and is not the cause of the symptoms which were attributed to it. Surgery is not needed, and the patient can be reassured that the position of the uterus is normal for her.

The *oviducts* (or Fallopian tubes) are two small, hollow tubes, one on each side, which stretch for about 10cm (4in) from the upper part of the uterus to lie in contact with the ovary on each side. The outer end of each oviduct is divided into long finger-like processes, and it is thought that these sweep up the egg when it is expelled from the ovary. The oviduct is lined with cells shaped like goblets, which lie between cells with frond-like borders. The oviduct is of great importance, as it is within it that fertilization of the egg takes place, and it is likely that its secretions help to nourish the fertilized egg as it is moved by the cells with long fronds towards the uterus.

The two *ovaries* are almond-shaped organs, averaging 3.5cm (1½in) in length and 2cm (¾in) in breadth. In the infant they are small, delicate, thin structures, but after puberty they enlarge to reach the adult proportions mentioned. After the menopause, they become small and wrinkled, and in old age are less than half their adult size. Each ovary has a centre made up of small cells and a mesh of vessels. Surrounding this is the ovary proper – the cortex – which contains about 200 000 egg cells lying in a cellular bed (the stroma), and outside again, protecting the egg cells and the ovarian stroma, is a thickened layer of tissue. The ovaries are the equivalent of the male testes, and in addition to containing the egg cells on which all human life depends, are a hormone factory producing the female sex hormones, which are so important.

As can be appreciated, the passage within the genital tract extends from the vestibule, along the vagina, through the cervix and uterus, and along the tubes to the ovaries. It is because of this that the male spermatozoa can reach the female egg for fertilization to take place within the body.

CHAPTER 2

How Human Life Begins

The human being, so complex in his behaviour, so different from his fellows, develops from a single fertilized cell. This cell – the fertilized ovum – divides almost at once into two identical cells. These two cells divide to make four identical cells, which then divide again, and so on. As they divide again and again, certain groups of cells become different, or differentiate, and form particular tissues or organs. For example, some cells form the bony skeleton, some the muscles, others the heart and blood vessels. Still others form the red blood cells which carry oxygen in the blood to the tissues, and others form the white blood cells which protect us against infections. Yet another group of cells multiplies to form the nerve cells of the brain and the nerves.

All these groups of cells with different functions have come from the single fertilized egg cell, and each and every cell has in its substance the information needed to perform the functions of any other cell, although once it has differentiated, it never does. Half of this information comes from the father's side of the family, and is transmitted in the speramatozoon which fertilized the egg. The other half comes from the mother's side, and is transmitted in the substance of the egg itself.

The information needed for the cell to perform its particular function is contained in the twisted strands of a substance found in the centre (or nucleus) of every cell. These strands are called chromosomes, and themselves are formed of long strings of several million beads, which are more properly called genes. The gene is the smallest unit of information, and is itself composed of twisted strands of a chemical called DNA (deoxyribonucleic acid). If you can imagine an ultrasophisticated computer, which responds to requests fed in by giving out information, you have a pretty good idea of how the genes work in the cell. In any cell a few genes operate to control the functions of that cell, the rest being covered over and inactive.

Each cell in the human body, with the exception of the egg cells in the woman and the spermatozoa in the man, contains 46 chromosomes. Forty-four of these chromosomes control all our physical characteristics and our body functions. These are called autosomes. The other two determine our sex. Recently it has been possible to take photographs of the chromosomes in the human body cells. In this way they can be displayed and measured. The two sex chromosomes can be identified easily. The smallest one has the shape of a Y, and is called the Y sex chromosome; the other has the shape of an X, and is called the X sex chromosome. Each of the millions of cells which make up a woman's body has 44 autosomes and two X chromosomes. A man's body cells have 44 autosomes, an X and a Y chromosome. You can see that even in the smallest body cell, a man is different from a woman because his cells alone have the Y chromosome.

As I have noted, the only cells in the body which do not have 46 chromosomes are the egg cells in the woman and the spermatozoa in the man. These two kinds of cells have only 23 chromosomes, and develop in special ways.

The development of the egg cells (ova)

Very early in life (about 20 days after fertilization) certain cells develop in the wall of the gut cavity of the embryo. These cells then migrate through the tissues to reach a thickened area lying in a ridge at each side of the midline of the gut cavity. This is the tissue from which the ovary will develop. By the 30th day after fertilization, the cells have settled in the tissue (which is now called a gonad), and have begun to multiply. By 140 days after fertilization (the 22nd week of pregnancy), a total of 7 million cells are found in the gonad, and many of them have acquired a coating of cells derived from it. They develop within this protective coat and fluid appears in many of the cells. These are the egg cells (or *oocytes*), and the cells which contain fluid are called *follicles*. The cells which do not have the coating are destroyed, and by birth only 2 million oocytes remain. In the childhood years, many more oocytes are destroyed and by puberty only 200 000 remain. Each month from puberty to the menopause between 12 and 30 of the oocytes develop further, and one which outstrips all the rest in growth is expelled from the ovary. This is the ovum which may be fertilized. Occasionally more than one ovum escapes from the ovary. If the additional ova are fertilized, twins, triplets or quadruplets will result, although twins may occur through another mechanism.

During its development in the ovary, the ovum divides into two daughter egg cells. This division is unequal, a large cell and a small cell being formed. Each of these cells has 23 chromosomes – 22 autosomes and an X chromosome. The large cell is the one which will accept the head of the spermatozoon into its substance at the time of fertilization, and will form the new individual. The small cell is pushed to lie just inside the zona pellucida (the 'shell' of the ovum), and has no further function. It is called a *polar body* (Fig. 2/4).

The development of the spermatozoa

It can be seen that all the egg cells in the ovary of the female are formed before birth, and none can be formed later. The male is different, spermatozoa are continually being formed in his testicles from puberty onwards, and into old age.

The spermatozoa are formed from parent cells found in the testicles. They undergo several changes before becoming mature, and during the changes the number of chromosomes in each spermatozoon is reduced by half. The mature spermatozoon therefore has 23 chromosomes. Of these 22 are autosomes and one is a sex chromosome. Since the parent sperm cell had 44 autosomes, an X and a Y chromosome, it follows that when it divides to form the spermatozoa, each will have 22 autosomes and an X *or* a Y chromosome (Fig. 2/1). In this way two equal populations of spermatozoa form, and when you remember that each time a man has an orgasm he ejaculates between 100 and 400 *million* spermatozoa, they are large populations of cells. One population of spermatozoa has 22 autosomes and an X chromosome, the other 22 autosomes and a Y chromosome. If a spermatozoon carrying the Y chromosome fertilizes the egg, the new cell will have 44 autosomes, an X chromosome and a Y chromosome. The baby resulting from this will be a boy. If the spermatozoon which fertilizes the egg is one with 22 autosomes and an X chromosome, the resulting cell will have 44 autosomes and two X chromosomes. The baby resulting from this will be a girl (Fig. 2/1). This means that the father determines the sex of the child, although, of course, as chance decides which type of sperm will fertilize the egg, the sex of the child depends on luck.

Because of the desire of many couples to obtain a male or a female baby scientists have tried to manipulate nature so that the couple conceives a child of the sex they desire. In spite of considerable 'hype'

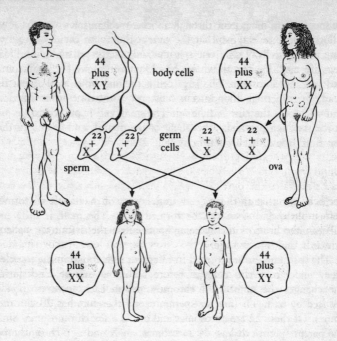

FIG. 2/1 The chromosomes of the ovum and spermatozoon.

in newspapers, none of these methods has proved more effective than chance.

The fertilization of the egg

A new life begins when a single spermatozoon, out of the millions which were deposited in the upper part of the vagina during intercourse, fertilizes the egg (or ovum). Of the millions of spermatozoa deposited in the vicinity of the cervix, only a few thousand manage to negotiate the twisting mucus tunnels of its canal to reach the cavity of the uterus. Of these only a few hundred get through the narrow cornu of the uterus to enter the oviduct, and only a few dozen swim up along the oviduct, against the current made by the moving fronds of its lining, to reach the ovum. Only one penetrates through tough, glistening, transparent 'shell' (the zona pellucida) which surrounds the egg. Once the spermatozoon has penetrated the 'shell' of the egg, it alters the zona pellucida in some way, so that no other spermatozoa are able to penetrate it. In this way only one spermatozoon fertilizes the ovum. The new life actually begins when the chromosomes of the ovum and those of the spermatozoon fuse together. Under the control of the genes, the cell then divides again and again until a human being is formed, as was described in the opening paragraph of this chapter.

The spermatozoon has a head, a middle piece and a tail (Fig. 2/2). The head contains the chromosomes, the middle piece supplies the energy, and the tail propels it on its journey through the woman's genital tract (Fig. 2/3). When the spermatozoon reaches the ovum, its head penetrates the outer shell, and enters the substance of the egg. The head then separates from the middle piece and tail, which remain stuck in the shell and are destroyed.

When the head of the spermatozoon enters the ovum, its nucleus (which is the part containing the chromosomes) loses its covering and the chromosomes are exposed. Simultaneously, the covering surrounding the nucleus of the ovum disappears. The two sets of 23 chromosomes move together and fuse, so the number of chromosomes in the cell is 46 once again (Fig. 2/4). In this way the number of chromosomes in the human body cell is kept constant at 46.

A woman is a woman because each cell in her body (with the exception of the egg cells) has 44 non-sex chromosomes and 2 X sex chromosomes. Her femininity is further confirmed by the fact that none of her body cells contains a Y chromosome. In the absence of a Y chromosome her internal and external genitalia will develop in a feminine way. There is also some evidence that the absence of a Y chromosome tends to make her 'psychologically' feminine. The effect of this is small, however, compared with the very considerable psychological pressures during childhood which confirm her in her feminine role. From the time she can notice anything she is treated as a girl; she

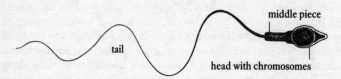

FIG. 2/2 The spermatozoon. The length is 0.05mm and the thickness of the tail is about half that of a fine hair. It is only visible under a microscope.

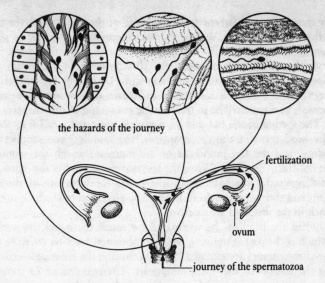

the hazards of the journey

fertilization

ovum

journey of the spermatozoa

FIG. 2/3 The journey of the spermatozoa through the genital tract.

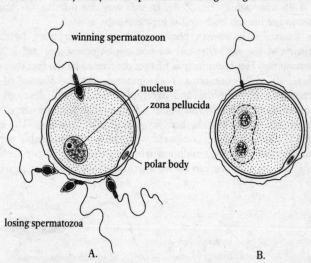

winning spermatozoon

nucleus

zona pellucida

polar body

losing spermatozoa

A.

B.

FIG. 2/4 Conception. The sperm head is seen in the substance of the egg in **A**, and the two exposed masses of genetic material are seen in **B**. Almost immediately they fuse and a new individual is formed.

is shown to be different from boys; she performs different tasks; is expected to behave differently, and so rapidly realizes that she is female.

In recent years the emphasis on the differences in the roles that females and males play has been reduced. Women in today's society can perform nearly all the activities previously reserved for men, although women continue to suffer from disadvantages compared with men.

Many problems of sexual discrimination will be reduced when the sex roles into which children are socialized become blurred, and boys and girls are expected to perform similar tasks in the home and outside it.

Such changes will be beneficial to the growth and development of girls, without diminishing their unique attributes.

CHAPTER 3

The Start of Femininity

The moment that the newborn baby is breathing properly, the doctor examines it to make sure it is normal in every way, and hands it to the mother to fondle and cuddle. She has done something no man can do – she has matured a new life in her uterus for 40 weeks and her baby has been born.

The newborn baby is totally dependent on others for all its needs, and forms its first physical contact with its mother. If she is going to breast-feed the baby, its first real tactile contact is the soft, warm breast, which provides a pleasant food. Even if she does not breast-feed her baby, it is she who cuddles the infant, lavishes affection on it, and performs the many tasks needed to sustain its life. The emotional links between infant and mother are strong, and a bond can also develop between infant and father if he plays a proper role, sharing with his wife the care of the child. But the bond between the infant and mother is so strong that the development of the growing child is influenced considerably by its character. If the mother is a warm, friendly person, the chances are that the child will develop in a similar way. If the mother is hard and unyielding, the child may reflect these characteristics, and find it difficult to adjust to a more normal human relationship in adult life. The sexual implications of this are no less important for the female than for the male.

The first sense an infant develops is touch, and although the warmth it obtains from cuddling is pleasurable, the infant soon begins to explore. The first explorations are necessarily confined to his own body, and the infant finds that touching the gential area produces pleasurable sensations. Similar pleasurable sensations are produced when the baby is bathed or the nappies (diapers) are changed. These explorations are completely normal. It is now known that most small children masturbate. This is easier to see if the child is a boy, but girls masturbate by 'rocking', which stimulates the area around their clitoris.

As the infant becomes a small child, its curiosity about its body increases. Most children explore each other's bodies and interact with each other (including sexually) in play. We do not know when this body exploration is interpreted by the child as erotic. By the age of 3, genital comparison is normal, as is body exploration. This sex play is valuable for it helps the child become familiar with its own body and that of others.

The attitude of parents towards sexuality and their comfort in answering a child's questions honestly are crucial in preventing sexual impairment when the child grows up.

Many small children assume that sex is evil; that the noise they may hear from their parents' bedroom is due to their father assaulting their mother; that babies are born through the mother's abdomen which has to be cut, and that girls once had a penis, but it was cut off.

Unless parents can reassure the child and answer its questions without embarrassment, it may get the message that sex is shameful or improper. If parents treat sex as 'dirty', and threaten to punish a child found engaged in sexual play, the child may develop attitudes to sex which may mar his or her adult life.

The female role

Parents behave differently towards their infant sons and their infant daughters and the different behaviour begins soon after the baby is born. The way in which parents (and others) behave to the child and the different expectations they have of the child depending on her or his sex, 'imprints' a distinct pattern of behaviour in the first three years of the child's life. This 'imprinting' induces the child to behave in a feminine or in a masculine way. Once the child's brain is conditioned in this way it is difficult to reverse it.

A child's masculine or feminine behaviour, depending on its sex, has two components. The first is its sex-typing or its gender-role. This is the way a person behaves to others to demonstrate he or she is a male or a female. The second is even more important. This is the person's own awareness that he or she is a male or a female. This is the person's gender-identity. Until a child has developed a gender-identity it is confused about its sexuality, and about its gender-role.

In Western societies a complete reversal of gender-identity can be made with relative ease before the age of 4, but after this time the change is only possible in highly motivated individuals who have had doubts about their real sex induced by the doubting attitude of their parents, or who are exceptionally insistent upon the change, such as transsexuals.

The gender-role of the child is fostered so assiduously by the parents that the girl is induced to behave as a girl is expected to behave in our culture. When she behaves in this way she has developed a gender-identity. This means that she knows that she is a girl, and knows that she should behave in a specific female manner. This process takes some time. Up to the age of about 2 or 2½ the child does not know his or her own sex. By 3 to 3½ years old, a girl-child is able to answer correctly 'I am a girl'. She knows what a boy is and she knows in what ways a boy is different from a girl. By the age of 4–5, the girl is able to identify boys as boys and girls as girls, and knows that her sex is unchangeable. She will always be a female.

In our society the female gender-role is still based on that needed for a less sophisticated society. In primitive societies, the survival of the tribe depended on the clear separation of male and female roles. The men were hunters, the women nurtured their children (breast-feeding for 2 years or longer), gathered fruits and grains and cooked. Women were inferior to men and were excluded from 'important' events, except the mysteries of menstruation and childbirth, which were women's secrets.

Today, in pre-industrial societies, survival is largely dependent on women and men filling different roles. These societies are based on male aggressiveness and competitiveness and female submission, sub-ordination and compliance. In Western post-industrial society today, women have greater choices. Women may choose to have fewer chil-dren and so need to devote less time for a shorter period to child-rearing. This gives women the choice of escaping from the traditional female role if they wish. But there are problems.

At present, women are disadvantaged in opportunities for jobs. They obtain less interesting jobs, get less pay, and achieve lower levels of promotion. This is not due to lack of ability or desire, but to the patriarchal structure of society. In a male-dominated society, women have to expend more effort, more time and more skill to achieve a position a less qualified man achieves more easily. This biases the competition strongly in favour of a man; it ceases to be true competi-tion. The lack of success of women in high-status jobs may also be affected by the way girls are reared. Females take orders from authority more easily and comply with them more readily, they are less likely to protest and are slower to become angry, so they are easier to exploit by men and more ready to take less interesting, lower-status jobs.

In spite of these problems many women who are married, or in a long-term relationship, work outside the home, usually to enable the family to achieve a higher standard of living. As well as working to add significantly to the family's income, most women continue to undertake nearly all the housework. Surveys in Australia and in the USA show that a working wife spends an average of 25 hours a week on household chores. In Britain only 2 per cent of men undertake any housework which involves more than doing household repairs.

The subordinate position of women to men, which is initiated by the way the two sexes are reared, tends to be self-perpetuating. Women brought up in this way believe they are inferior to men in both intelligence and ability. Even when the work of men and women is of identical quality, women tend to denigrate that of their own sex and to rate a man's work more highly.

Why women perpetuate their sense of subordination is not an easy question to answer. Anthropologists have found that many repressed minority groups tend to adopt the attitudes of the stronger dominant group towards themselves. Women may do the same by accepting the submissive stereotype, and by this device are able to escape some of the anxiety which arises if they feel themselves to be oppressed. It is easier to accept the status quo than to rebel against it, particularly if you rationalize that because of your sex you can never achieve as much as a man, but you are better at nurturing activities, and have an important role to play in caring for children and looking after your husband.

Changes are occurring, although slowly. More men are now prepared to shop at the supermarket, to cook, to clean and tidy the house. More women are doing household repairs and washing the car. But these couples tend to be more highly educated than average and are more adaptable in their sex roles.

There are those who fear that any reduction in the differences between how the sexes look and behave and what they do in sexual encounters, in work, or in play, will lead to a destruction of the fabric of society. This is a false fear; equality of opportunity for women in all spheres of activity will not reduce the gender-identity of women, but rather will permit women to develop as freer human beings. The reduction in a man's competitiveness and aggression and the social permission for him to show emotion and affection will not reduce his male gender-identity but will enable him to relate more freely and equally with other human beings, irrespective of their sex.

Gynaecological conditions in childhood

Since the genital organs are immature and have not been stimulated by the sex hormones which will be produced by the ovary at puberty, gynaecological problems in infancy are uncommon. However, two require mention, as they may cause distress.

The 'genital crisis'

A few female infants either bleed slightly from the vagina, or develop enlargement of the breasts which secrete a watery solution in the first weeks of life. These conditions are called the 'genital crisis' and are due to the passage from the mother to her baby of certain hormones. Following birth, the hormones no longer pass. The symptoms are without significance; no treatment is required as they settle down and disappear within a few days.

Inflammation of the vulva and vagina

In small children the vulva and the vagina may become inflamed and sore. The inflammation may be due to irritation from soaps used for washing, to lack of washing and poor hygiene, which permit bacteria to grow, or to the introduction into the vagina of some object.

The condition is very painful, and medical help should be sought. Meanwhile, certain general principles of treatment can be adopted. These are: (1) general cleanliness, using only a mild soap, or none at all, for washing the child's vulva, (2) careful drying and powdering after vulval washing, and (3) the wearing of light, cotton panties day and night to prevent the child from scratching the area.

CHAPTER 4

Adolescence

The period of life between childhood and maturity is adolescence, which biologically extends from the age of 10 to the age of 19. The most important event in adolescence, as far as the girl and her mother are concerned, is the onset of menstruation, which may occur at any time between the ages of 10 and 16. The time of onset of menstruation is called the *menarche*. In rural societies the menarche was a mark that the girl was now a woman, and could take up the duties and obligations of womanhood. This cultural attitude is retained in many societies today. For some reason, which may be concerned with better nutrition, the age of the onset of menstruation has become earlier. In Britain the average age of the onset of menstruation is now 13 years, compared with 15 years a century ago. It seems that the daughters of better-off parents tend to start menstruating a little earlier than those whose parents are poor, but the average difference is no more than 6 to 9 months. The old belief that the menarche occurred earlier in girls living in the hot tropics does not appear to be true, and the average age of onset of menstruation depends more on the socio-economic status of the parents than on the climate.

The menarche, however, is only the culminating change in a sequence of events which change the girl into a young woman. These changes are due to a series of interactions between several glands in the body. The controlling gland is a special part of the brain called the *hypothalamus*, which, working with the pituitary gland, controls the subsequent events. For reasons which are not yet clear, the hypothalamus begins to secrete substances called releasing hormones about four years before the menarche. The releasing hormones pass down the blood vessels connecting the hypothalamus to the pituitary, where they cause the release of several hormones. One of these hormones is the growth hormone which causes the spurt of growth that precedes the menarche. The girl begins to grow about four years before the menarche, and the rate of growth is greatest in the first two years, slowing down as the menarche approaches.

About the age of 12, another releasing hormone, the gonadotrophin releasing hormone (GnRH) begins to be secreted by the pituitary gland in surges which occur every 90 minutes. These surges of GnRH have a profound effect on the girl's sexual maturity. The hormone reaches the pituitary gland where it causes certain specialized cells to produce two hormones which act on the girl's ovaries.

In Chapter 2 it was noted that by the time of birth, fluid had appeared in many of the egg cells, which were then called egg follicles. The first of the hormones which affects the egg cells is called the follicle-stimulating hormone (or FSH), because it stimulates the growth of some of the follicles. At first only a very few follicles grow, and as they do their surrounding mantle of cells manufactures a hormone called *oestrogen*. This hormone is the one which makes a female child become a woman. The stimulated follicles produce oestrogen for about a month, and then die. But by this time other egg follicles have been stimulated, and these secrete oestrogen in their turn. As time passes, more follicles are stimulated each month (eventually between 12 and 20 being stimulated), so that there is a gradual rise in the amount of oestrogen produced by the ovaries. Oestrogen has many effects. It stimulates the growth of the ducts of the breasts and the area under the nipples, so that this becomes enlarged. It stimulates the growth of the oviducts, the uterus and the vagina. In the vagina it thickens the vaginal wall, and causes increased vaginal moisture. It causes fat to be laid down on the hips. It slows down the growth spurt which was started earlier by the pituitary growth hormone, so that a mature girl is generally not as tall as a mature boy.

As time passes, the amount of oestrogen in the circulation rises more rapidly, and the menarche is near. The rising levels of oestrogen stimulate the growth of the lining of the uterus, the *endometrium*, but at the same time 'feedback' reduces the quantity of follicle-stimulating hormone secreted by the pituitary. Once the level of follicle-stimulating hormone begins to fall, the growth of the follicles in the ovaries and the secretion of oestrogen are reduced. The blood vessels supplying the lining of the uterus become kinked and break, so that bleeding occurs in the uterus. The endometrium crumbles. Blood, tissue fluid and endometrial cells collect in the uterus, and then escape through the cervix into the vagina. Menstruation has started – the menarche has arrived. The description given fails to answer the question: What factor activates the hypothalamus to start the sequence of events which leads to menstruation?

Recent information suggests that the activating factor is the amount of body fat. Until the body fat reaches a specific proportion of bodyweight menstruation is delayed. This is the reason that thin girls, and particularly ballet dancers who are not only thin but do a great deal of exercise, tend to have a delayed menarche.

The average age at which various changes occur is:

Age 9–10   The bony pelvis begins to grow and to attain a female shape.

Fat begins to be deposited, commencing the changes in shape to that of a woman.

The nipples bud.

Age 10–11   The nipples increase in size.

Hair begins to appear over the pubis.

Age 11–13   The area beneath the nipples develops.

The internal and external genitals grow and develop.

The vaginal wall thickens, and vaginal secretions may appear.

Age 12–14   The breasts develop further, and the nipples become darker in colour.

Age 13–15   Hair increases over the pubis, and appears in the armpits.

Acne appears on the face of about half the girls.

The menarche occurs, but the first few periods occur at irregular intervals.

Age 15–17   Increased fatty deposition occurs on the hips and the breasts.

The periods become more regular.

Age 16–18   Growth of the skeleton ceases. The girl has now reached her maximum height.

Menstruation

At intervals from the menarche – irregularly at first but with increasing regularity as time goes by – the girl 'has her periods', or menstruates. Within 4 to 6 years of the menarche (by the age of 17 to 19), her menstrual pattern will have become established. Each individual has her own pattern, but in most women menstruation occurs each month (unless pregnancy intervenes) until about the age of 45, when it becomes increasingly irregular once again. For convenience, the menstrual cycle is considered to start on the first day of menstruation (day 1), and to end the day before the next menstruation starts. The menstrual cycle therefore includes the days when bleeding occurs and the interval between each menstrual period. In most women the cycle varies in length from 22 to 35 days, averaging 29 days. But even the woman who says she knows exactly on what day menstruation will start is often a few days out either side. In adolescence, until the pattern has been established, menstruation tends to occur at irregular intervals, usually of longer duration than normal, but occasionally more frequently. In the first year or two after the menarche, the periods may only recur twice or three times a year, and when they do occur may be heavy. Sooner or later, however, a regular rhythmic pattern is established.

The menstrual cycle

It has been said that menstruation is 'the uterus weeping because pregnancy did not happen'. Bleeding from the crumbling of the lining of the uterus is the culmination of a series of interlocked events which prepare the uterus to accept a fertilized egg. If pregnancy does not occur, this prepared lining is shed from the uterus, and the whole cycle of events begins again.

The ultimate 'controller' of these events is the hypothalamus, and even this part of the brain is affected by emotions and upsets. This is demonstrated by the fact that menstruation may cease after a particularly strong emotional upset, or if a girl leaves home and changes her occupation. The duration of time during which menstruation ceases is variable and the periods usually return after two or three months; but in some women the absence of the periods, which is called amenorrhoea, may last for more than a year. Such women require careful investigation to exclude an underlying disease which may cause amenorrhoea. Luckily the cause is not usually a disease, and menstruation can be restored with certain drugs if this is considered desirable. It should be stressed that if there is no underlying disease, the absence of menstruation is of no importance. Contrary to a popular myth, menstruation does not clean the body, and the absence of menstruation does not mean that 'dangerous substances' are dammed up within the uterus.

As the sequence of events leading to each menstrual period is complicated, it is perhaps best to start at the time of menstruation and trace what happens up to the time of the next menstruation.

During menstruation the hypothalamus sends quantities of the gonadotrophin-releasing hormone to stimulate the cells in the pituitary gland which manufacture FSH. The amount of FSH in the blood rises and stimulates a number of egg follicles in the ovary, usually 12 to 20. These follicles grow, and as they do so they manufacture oestrogen, so that the amount of this special female sex hormone increases in the blood. As has been noted earlier, oestrogen has several effects upon the tissues which make up the genital tract, but the one in which we are particularly interested is its action on the lining of the uterus. Oestrogen stimulates the lining to grow. At the end of menstruation most of the lining has crumbled away and, mixed with blood, has been shed as the menstrual flow. The lining is made up of narrow tubes, called endometrial glands, set in several layers of cells, called endometrial stromal cells. Oestrogen makes the glands grow, and the layers of stromal cells increase, or proliferate. Because of this, the changes in the uterus are called proliferative, and this part of the cycle is called the proliferative phase of the cycle.

As the follicles grow, the amount of oestrogen in the blood continues to rise, and by 13 days after the onset of menstruation, it has increased six-fold above the level found at its onset. The rising blood levels have an effect called a 'feedback' on the hypothalamus, causing a reduction in FSH-releasing hormone, but making the hypothalamus release another substance called the LH-releasing hormone. This factor is carried down the blood vessels which connect the hypothalamus to the pituitary gland, where specialized cells produce a substance called luteinizing hormone, or LH (Fig. 4/1). This hormone is so-called because it induces one of the egg follicles to burst and expel its contained egg, and it then changes the cells which make up the follicle to a bright yellow colour. The Latin word for yellow is '*luteus*' – hence the luteinizing, or yellow-making hormone. On about the 14th day after the onset of menstruation (in a girl with a normal cycle, or later if the cycle is prolonged unduly) a sudden surge of luteinizing hormone sweeps through the bloodstream. It reaches the ovary, where it induces 'bursting' of the egg follicle which has grown the most, and which is blown-up and tight like a tiny balloon. During growth, this particular follicle has swollen and moved through the ovary to reach its surface, where it makes a tiny bulge that can be seen by the naked eye.

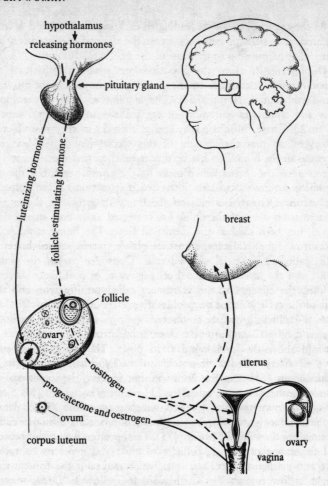

FIG. 4/1   The control of menstruation.

Suddenly, under the influence of the luteinizing hormone, the follicle bursts and the egg is pushed out, together with the fluid in which it lay. The egg is caught in the finger-like ends of the oviduct which caress the ovary at this time, and is moved slowly but gently into the cavity of the oviduct tube, where fertilization takes place, if this is to happen (Fig. 4/2).

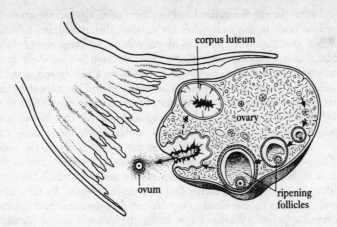

FIG. 4/2 The growth of stimulated follicles in the ovary during a menstrual cycle.

Once the egg (or ovum) has been expelled, the now empty follicle collapses, and the luteinizing hormone acts on the cells of its wall, turning them yellow. The collapsed follicle is called a yellow body, or, in Latin, a *corpus luteum*. The change in colour of the cells of the corpus luteum is due to a change in their activity. Now not only do they continue to secrete oestrogen (along with the other 11 to 19 stimulated follicles which failed to grow so quickly), but uniquely they also manufacture a new hormone called progesterone. The name is apt, for the hormone prepares the uterus for pregnancy (*progestos*) – hence pro-gest-erone (-one indicates the kind of chemical substance). Progesterone is the second main female sex hormone. It has many actions, but the main ones are that it relaxes smooth (involuntary) muscles; increases the production of the waxy secretions of the skin; and raises the temperature of the body. This is why it is normal for women in the second half of the menstrual cycle to have a temperature up to 37.4°C (99.5°F). The most important progestational effect of progesterone is its action on the uterus. Progesterone thickens the lining of the uterus, and induces the glands to secrete a nutritious fluid and become succulent, so that the fertilized egg may be nourished during the time it needs to take root or implant in the lining of the womb. The part of the menstrual cycle after ovulation is called the luteal or the progestational phase.

Unless the egg is fertilized and implants on to the endometrium, the yellow body in the ovary dies (as do the other stimulated follicles). When this happens, the level of oestrogen and progesterone in the blood falls. This has two effects: first, the restraint on the gonadotrophin releasing hormone by the hypothalamus is removed, and FSH production by the pituitary gland increases. Second, without the stimulation of oestrogen and progesterone, the now thick, juicy lining of the uterus begins to shrink, and in doing so kinks the tiny blood vessels which supply it. The kinked blood vessels (really blood capillaries) break, and patchy bleeding occurs in the deeper layers of the lining. This separates the lining above the blood; it crumbles and is shed into the uterine cavity, together with blood and fluid which has seeped into the cavity of the uterus from the endometrium. In fact, blood only accounts for one-third to one-half of the total menstrual discharge during a period. Within a few hours the amount of the menstrual discharge in the uterine cavity is such that the uterus contracts, expelling the blood through the cervix in to the vagina. Menstruation has begun.

Attitudes to menstruation

Most girls learn about menstruation from their mothers. Unfortunately some mothers do not give their daughters sufficient information, and some do not talk openly about menstruation before the girl has her first menstrual period. This worries some girls and often leads them to the belief that menstruation is unpleasant or serious. In other words, the girl has a negative attitude to menstruation. She may feel embarrassed about menstruation and see it as an 'illness', particularly if she becomes tired or irritable about that time. The negative view of menstruation persists into, and after late adolescence. In a study made in Sydney in 1984, over three-quarters of the 1200 adolescent women surveyed said that if there were a safe reversible method they would prefer not to menstruate.

Facts about menstruation

During the two days before menstruation starts, many women feel 'off colour'. The woman may have a headache, her stomach may feel swollen, she may feel tired or irritable and may have a pressure feeling in her pelvis. Most of these symptoms disappear when menstruation starts.

Menstruation usually lasts from 3 to 7 days and the average amount of menstrual discharge is 30ml (1 fluid ounce) although some women lose less and some more. A loss of more than 80ml (2¾ fluid ounces) is abnormal. Usually this is accompanied by the loss of blood clots. Menstruation normally occurs every 22 to 35 days, but each woman develops her own pattern.

'Protection' during menstruation

No woman wants to discolour her clothes with menstrual blood. In the past a rag was used which was placed over the vulva, and which is the origin of an English name for menstruation, 'the rags'. Today clean, absorbent, easily disposable materials are used to make sanitary pads and intravaginal tampons, the two usual ways of dealing with menstrual loss. The sanitary pad has the disadvantage that it may chafe the upper thighs as it lies applied to the vulva, and may be apparent, particularly in sports clothes. The latter objection is more often in the mind of the wearer than of the observer, and if menstruation is considered a normal function (which it is), it is surely unimportant if others know that a menstrual period is in progress. It is only in communities which consider menstruation something of which to be ashamed and to be hidden that these attitudes apply. In recent years slim mini-pads which are made to adhere to the woman's panties or pantihose have become popular, as they protect the woman against menstrual staining and are inconspicuous.

An intravaginal tampon has the advantage that it is convenient, inconspicuous and efficient. A tampon can be used by women of any age, provided it can be introduced into the vagina without discomfort. Special slim tampons are available for women who have not had sexual intercourse. Many young women prefer to use a tampon rather than a sanitary pad. Women who have profuse periods, however, find that the tampon is inadequate to mop up the blood loss, and may find a sanitary pad more satisfactory. The choice is that of the woman – neither method is superior to the other, both being satisfactory.

A tampon should be changed every 4 hours during menstruation. It should be removed if the woman chooses to have sexual intercourse. The reason for changing tampons at regular intervals is that an offensive vaginal discharge may result and in a few cases a serious illness, called toxic shock, has occurred.

Toxic shock

This uncommon condition (less than one case occurs each year for every 25 000 menstruating women) has been given considerable publicity. A woman developing toxic shock suddenly has a high temperature, sore throat, headache, aching muscles and, sometimes, watery diarrhoea. A sunburn-like rash covers her skin, her eyes become reddened. Three days later, the skin begins to flake, like dandruff. In a number of cases the blood pressure falls and the woman develops 'shock'. Toxic shock is due to the release of a toxin from a bacterium called *Staphylococcus aureus* (the 'golden staph') which lives in the vagina.

Women who choose tampons have an increased risk of developing toxic shock, and should choose a cotton or 'non-enhanced' rayon tampon, of the lowest effective absorbency. A proposal in the USA is that all tampon packages should have the absorbency 'rates' of the various tampons printed on the package, so that a woman can choose the tampon with the lowest absorbency which works for her. As well the woman should change her tampon every 4 hours and use a pad or a mini-pad at night, rather than a tampon.

Myths about menstruation

In primitive cultures, menstruating women were regarded not as dirty, but as evil and dangerous. To primitive races the loss of blood was a loss of life. As menstrual blood emerged from the same passage as did the baby, but seemed in some way to prevent pregnancy, it was felt to be a danger to growing things. A menstruating woman therefore could damage crops, cause animals to abort, turn wine into vinegar and turn milk sour by her presence. These primitive beliefs are still accepted in parts of Europe today, and it is believed that if a menstruating woman makes jam it will not keep: if she touches wine, beer or milk it will go bad; if she touches buds they will wither; and if she rides a pregnant mare it will miscarry. In most societies it was therefore felt imperative that a woman, at the time of the menstrual period, withdraw from the life of the community, and remained secluded and hidden from view in the house. While menstruating, she could not touch food or cook, nor should her shadow fall on another woman, particularly if she was pregnant. These strange prohibitions are found in Australian Aboriginal tribes, and among the highly intelligent but superstitious

Hindu cultures. Almost all societies have surrounded menstruation with myth and ritual. Both the Jews and the Muslims have elaborate rituals for purification following menstruation, and even in modern Western society strange traditional beliefs persist. Certain foods, especially pineapple and raspberries, are thought to be 'bad' if eaten during menstruation. Washing the hair is believed to lead to an increased menstrual loss, and to the development of a cold or pneumonia.

Of course there is no basis of truth in any of these beliefs. Provided the menstrual flow is not too heavy and the girl wishes, she can take part in any activity. She can ride, swim, work or walk, wash her head or her feet, eat what she likes, bathe or shower, dance or drive. It is also a myth that menstruation is necessary for a woman's health. The basis of this myth is that the menstrual blood, in some obscure way, washes 'bad substances' from a woman's body. This is quite untrue. Menstruation has two psychological functions. It indicates to a woman that she is still in the period of life when she can conceive children and it indicates to her that she has not conceived. If she has no desire to have children, or has completed her family, there are no physical or psychological reasons why she should menstruate. But unless she takes drugs (such as the injectable hormonal contraceptives) or has had her uterus removed surgically, her biological rhythm will ensure that menstruation will continue.

Menstrual irregularities in adolescence

The menstrual cycle is repeated throughout the reproductive years, unless pregnancy occurs. At each extreme – that is in adolescence and near the menopause – the cycles are less regular, and ovulation may not occur. In these cycles the endometrium is only stimulated by oestrogen, and only FSH is secreted (in any quantity) by the pituitary gland. The menstrual cycles tend to be irregular in duration: they may be as short as 12 days, or as long as 3 or 4 months. The duration and amount of menstrual bleeding is also variable: it may be scanty and of short duration, or heavy and long. If the bleeding is too heavy or too prolonged, the girl should consult a doctor who can give hormonal treatment for a few months to regulate the periods. During this time, the girl's own rhythm is established. In most cases, the irregularity is not too inconvenient, and the knowledge that normal cycles will eventually appear is sufficient reassurance. But if there is any doubt, the girl should consult a doctor.

A few teenaged women (and other women) deliberately starve themselves, either because of a desire to be slim, or because of a deeper psychological disturbance. The condition is called *anorexia nervosa*, and it is usual for menstruation to cease. The menstrual periods will only return when the woman can be persuaded to eat sufficiently to restore her body-weight to normal.

Delayed onset of menstruation

Of even more concern to the girl, and more particularly to her mother, is when the periods fail to start. If menstration has not started by the age of 16, and particularly if the girl is of short stature, a doctor should be consulted. He will take a careful history, will require to make a full physical examination, and finally will need to make a pelvic examination (although in some cases an examination by inserting a finger into the rectum will give sufficient information). If at the end of this time the doctor has not been able to find out why the periods have not started, the girl should be referred to a gynaecologist so that special investigations can be started. The investigations are fairly simple and include the examination under a microscope of cells taken by a swab from the inside of the cheek. A sample of the girl's blood is taken and the levels of FSH, oestrogen, progesterone and a hormone, called prolactin, are measured. Some of the blood is treated in a special way so that the chromosome pattern of the body cells can be determined. The result of the tests enables the doctor to give advice and, if necessary, treatment. If the tests show that there is no abnormality, it is usual to await the spontaneous onset of menstruation. Drugs are usually given only if the woman's lack of menstruation persists until such time as she wishes to become pregant.

Menstrual cramps (dysmenorrhoea)

Many girls suffer from painful crampy periods. This is called dysmenorrhoea. Dysmenorrhoea does not usually start until two or three years after the menarche, and usually only occurs if the menstrual period follows a cycle in which ovulation occurred. Occasionally dysmenorrhoea occurs in a period in which ovulation did not occur (called an 'anovulatory cycle'), particularly if the menstrual blood clots in the uterus, and the small clots are then expelled.

The pain is cramplike in character, felt in the lower abdomen, and usually starts in the 24 hours before the menstrual period and lasts for the first 12 to 24 hours of bleeding, when the discomfort goes.

The cause of dysmenorrhoea is now believed to be due to an extra sensitivity of the body to, or an accumulation in the body of, substances called prostaglandins. Prostaglandins cause spasm of the uterine muscle. The cause of the pain is therefore similar to that which occurs in your arm if you tie a tight band around the upper part. Cultural beliefs, and the concept that menstruation is the discharge of waste products, have the effect of increasing the pain sensation. Thus adolescents in 'primitive races' are said to suffer less dysmenorrhoea than girls in more sophisticated Western societies. It is by no means certain that this is true, but Western society in calling menstruation 'the curse', the 'poorly time' and the 'unclean time' (as in the Bible) only intensifies the erroneous belief that menstruation is something of which to be ashamed, and not the naturally-occurring shedding of the uterine lining prepared for a pregnancy which failed to occur.

Probably 50 per cent of women complain of dysmenorrhoea at some stage of their life. Usually the peak years are between 17 and 25, and the condition is relieved or cured by pregnancy. Because of this high incidence, a bewildering variety of treatments have been prescribed in the past, and continue to appear today. Some of the more bizarre methods, such as exotic spinal and pelvic exercises, Sitz baths, cold showers, and surgical operations for removing the nerves of the pelvis, are now of only historical interest, but others which are equally wild appear from time to time.

The great majority of girls need no more than an explanation of what dysmenorrhoea is, a sympathetic attitude from parents which is neither too hard nor too pitying, and the use of aspirin or other pain-relieving drugs. If the pain is more severe, more potent medications are available. As the cramps are caused by prostaglandins, drugs which prevent prostaglandins being synthesized in the body should relieve the pain. There are several anti-prostaglandin drugs available on prescription. The drugs are taken from the onset of the pain for 2 or 3 days. An alternative is for the woman to take 'the Pill'. 'The Pill' usually prevents dysmenorrhoea (by preventing ovulation) and, as well, prevents an unwanted pregnancy if the woman is sexually active. She should choose one of the older Pills available, as the new low-dose Pills do not always prevent menstrual cramps.

Emotional changes in adolescence

With the hormonal tides which ebb and flow before and after the menarche, with increasing knowledge and with increasing information (and misinformation) received from her peer-group, the adolescent has to adjust to a new identity – that of a young woman. In the adolescent period of transition, she has to emerge from the family-orientated dependent tranquility of childhood and enter the frustrations, competitiveness and trauma of adult life. Successful adaptation demands that she matures not only biologically but emotionally and socially as well. In the initial period of biological development she begins to become much closer to other teenagers than to her family. From them, she learns of different attitudes to morality and to sexuality. She now has to resolve a conflict. She has to decide which set of values she should adopt, or more accurately, how many of her parents' values she will reject. And at this time she begins to feel the force of new, ill-understood heterosexual attractions.

The great majority of adolescents adjust with little trouble, but during the period of adjustment are moody, irritable, apparently irrational and 'difficult'. These are outward expressions of inward conflicts, of frustrations, of doubts, even of despair. The adolescent resents adult criticism, particularly when she is told to behave one way by parents who are quite clearly behaving in an entirely different way.

Adults complain about the irresponsibility of teenagers, about their lack of respect, about their morals and about their promiscuity. Yet it is difficult to ask teenagers to develop responsibility when adults seem to be rejecting it, and when society seems to be fragmenting. It is particularly difficult to ask young people to maintain sexual responsibility, when the mass media constantly emphasize that all wants can be instantly gratified. The adolescent needs understanding and love. And she needs to be able to talk to someone close to her, not to have to talk to her parents as strangers. If parents are unable to answer her questions regarding social, moral and sexual attitudes, they have failed as parents, and should not blame their child if she appears to have failed them.

As I shall mention in the next chapter, sexual problems arise in nearly 50 per cent of marriages and, although many are apparently only minor, they can and do much to cause marital discord. It is now clear that many of the problems occur because one or other partner thinks that sex is 'dirty' or 'indecent' or something to be hidden. The importance of a healthy attitude towards human sexuality in childhood and adolescence is crucial, and this is mainly the responsibility of the child's parents. Parents should be aware of their important function in educating their children to a healthy sexuality by their words and their 'non-verbal cues', that is, by the way they behave themselves in sexual matters. Both are important.

In childhood, a boy or a girl should be able to say with conviction by the age of 3 'I am a boy' or 'I am a girl'. As the child grows older its interest in sex increases. Young children, for example, explore their own and their playmates' bodies in games such as 'playing doctors' or 'mothers and fathers'. Young children find that stimulation of their genitalia is pleasurable: boys fondle their penis, girls 'rock', indirectly stimulating their clitoris and stimulate their clitoris directly with their fingers. These preliminary explorations should be treated by parents with respect and acceptance and neither condemned nor punished. When children ask questions about sexual matters, their questions should be answered factually and the child should be given access to accurate printed information, including pictures. Parents should always stress that sex is a natural function but that it carries responsibilities to another person.

In adolescence, the needs for privacy, for intimacy and for erotic expression should be recognized by the child's parents; and parents should try to stress that there are satisfying, non-exploiting ways of meeting these needs. They should also accept that much information (and misinformation) comes from other children in the child's group. To put it in a sentence: an adolescent should have been helped to be aware of her own body, to be able to touch it joyfully, and to see it as a uniquely personal possession, so that later she will be able to respond when in close joyous touch with another person's body. If she can achieve this contact she will also be able to communicate her needs to the other person, as you will see in Chapter 5.

Edward Brecher, in *The Sex Researchers*, has put the matter very clearly.

'The moral for parents of the next generation of little girls seems to me crystal clear. The repression of masturbation and other forms of childhood sexuality is not going to lead your daughter to maintain her chastity until marriage, or to remain faithful and monogamous there-after. But if your intention is to spoil your son's and your daughter's *enjoyment* of their future sexual experiences, including marital coitus, then the castigation of childhood masturbation and other forms of sexuality as shameful and filthy is almost guaranteed beyond your expectations.'

Eating disorders in adolescence

Most adolescent young women want to be more slim and most diet at some time. A few binge-eat between periods of dieting or use quantities of laxatives to 'hurry' the food through their intestines. These episodes of disordered eating appear to be normal in adolescence.

A few young women (and a very few young men) develop an eating disorder. The two eating disorders are anorexia nervosa and bulimia nervosa (or persistent binge-eating). These illnesses affect about 5 women in every 100 in late adolescence or early adulthood.

Anorexia nervosa

A young woman who has anorexia nervosa relentlessly pursues her desire to be thin. She fears becoming fat, and may exaggerate the size of her body when she looks in a mirror. Her menstrual periods cease. She may exercise excessively. As her weight falls so that she becomes emaciated, her body functions alter and she may become seriously ill. Treatment is to help the woman regain weight. If she is very ill she will have to be re-fed in hospital, but in less severe illness, it is better to treat her outside hospital. The treatment of anorexia nervosa is by counselling, and she frequently needs to talk with her therapist during a period of months or years.

Bulimia nervosa

Women with bulimia nervosa binge-eat two or more times a week, sometimes eating 10 or 20 times the amount they normally eat. Because they know that binge-eating this amount will make them fat, they starve between binges, learn to induce vomiting, or abuse laxatives. Most binge-eaters are secretive about their eating behaviour. Their weight is within the normal range but may fluctuate widely. About 1 anorexia nervosa patient in 5 also binge-eats. The treatment of bulimia is the same as that of anorexia nervosa.

Interested readers may care to obtain a book by Suzanne Abraham and myself called *Eating Disorders – The Facts*, 3rd Edition 1992, in which anorexia nervosa and bulimia are discussed at greater length.

Acne

Acne affects between 60 and 80 per cent of teenagers, and 15 per cent are severely affected. Severe acne can cause psychological problems, the young woman either withdrawing from her peers or seeking many treatments.

Acne is due to an increased sensitivity of the sebaceous glands in the skin to the hormone, *androgen*. This 'male hormone' is secreted by the ovaries and by the adrenal glands. Androgens cause the overgrowth of the cells which line the duct leading from the sebaceous gland to the surface of the skin. This 'blocks' the duct and a pimple or pustule forms.

Acne is not due to dietary indiscretions, to poor hygiene or to lack of exercise. In women it often becomes more apparent around the time of menstruation. Mild acne often responds to removal of skin 'grease' by washing, or if the woman takes one of the oral contraceptives. In more severe cases, particularly if there are pustules, antibiotics are often prescribed by doctors. Recently success has been achieved if the young woman takes a mixture of a drug which opposes androgen, called cyproterone, and an oestrogen for 21 days each month.

If the woman has severe disfiguring cystic acne another drug has proved very successful in clearing the acne. The drug is called isotretinoin (Roaccutane). It must be prescribed by a doctor and should not be taken unless the woman is protected against becoming pregnant as it causes severe deformity to the baby.

Sexuality

In the past 12 years there has been a significant increase in the number of teenaged women who have experienced sexual intercourse. Several investigations about teenage sexuality have been made in Britain, the USA, Canada and Australia in the past two decades. These studies show that increasing numbers of teenaged girls are becoming sexually active and they are having sex at an earlier age. The most recent studies show that between 25 and 35 per cent of girls have had sexual intercourse before they reached the age of 16; and between 40 and 70 per cent of girls aged 16 to 19 have had sexual intercourse. By the age of 20, over three quarters of teenaged women have had sexual intercourse at least once.

There does not appear to be much difference in the proportions of teenagers having sex between the countries, but within countries there are differences. For example, black Americans are more likely to be sexually active at an earlier age than white American teenagers.

Although more young women are experiencing sexual intercourse, they are not as 'permissive' as many older people might suppose. Most teenaged women have sexual intercourse infrequently and usually only have sex with one partner. Fewer than 15 per cent of teenaged women are 'sexual adventurers', which means that they have sexual intercourse with three or more partners in any one year.

Teenaged women today, despite popular mythology, are not sexually promiscuous, but more of them experience sexual intercourse, usually at their partner's home or at their own home. The popularity of the automobile for sexual experience seems to have waned.

It is interesting that most of the British teenaged women, or their partners, were aware of the possibility of pregnancy and used some form of contraception, although one couple in three used an unreliable method, usually withdrawal. The older the teenager, the more likely were the couple to use reliable contraceptives. Those most favoured were the condom and the Pill. In the British survey, 8 per cent of the teenaged women had become pregnant, and one in four had had an abortion. Of those who had had a child, most were married, but two-thirds of them had married because of the pregnancies.

The evidence of this British study is that abortion is not as widespread among teenaged women as is sometimes stated. Only 2 per cent of the women said they had had an abortion.

The information from the USA is less satisfactory. Over 9 per cent of teenagers became pregnant, as shown in a study made in 1985. This investigation suggests that over 1 000 000 pregnancies occur each year among the 3.5 million sexually active teenaged unmarried women.

It seems obvious that as premarital sexual intercourse is now common among teenagers, parents and society have an obligation to make sure that young people have sexual knowledge and have the opportunity to obtain efficient contraceptives without difficulty or embarrassment. The alternative to this is an increase in requests for abortion or in the number of teenaged mothers.

If teenagers are to become responsible about their own sexuality, they need to understand their sexuality and to have contraception accessible to them. This will not increase their sexual activity; rather it will reduce the potential consequences of this activity.

CHAPTER 5

About Sexuality

In these days of change – social, education and sexual – the differences between men and women have been reduced considerably. Although a woman tends to have less well-developed muscles than a man, she can equal him in physical and mental stamina, and is able increasingly to perform jobs which have been reserved for men in the past. The degree to which this change has occurred varies between countries but, more and more, the two sexes are peforming the same work and are sharing responsbilities previously reserved for one or the other. Political power, industrial power and military power – the three props which support Western society at present – are still predominantly male preserves, but even here increasing numbers of women are playing a significant part and sharing power with men.

In the earliest tribal societies, the culture was predominantly feminine, centred around childbearing, food-getting and home-making. The women tilled such fields as there were, and cultivated the edible vegetables. The men had far less responsibility; they brought in food from hunting, they took part in certain rituals necessary to bring rain or deflect the anger of the gods, and they occasionally helped with certain limited duties. Once nomadic tribes settled, cultivated fixed fields and domesticated animals, man began to dominate society. Man's status in his tribe could be measured by the number of his cattle or goats, and women became debased to be possessions of man, ranging only a little above his cows. In the West, by the Middle Ages, women of the peasant class had lost all of their traditionally dominant duties and now worked in the fields and in the house under the guidance and dominance of the man, who considered woman his chattel. If a woman was born into the upper classes, she did little except grace the house, organize the servants and act chiefly as a toy or pet for her husband. Even so, her position was not without merit. The organization of a great establishment, many of which were self-contained communities, took skill and knowledge. Educated women of the seventeenth and eighteenth centuries took the same pride in the way they managed their households as they did in learning to play musical instruments, or embroider intricate pieces of needlework and to paint.

In India, Hindu society had strict rules for the conduct of the sexes, which hardly changed over 1000 years. The women entered her husbands's family at marriage and the primary object of marriage was the birth of a son so that the family line might continue. The woman was therefore totally subordinate to her husband, who believed that she was inferior to man, less able to resist temptation and therefore weaker. Because of this, it was his duty to protect his wife with 'the respect due to his mother' but also to regulate her behaviour to his desires.

The Christian cultures of the West also held that woman was inferior to man and, following St Augustine, believed that sexual intercourse was permissible only for the purpose of producing children, a belief similar to that of the older Hindu religion. The pronouncements of the early Christian theologians were further codified during the turbulence of the Reformation, when male dominance and female subjugation were confirmed. In such an environment men were able to insist on their exclusive right to the women they owned. The woman was to be a virgin at marriage and monogamous after marriage, so that the man could be certain that any child she conceived was his. This encouraged the belief that only heterosexual intercourse was normal, and that only orgasm achieved during heterosexual intercourse was proper. Other forms of sexual pleasure, such as masturbation, clitoral or penile manipulation, or homosexual relationships were evil. A 'double standard' of sexual behaviour was established, in which the male was permitted to seek sexual satisfaction with women and even encouraged to do so, while the female was expected to avoid sexual relations until marriage and then submit to the dominance of her husband.

This rigid pattern of male dominance and female submission was changed to some extent by the influence of Sigmund Freud towards the end of the nineteenth century. He insisted that sex was a basic instinct which should be enjoyed by both men and women. Other psychologists amplified Freud's original work by confirming that sex should extend beyond the mere physical act of copulation to involve the emotional responses of both partners. In other words, both partners needed to have a knowledge of, and involvement in, sex for the further development of their relationship.

Despite the evidence, the double standard remains remarkably strong in much of Western society. People, both men and women, are conditioned by their upbringing, and by the prevailing cultural attitudes, to believe that men, by virtue of being men, are sexually knowledgeable, aggressive and have an urgent, highly demanding sexual drive. Many people are taught that sex is a man's 'responsibility'; he should always take the initiative for sex, and in sexual encounters he is the master, the woman the passive servant. Many people think that women should be sexually innocent, relatively inert, rarely initiating sex and never obviously pursuing the man. It is also thought that a woman should value her sexuality as a necessary precursor to reproduction, rather than something deeply pleasurable in itself, and that a woman is expected to suppress her sexual feelings or to perceive them as something not 'quite nice'. Many women brought up to expect that their sexual arousal will be slow, will depend on their partner to be aroused and believe that they do not need to be aroused as often and as much as a man. Because of all this, in many relationships, a woman is treated as, and accepts the role of, a sexual puppet, available for a man when he requires release of sexual tension. She may be regarded by him lovingly, valued for her qualities as a housewife and mother, accorded respect when she adds to the family income by working, but he never treats her as a human being who has equal sexual needs.

Unfortunately, if a man believes that a woman has a reduced sexuality, compared with his, and if he treats her as his sexual possession, he will 'use' her sexually. He may condescend to stimulate her sexually in a perfunctory way, but his real objective is to reach his orgasm at his speed without really considering her sexual needs. If 'his' woman manages to reach an orgasm during sexual intercourse that is great. If she does not, he need not worry unduly, as woman are 'known' to be less sexually responsive than men. But, paradoxically, a man may expect a woman to reach an orgasm during sexual intercourse, preferably simultaneously with his orgasm. If a woman fails to reach an orgasm, the man may feel sexually inadequate, his masculinity suspect, as he has learnt that a man 'gives a woman her orgasm'. So that he will not feel disappointed, or to protect his masculine self-image, many women attempt to 'fake' orgasms.

This attitude is beginning to change as women obtain emancipation politically, socially and sexually. But the majority of women are still confused about their sexuality, because parents, by their behaviour to each other and within the family, reinforce the 'double standard' of

43

sexuality. This behaviour may convince the girl that human sexuality is something which cannot be discussed and which is a taboo subject. Such conditioning can cause a woman to suppress her sexuality; not necessarily her desire for sex but certainly her full enjoyment of sex.

A woman will only obtain full sexual pleasure when she and her partner have equality in sexual matters, and when the sexual pleasure is mutually shared, something that is done together, rather than to the other person; something done with each other, rather than for the other. Women will only be sexually equal when men accept that a woman is not merely a sexual receptacle, and when women accept that a man is not merely a sexual instrument.

Many groups within our society resist the idea of a woman having sexual equality. Some people fear that the change will diminish the status of those women who prefer to remain 'mere housewives'. Some men fear it will place heavy burdens on them to prove their masculinity. As long as a man has only to express to the woman, by word or gesture, that he wants sex, so long as he only has to obtain an erection and reach an orgasm at his desired pace, he is in control of the situation. But if he has to consider the woman's sexual needs, he has to be more perceptive and more receptive. He may even feel that a woman's sexual equality is a threat to his sexuality. Some men and women resist the change to sexual equality because of inhibitions towards sex which they acquired during their early upbringing. One such inhibition is that sex is dirty and should be 'indulged' in secretly rather than enjoyed mutually. Some men and women also fear that women's sexual equality will diminish her 'femininity'. These fears are all groundless. All have the effect of reducing the right of women to equality with men in all spheres of life and particularly in the sexual sphere.

Sexual and socio-economic emancipation place additional burdens on a woman, particularly if she is sharing her life, whether married or not, with a man who rejects her views. Because of cultural attitudes, rather than biology, a woman is expected to manage her home and rear her children without necessarily receiving help. Biologically, it is true that only a woman can breast-feed a baby, but there is no reason why a man should not share in all the other home-making and child-rearing functions. As more women prove themselves the equal of men in practically every field of human endeavour, it is extremely galling to discover that many men expect their women to give up their careers on marriage, or, if the woman has to work to supplement the family income, refuse to help in the house. This can place an intolerable strain on a woman and, so far, Western society has done little to help women solve this problem. A new approach to the partnership between a man and a woman is needed and this should start in childhood. Children should be brought up to accept that domestic chores should be shared, that the kitchen and the nursery are as much the joint responsibility of the father and mother as is the bedroom.

It is equally important to women's dignity that society accepts the idea that not all women believe that the 'be-all and end-all' of their life is marriage. Only a woman can conceive and bear a child, but this in itself does not mean her life can only be fulfilled if she carries out this biological function. To bring up a girl to believe that she is unfeminine unless she marries and becomes a mother, is probably one of the more dangerous heresies of this century. Some women may never have the opportunity to marry, others have no desire to do so. They can still live full, active and stimulating lives as single women, as personalities in their own right. Once this fact is accepted, many outmoded conventions will disappear from our society.

Meanwhile, convention still requires that a woman must display a willingness to be a housewife, a mother and have the capacity to be sexually attractive to a man. A woman is also taught to be sexually available to a man, paticularly if she is married to him. Some women who do not enjoy sexual intercourse, make themselves 'available' for their man to have sex with because they are afraid that they will lose the man's love if they challenge his sexual expertise by suggesting ways in which they might enjoy sex more. Some women 'trade sex for love' and believe their man gives love for sex. Other women trade sexual intercourse for body contact and the close touch of another human, rather than for the emotional and physical sensations of intercourse, and especially of orgasm which, because of the man's insensitivity, may be minimal. It is becoming accepted, at last, that women have no less enthusiasm for sexual intercourse and no less enjoyment of sexuality than men. It is true, however, that some women take longer than men to reach their full sexual response; but a woman's total sexual response exceeds that of a man and, once aroused, women can often have orgasms more frequently than men.

In our society, a woman will only achieve her full potential for sexual pleasure if she is able to let her partner know her sexual needs and desires, confident that he will respond understandingly and lovingly. Equally, she must be just as responsive to his sexual needs and desires.

Unfortunately, because of the way children are reared in our society and our 'hang-ups' about expressing emotions, many couples are unable to let each other know how they feel and what their emotional needs are. One of these emotional needs is the need to be sexually fulfilled. What stimulates a person sexually, what 'turns them on', is an individual matter. It is based on the person's memories and experiences. If you are unable to express your special needs to your partner and he, or she, is unable to guess them, your sexuality will be less enjoyable than it should be. Your partner may 'know' what you want, but often this 'knowledge' is based on myths, not on the reality of your sexuality.

Sexual desire (the sexual drive)

At puberty, the sex hormones, testosterone and oestrogen in girls and testosterone in boys, increase in quantity and 'stimulate' the person's sexual drive, which has been developing slowly since infancy, so that his or her desire for sexual pleasure increases.

Your sexual drive is not your capacity to have sexual relations but your desire or urge for sex. It is determined largely by the attitudes towards sexuality you have acquired during your upbringing. Your sexual beliefs and attitudes are formed by what you have learnt from your parents and other adults, which in turn depends on their attitudes and beliefs. In late childhood and in adolescence these attitudes may be influenced by the sexual values of your peer-group from whom you 'learn' a good deal about sex. Some of this information is inaccurate, some is not, but you form your sexual values from these examples and from your own experience.

In our kind of society, girls are thought to be more inhibited about sex than boys, because girls are given different values about sex. This has led to the belief that in adolescence and when adult, women are less sexual; they 'demand' and 'need' sex less often than men; they respond sexually more slowly, and they reach orgasm less rapidly and less often than men. Because of this, many women still believe that they have a lower sex drive than men, which is not true. Biologically, a woman's sex drive is no different from that of a man, but if a mother has taught her daughter, by example or by words, that sex is 'dirty', that sex outside marriage is 'sinful' and that it is a wife's 'duty' to submit passively to her husband's sexual 'demands', rather than enjoying sex, her sexuality may be impaired. As I mentioned in the last chapter when I quoted Edward Brecher, the importance of sensitive sexual upbringing by informed parents and teachers is obvious, if a person is to achieve his or her full potential for sexual pleasure.

The intensity of a person's sexual drive is not only influenced by their upbringing but also varies at different times during their life. It is believed that it decreases in intensity as people grow older. This is untrue and many people have a high sexual drive well into old age. A person's sexual drive is influenced by many factors. For example, pressure of work, fatigue, chronic pain, anxiety about a job, excessive alcohol or a defective relationship with one's sexual partner can reduce the drive of men and women, while the demands of child-rearing (see p. 260) can reduce it in women.

There are many ways in which you may solve the problem of having a different sexual drive compared with that of your partner, if this occurs, as it may, from time to time. One of these ways (and you may have found others), is for you to share your feelings, so that your partner understands the kinds of feelings you have about your sexual desires. If you can do this, your sexual relationship is likely to be enhanced, as each of you will understand and accept that sex is not something done to the other, but a pleasurable activity enjoyed together.

Unfortunately, because of the inhibitions about sex we acquire from our parents and others during our upbringing, and because of our own 'hang-ups', many of us do not have a sexual relationship in which each partner is considered to have equal needs. Many people find it difficult to talk openly about their sexual desires and needs, so that they do not find out what is right, sexually, for each person in the relationship. Your unwillingness, or inability, to talk openly with your partner about your sexual needs, may be one facet of an inability to relate to each other emotionally in other matters. If you have emotional barriers, sexual or other, your relationship may be unequal and perhaps fragile, and frustration can mount.

Women in our society seem to be especially affected by the inability to express sexual and other emotional needs, and the resulting frustrations can be damaging to health. The frustrations may be pushed deep into the woman's unconscious mind to emerge as depression, fatigue or irritability, or they may be expressed in a bewildering variety of gynaecological disorders, such as pain in the lower abdomen, backache, increased vaginal discharge or changes in the quantity and duration of menstruation. In all of these conditions, the problem originates in the mind, not in the pelvis, they are psychosomatic in origin, but that makes them no less real.

It is interesting to speculate on the extent to which sexual problems are present because of the 'work-ethic' of Western society. A man will spend long hours attending to his business, or working at his job. He may come home tired and frustrated, and expect his wife to console him; but to him sex, like work, has its special place and special time. It may be subordinate to work, and the time spent on establishing a warm, mutually pleasurable relationship is thought to be less important than the time spent at work, at sport or in the pub. The man may be insufficiently sensitive to realize that his wife has also had a tiring, frustrating day. He needs sex for consolation; but because of the double standard of sexuality he can only envisage sex as something to be 'indulged' in, rather than something to be shared. In this type of situation the resolution of the couple's sexual problems will depend on their ability to give time to the pleasure of their sexual relationship, and to know that both of them have sexual and other emotional needs which they want to share with the other.

Sexual arousal and excitement

What is it that attracts one person to another, while both ignore a third person? The answer is not yet known, but it seems likely that each person begins developing his or her own pattern, or scenario, in childhood. In the scenario, the person, who is the 'writer' of his or her own sexual arousal script, builds it up from childhood memories and fantasies obtained from parents and peers. The scenario is added to, modified, expanded and rewritten again and again as the person grows up, until he or she creates a unique, individual pattern of sexual arousal. In the scenario, the 'writer' has created and identified the type of person by whom he or she is sexually excited. When he or she meets such a person, sexual arousal occurs, and if this is reciprocated by the other person, who has his or her own scenario, the couple make closer contact. The contact may be emotional, or physical, but is usually both. With the contact, the couple explore each other's personality and become closer, or separate, as they learn more about each other.

If the contact becomes closer, their sexual arousal and excitement increase. All the senses – sight, sound, taste, smell and touch – may be involved in increasing your sexual arousal. Sight appears to be a potent stimulus for men, and both advertisers and publishers of erotica play on this by using women's bodies as sexual symbols. In Western nations, a woman's breasts, suggested through clothing, or naked, and her buttocks are considered to be sexually arousing to men.

The smell of a clean body is stimulating to both sexes, and in many cultures including our own, perfume, usually sold under a sexually provocative name, is used by women for their own pleasure and is sexually exciting to men. Unpleasant odours can be sexually repellent. Women have a more precise sense of smell than men, so that an unpleasant smell from a man can depress them sexually. Sound, of voice or of music, can be sexually arousing, as can the taste of a partner's hair, lips or body.

For many people, the touch of body contact is the most sexually exciting of all the senses. Most men and women become sexually excited when they kiss or hug each other, particularly when those parts of the body which they find most erotically arousing are caressed. Each person has his or her own erotically arousing parts of the body. Most men are aroused by the sight and feel of a woman's breasts, buttocks and vulva, and most women are aroused by the buttocks and genitals of a man. Other people are aroused by different areas of their body. Only you can find out what part of your body, and your partner's body, arouses you the most.

The emotional and physical components which cause sexual arousal lead in turn to sexual desire. Sexual desire is the feeling that you want to touch and explore the other person's body and probably to have sexual intercourse, or to be sexually stimulated in some other way. Sexual desire causes a feeling of excitement, which, in turn leads to physical changes, which have been observed and described. Some of what follows has been known for centuries, but some was only reported by Dr Masters and Dr Johnson in 1966.

Since human sexuality is a shared experience and each partner obtains, or should obtain, pleasure and fulfilment, I think it appropriate to describe what happens to each sex if sexual excitement continues and is not suppressed.

The sexual response of men

The most obvious sign of sexual excitement in a man is the erection of his penis, which enlarges both in length and in diameter. With further excitement, a clear secretion, which may be scanty or profuse, emerges from the 'eye' of his penis and lubricates the glans, whether he has a foreskin or not. Once the man's penis is erect, he is in a state when additional sexual excitement will make him want to have sexual intercourse, or to have his penis stroked so that he can reach orgasm and ejaculate. In erection, the penis approximately doubles its length and measures 9.5cm (4in). There are several fallacies connected with the penis. The first is that the larger the penis, the better is the man as a lover. This is not true, as the size of the penis is not related to its function. A man with a small penis is as sexually adequate as a man with a large penis, and can provide as much sexual satisfaction. A second fallacy is that the circumcised male takes longer to reach orgasm, and so may more readily help a woman to reach an orgasm. The evidence is that there is no difference in time to reach an orgasm between circumcised and uncircumcised men. There is, of course, a considerable difference between men in the time they take to reach an orgasm, but circumcision or its absence is not a factor.

Once penile erection has occurred and the arousal stimulus continued, the man either seeks to have sexual intercourse or masturbates. In essence, there is little difference as far as the penis is concerned. During sexual intercourse he thrusts his penis in and out of his partner's vagina; during masturbation he stimulates his penis by grasping it lightly and stroking the length of the entire organ.

As orgasm approaches, a time is reached when the man knows that within a few moment ejaculation will occur. The phase lasts about 3 or 4 seconds, and even if he ceased all movements of his penis, he knows that ejaculation is inevitable. There is nothing he can do to stop it. This time of 'suspended animation' is followed by a warm feeling along the shaft of his penis as the seminal fluid moves from the collecting area deep in his pelvis, to the top of the penis. Then, spasmodically, three to six expulsive contractions of the muscles at the base of his penis lead to spurting of seminal fluid, and simultaneously the muscles of his thighs and lower abdomen jerk and thrust convulsively. During his explosive, expulsive period, he may clasp the woman tightly to his body. The 'crisis' or 'climax' passes with smaller contractions fading away. Immediately after ejaculation, the glans of the penis becomes momentarily exquisitely tender, and a feeling of warm well-being envelops the man. It is usual for complete relaxation and short sleep to occur, the 'little death' of the French, during which time the penis becomes limp.

As a man grows older, certain changes in his sexual response may occur. He may take longer to get an erection, during foreplay his erection may disappear and return several times; his penis may not become as hard; he may take longer to ejaculate, and the period after ejaculation before he desires sexual intercourse again may increase, often to 24 hours. These changes vary in degree: some men experience no alteration in sexual response while in others the changes are considerable. It is important for a woman to know about these changes as she may feel that because her partner is slower to respond sexually, he no longer loves her, or that he finds her ageing, less firm body no longer sexually stimulating. Of course, this is possible; but it is equally possible that the changes are only due to increasing age, and that if she makes allowance for this, their relationship will be enhanced. This is more likely to occur if the partners are able to communicate with each other.

The sexual response of women

The sexual response of a woman can be divided into four phases, which Masters and Johnson have called (1) the excitement or arousal phase, (2) the plateau phase, (3) the phase of orgasm, and (4) the phase of resolution. The phases are useful to describe the sexual response but of course one merges into the next in real life.

Excitement phase: This is initiated more by bodily contact with the male than by visual stimuli, although the sight of an attractive male may play some part. Sexual arousal varies in women depending on the time of the month. Many women have a heightened sexual interest at certain times, often at midcycle or just before and during menstruation, but no consistent pattern can be determined. Tradition has held that sexual intercourse during menstruation is dangerous because the tissues are more fragile and liable to infection, but probably really because of the old Jewish law which held a woman to be 'unclean' during menstruation. This is unfortunate because some women are particularly aroused sexually at this time. There is no medical reason why a woman who desires sexual intercourse during menstruation should not have it. The tissues are not more fragile, nor is infection more likely to occur. There is no danger and the woman is not unclean.

The excitement phase of a woman tends to be slower to reach its peak, and to last for longer, than that of a man. During it her nipples become erect, and the areola around them becomes swollen and dusky. Her clitoris increases in size, mainly in width, and the 'lips' around the vaginal entrance become softer and thicker as they become congested with blood, forming soft swellings. These changes vary in degree from woman to woman.

At the same time as these events are occurring, fluid is entering her pelvic tissues, her vagina is becoming softer and some of the fluid seep through the layers of tiny cells which make up the vaginal wall, so that the vagina becomes lubricated. Two small glands which lie near the opening of the vagina also secrete fluid, so that both the vagina and the entrance become moist and slippery. If the man attempts to introduce his penis before the fluid has been secreted and the area has become lubricated, coitus may be painful. This is one reason, but not the only one, for a woman's partner to stimulate her by kissing and caressing her, until she is sexually excited. Simultaneously the tissues surrounding the lower one-third of the woman's vagina become swollen with blood, so that soft, warm, 'cushions' form which will caress the man's penis as it enters the vagina.

Plateau phase: The woman is now in the plateau phase and if she has a sensitive, relating partner will want to feel his erect penis in her lubricated vagina. Even if he is not sensitive to her sexual needs, she is physically able to accept his penis without pain, although she may be resentful, or trade her vagina for the favours he gives her.

In a recent survey, many women said that the most pleasurable part of sexual intercourse, apart from the orgasm itself, was the feeling of the man's penis entering the vagina. Also, the closer contact of the couple's bodies may stimulate her clitoral area directly, while the movement of the man's penis, by moving the lips around the vagina, stimulates it indirectly. This stimulation may bring her to orgasm. About one women in three reaches an orgasm while the man is thrusting in her vagina, either before he ejaculates, simultaneously with his orgasm, or very soon after. But if a woman does not have an orgasm at this time, she may wish the man to help her have an orgasm by gently manipulating her clitoral area at her direction, or by caressing it with his tongue and lips. This is called cunnilingus. She may prefer to have an orgasm before they begin coitus, or after the man has ejaculated depending on her mood and that of her partner.

Whatever the timing, she is in control and should let the man know what movements of his fingers or tongue stimulate her most and what movements distract her. Most women prefer to have the shaft of the clitoris stimulated rather than the tip (or glans), and finger stimulation is more comfortable if the area is moist. The man can obtain lubrication from her vaginal secretion or from his saliva. The woman should let her partner know what she wants, and he should accept that she knows what is most pleasurable to her, instead of doing what he assumes will give her most pleasure.

Orgasm: It is difficult to describe an orgasm as it is something each person feels and perceives in a unique way. Descriptions given by women suggest that an orgasm is a feeling of intense pleasure which is the peak of sexual arousal. Initially, the feeling is usually located deep in the pelvis, but later it spreads over the whole body. During the orgasm the person's feelings are concentrated on the sensations, largely to the exclusion of anything else. It begins with moments of stillness which are followed by uncontrollable muscle movements, a general tingling, a floating feeling, warmth, well-being, a release of mental tension, and exhilaration.

An orgasm is due to a reflex. Stimulation of the clitoral area, either directly when a woman masturbates or is caressed, or indirectly by the movement of the man's penis as he thrusts in her vagina, sends a message to her spinal cord. In the spinal cord, the reflex occurs and the message is relayed to the nerves which control the muscles of her pelvis. But whether the message is relayed at all, is increased in its intensity, or is inhibited, depends on the degree of control by her brain over the reflex. A woman who has no inhibitions about sex will probably enhance the strength of the message and will have an orgasm. If she has inhibitions or does not like the feeling that the man is 'using' her, she may fail to have an orgasm during coitus, although she can reach an orgasm by fantasizing when she masturbates.

A woman's orgasm is usually associated with the same jerking thrusting movements of the thigh and pelvic muscles, as those of a man, but some women remain still and rigid during the orgasm. A woman's orgasm only differs from a man's orgasm by the absence of ejaculation. Contrary to popular belief a woman does not have to arch her back or 'writhe' in ecstasy during her orgasm. The muscles of her womb and her vagina contract, and some women have a more intense orgasm if the erect penis is deeply inside the vagina at the time, so that it can be rhythmically gripped and released by the contracting vaginal muscles. It was believed until recently that women had two types of orgasm: the 'clitoral orgasm', and the 'vaginal orgasm'. An error of observation and of deduction by Freud is responsible for this. He maintained that the clitoral orgasm was an immature form, which was obtained by masturbation, and that vaginal orgasm only developed with sexual and psychological maturity, when the centre of sexual sensitivity was transferred from the clitoral area to the vagina. The deduction from this was that masturbation was immature, and a woman who could only reach an orgasm by masturbation was sexually and psychologically immature, while the woman who had a vaginal orgasm was sexually and psychologically mature. This error, although suspected for some time, was finally laid by Masters and Johnson who showed that an orgasm is an orgasm, and there is no difference in how it is produced, whether as a result of clitoral area manipulation, by movement of the penis in the vagina, by simply fondling the breasts, or even by listening to music.

In nearly all orgasms, the 'trigger' which starts the orgasm reflex is the stimulated clitoris, although additional messages may come from stimulation of the vagina. In all people an orgasm is expressed by contractions of the deep pelvic muscles, including those of the vagina, and is felt as pleasure by a special area of the brain. Many women believed, until recently, that men 'gave' them orgasms and if a woman failed to have an orgasm during coitus she was deficient in femininity and would make the man feel sexually inadequate. Because of this woman 'faked' orgasms so that the man would not feel inadequate or she unfeminine. With a more open approach to women's sexuality, it is now known that women who fail to reach an orgasm during coitus are not deficient in sexual drive, and that to 'fake' an orgasm is folly.

Almost every woman can have an orgasm either by masturbating, or by being sufficiently relaxed and confident in her relationship to let her partner know her needs, so that he helps her reach an orgasm by stimulating her. In a fulfilling relationship the man must be willing and happy to stimulate the woman sexually in the way she wishes. Ideally, no woman should be embarrassed about asking her partner to do this, nor should a sensitive lover be resentful if asked. But many women are ashamed to ask, and because of this reduce their sexual pleasure.

Resolution phase: In both sexes, the convulsive muscle contractions and the deep pleasure of orgasm are followed by relaxation. But in contrast to a man's penis, the clitoris usually is not tender and some women can have one orgasm after another without intermission. Other women find one orgasm is all that they want. In the first five to ten minutes of the resolution phase the tissues of the vagina and the vulva lose the fluid which had seeped into them; but if re-stimulated sexually a woman can be aroused and have other orgasms at shorter intervals than a man.

On the other hand, if a woman is stimulated to the plateau phase but is not helped to have an orgasm, or does not masturbate to give herself an orgasm, the resolution phase is often prolonged and the congestion of the tissues is slow to resolve. Repeated stimulation and failure to achieve an orgasm may lead to physical and mental frustration, and may be an underlying cause of several psychosomatic gynaecological complaints. For this reason, as well as for reasons of love and affection, the man should help the woman to reach a climax if she desires this.

About 40 per cent of women reach an orgasm with every, or nearly every episode of sexual intercourse and one woman of every three in this group is able to have multiple orgasms. About 50 per cent of women occasionally reach a climax during sexual intercourse and consistently do so if the clitoris is stimulated with the man's finger or his tongue before or after he has had an orgasm, or if the woman masturbates. Only about 10 per cent of women reach an orgasm very occasionally or never.

Masturbation

Stimulation of the genitals by the fingers is almost universal in childhood, and in adolescence masturbation is general. Studies in several countries have shown that almost all young males masturbate, and three-quarters of females have masturbated by the age of 21. As the person gets older and heterosexual contacts are more readily available, the frequency of masturbation diminishes, although it continues throughout life. Masturbation is a normal part of sexual development, and does no physical harm whatsoever, however frequently or infrequently it takes place. The only harm which may result from masturbation are feelings of guilt, occasioned by the Judeo-Christian religious disapproval of masturbation.

Strange, nonsensical myths are still perpetuated: masturbation is said to make a person weak, to damage the eyesight and, in excess (whatever that is), to cause brain decay or insanity. Masturbation does none of these things, but these particularly pernicious ideas are still spread by ignorant people. In women, masturbation has been said to lead to enlargement of the inner lips of the vulva, to 'congestion of the pelvis', and to venereal disease. Again, all these ideas have no foundation. Masturbation has been declared as evidence of immaturity, which is clearly not true, as people who are sexually well-adjusted and mature obtain sexual pleasure from masturbation, when married or when single. Masturbation is said to lead to sexual frustration and frigidity, but as other equally distinguished investigators declare that it leads to sexual excess, it is obvious that these objections are emotional not factual. It has been said that one cannot possibly get full emotional gratification through masturbation. Recent research has shown this to be false, and many people obtain as much, or more pleasure from masturbation as they do in sexual intercourse.

Masturbation has several positive values. Through it, in childhood and adolescence, a girl may learn to explore her body and not to feel shame or guilt about touching her genital area. It may help a girl become aware of her response to stimulation, and to recognize the stages of her sexual arousal. It may also enable a girl to develop the physical aspects of her sexuality, which should contribute to her later sexual fulfilment. Despite the positive value of masturbation, many parents still condemn their children if they find them masturbating. The effect of this is to increase the child's guilt, as 95 per cent of boys and over 70 per cent of girls masturbate, whatever their parents say.

As adults, both men and women continue to masturbate, although less often than when adolescents. Within a sexual relationship the couple may enjoy masturbation as another way of making love. During periods of separation or if one's sexual partner dies, women and men may prefer to masturbate rather than seeking a lover, when they become sexually tense or excited.

Most people – both men and women – fantasize during masturbation; that is, the person imagines a sexual situation with a lover, or some other sexual situation. Some people can fantasize unaided, but others need the added stimulus of erotic literature or pictures to enhance the fantasy.

As sexual desires continue into old age; as women tend to live longer than men; and as, in our society, it is easier for an older man to find a new partner than it is for an older woman, maturbation may be an older woman's only way of obtaining an orgasm. No guilt should be experienced, as masturbation is a normal sexual outlet at any age.

Petting

Petting is an American term for love-making which reaches to, but stops short of, sexual intercourse. In other countries and at other times, other terms have been used; 'bundling', 'lolligagging', and 'smooching'. The activity is as old as tribal society, and is practised by tribes as primitive as those of New Guinea, or by people with a culture as sophisticated as that of the USA. In Western countries, petting seems to be confined largely to adolescence. In 'light petting' or 'necking', the couple kiss passionately, their bodies (usually fully clothed) are in contact, but certain zones are 'forbidden' by the girl, who may refuse to allow her breasts to be caressed, and will not allow wandering hands to reach for her vulva. In 'heavy petting', passionate kissing, love bites, breast stimulation, caressing of the clitoris to orgasm, and of the penis to ejaculation, are accepted in varying degrees; but the girl remains a technical virgin, as she does not allow a man's penis to enter her vagina.

'Petting' plays an important role in the development of sexual behaviour as it offers the opportunity for body exploration, for genital exploration and for emotional interaction. The body exploration which petting permits is important, particularly for those people who obtain a great deal of pleasure from touch. Since this is conditioned by childhood learning, it is likely that men would be more willing to touch, and would obtain more pleasure from touching were they not taught to believe that touching is 'weak' and 'feminine'. Many women enjoy body contact for long periods of love-making before they want sexual intercourse, and many men would find that they too would get sexual pleasure from touch if they could overcome their inhibitions.

Petting was until recently a socially acceptable way of releasing sexual tensions in a society in which sexual intercourse outside marriage was condemned – at least for women. This has changed to some extent in recent years, as the prohibitions of the 'double standard' of sexuality have diminished. Today, when there is a more open attitude towards non-marital sexuality the question, 'what intensity of petting should be permitted' has been replaced by new questions. These are: whether to have (or to allow) sexual intercourse; with which partner or partners, and in what circumstances.

Information from surveys of sexual behaviour in Western nations suggests that by the age of 17, 55–65 per cent of single men and 25–35 per cent of single women have had sexual intercourse. By the age of 24, 85–90 per cent of single men and 70–80 per cent of single women have had sexual intercourse. Even though sexual intercourse is increasingly usual among single people, so that petting as a substitute has become less common, the change should not diminish the importance of touch and of the arousal of sexuality by body exploration and contact, which was a feature of petting. To do so would reduce the pleasure women and men can obtain from sex.

Sexual intercourse

It is strange that there is no verb for sexual intercourse which can be used normally. Even the Latin term used in medical textbooks, *coitus*, is a euphemism. It is made up from the two words *co*, together and *ire*, to go, so that it means to 'go together'.

The delicacy in language about a universal pleasurable activity may be due to the Judeo-Christian belief that coitus should be practised principally for the procreation of children, and only secondarily permitted as an expression of the love that exists between the two sexual partners. Today, with efficient contraception, these two functions can be separated, and it is increasingly accepted that sexuality and its active genital component, coitus, form a physical and emotional bond holding two people together in warmth, security and mutual pleasure. Sexual intercourse should not be a competitive indoor sport, nor a virtuoso performance to be boasted about later, but a physical and emotional expression of a warm relationship between two mutually attracted people, which may last permanently or may be temporary.

A sexual relationship implies more than sexual intercourse. It also includes enjoyment of being with a person, touching and mutually pleasuring. In the early years of a sexual relationship, coitus commonly takes place frequently, often one or more times a day. The frequency falls off after one or two years, to two or three times a week up to the age of about 35. As middle age approaches, coital frequency often falls to once a week or less. But there are very considerable variations, and some couples only have sexual intercourse at infrequent intervals in the early years, while other couples enjoy sex frequently and satisfactorily well into old age.

It is sometimes asked, can coitus take place too frequently? The answer is a firm No! There is no such thing as 'excessive coitus'. Provided the male can obtain and maintain an erection of his penis, and provided that he can do this as often as he and his partner desire to have sexual intercourse, coitus can take place as often as they wish. Frequent coitus does not lead to any weakness of either partner. Occasionally, frequent coitus does cause irritation to one or other partner's genitals from over-stimulation or friction. In such cases, a period of a couple of days' rest will restore the function to normal.

How often a couple have sexual intercourse is a matter for their joint decision. 'Excessive' coitus does not exist, and 'infrequent' coitus is equally harmless provided that this pattern is acceptable and not frustrating to either partner. Nor is there any truth in the belief that to be healthy a woman or a man needs to have sex at regular intervals. Neither a woman nor a man can have too many nor too few orgasms. Each individual has different needs and desires for an orgasm at different times in his or her life. When a person has no sexual partner, orgasms can be produced as often as the person desires by masturbation. With a partner an orgasm may be the culmination of sexual intercourse, which is the way a man usually prefers; or can be produced by one partner stimulating the other's clitoris or penis with tongue or finger; or by masturbating either during sexual intercourse, or afterwards.

As I have mentioned, because of culturally-induced inhibitions, many women take longer to be aroused erotically than do men. For this reason, mutual pleasuring should take place before coitus is attempted. I prefer the term mutual pleasuring to the older word, foreplay, because foreplay has acquired a special meaning which is insulting to women. Many men believe that foreplay means that the man briefly fondles the woman's breasts and fumbles at her vulva while she caresses his penis. It is brief because it delays what he really wants; and that is to put his penis in her vagina, thrust and have an orgasm. Mutual pleasuring involves much more than that. It involves cuddling and exploring each other's body surface. It involves stroking, and it involves kissing and exploring other parts of the body with lips and tongue. It involves stimulating those parts of the body each person feels are erotic by fingers, tongue, lips, thighs and body.

The extent and sequence of mutual pleasuring are those which each couple evolve uniquely for themselves. They make their own formula, for what erotically stimulates a person is unique for that person, and has to be communicated to the partner either by using words or by body language. And in this communication each partner has to accept that the other knows what most excites him or her.

During the period of mutual pleasuring, both partners become increasingly stimulated by kissing, by bodily contact when they hug or cuddle each other, by stroking each other's bodies, especially the areas which arouse sexual desire – for example, the woman's breasts and thighs and the man's genitals. But each partner has to discover the erotic areas of the other. Mutual pleasuring goes on for as long as the couple wish, until each is aroused and ready for coitus. The man shows this by his erect penis, the woman by her lubricated vagina. Both acknowledge it by an increased sexual urge. Women, particularly, say that they can enjoy the closeness, the body contact and the intimacy of sexual intercourse, and obtain pleasure in 'pleasing' a man sexually. But the overwhelming pleasure occurs when sexual pleasuring comes to a climax in an orgasm.

The first time a couple have sexual intercourse, particularly if neither partner is sexually experienced, or if the man is unaware of a woman's sexual needs, can be clumsy and frustrating to both partners, or painful to the woman. The psychological dangers of forceful, clumsy attempts at penetration on a woman who is not ready for coitus have been exaggerated. Even so, a traumatic first coital encounter with an insensitive man may create anxieties in the woman which even her love for him cannot resolve, and their sexual relationship may be marred. The full establishment of sexual compatibility may take some time.

The period of sexual arousal during the first time the couple have sexual intercourse is important, as it may be painful to the woman if her vagina has not become lubricated before her partner's penis enters it. Once she is sexually excited and her vagina is moist, she may wish to feel her partner's penis in her body. She should guide it so that it lies against her hymen, making sure that no strands of vulval hair are in between. If she lies on her back, the man on top of her, her legs apart, her knees bent, she will find it easier to guide his erect penis. In this position, as he lies over her, he slowly and gently presses his penis into the vaginal entrance, and then withdraws slightly. This movement is repeated, and each time he presses his penis a little further into the vagina, always moving slowly so that the muscles which surround the vagina have time to relax, and the hymen to stretch. Slowly he moves, and soon he finds that his penis has been introduced fully into the vagina. If he tries to introduce it too quickly, he may cause the woman pain, which could cause her vaginal muscles to contract against him causing her more pain. With careful penetration, coitus can proceed normally, the penis deeply inside the vagina and its thrusting movements bringing the man to orgasm. Immediately after ejaculation of semen, the tip (or glans) of the penis is exquisitely sensitive, and the erection subsides. The sensitivity lasts only for a few minutes, but while this is occurring he lies relaxed and still.

The woman may reach her orgasm during the man's thrusting but if she has not, she may wish him to help her reach orgasm by stimulating her with his fingers or tongue. If they are aware of each other's needs and desires, there should be no problem about this. Embarrassment or resentment should have no place in a warm loving relationship.

Sexual adjustment between the two partners may occur quickly, may take time, or may never be fully achieved, depending on the sexual knowledge of the couple, their inhibitions towards sex and their ability to express their sexual needs to each other. The understanding between them required for the first coitus to be pleasurable to both partners, needs to continue into subsequent love-making. Unless a woman is sexually aroused and stimulated each time, so that her vagina is lubricated, intercourse may be painful because of soreness at her vaginal entrance. The cure for this is to improve the quality of the pleasuring, for the man to be sensitive when he inserts his penis and for the couple to use some other form of sexual expression, such as masturbation, until the woman's discomfort has subsided.

Coital technique

Sexual intercourse can take place in a variety of positions. These have been described in the literature of all cultures, and ancient Indian literature is particularly informative, as shown by Vatsyayana's *Kama Sutra*, written in 200 BC, and in the sculptures on the temples of Khajuraho. Basically, the positions can be reduced to about half a dozen, all of which are normal.

Face to face, the man on top: The man lies on top of the woman, either putting his weight upon her, or supporting most of his weight on his elbows or hands. She spreads her legs apart and, for variety may flex her knees, sometimes placing them around her partner's waist. She may place a pillow beneath her buttocks to lift her pelvis. There are many variations of this basic position. The woman may keep her legs stretched out, her partner's legs inside hers, or she may bring her legs together, so that her partner's knees are outside. She may flex her thighs more so that her legs are clasped around his shoulders.

The 'man on top' position is the most usual, and has the advantage that it makes penile entry into the vagina easy. The bodies of the two partners are in close proximity, so that they can kiss and caress each other during coitus; it permits the male to set the pace and slow or hasten coitus, to reach an orgasm at a desired speed; and it is probably the best position for pregnancy to occur, as after ejaculation the seminal fluid bathes the cervix. The disadvantages of the position are that it restricts the woman's movements and thrusts; male orgasm is often reached too quickly; penetration may be painfully deep, and the male is

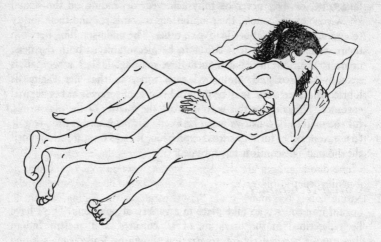

FIG. 5/1   Coital position. Face to face, man on top.

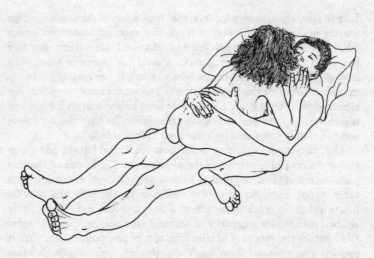

FIG. 5/2   Coital position. Face to face, woman on top.

unable to caress the woman's clitoris during coitus, which she may desire (Fig. 5/1).

Face to face, woman on top: The man lies on his back, the woman squats over him and guides his penis into her vagina. Once this has occurred, she may lie upon him, her weight resting on his body; she may support her weight on her arms, or she may sit upright across his thighs. The man may lie flat, raise himself on his arms, or clasp his legs around the woman's waist.

This position has an advantage if the man is heavy and his partner light in weight. In it the woman has the greatest freedom of movement, and the man can caress her clitoris and vulval area during coitus.

The disadvantages are that some women cannot control the depth of penile penetration too easily, and it may be too deep and so painful. During coitus the man's penis may slip out of the vagina, which is uncomfortable for both and spoils smooth coital sequence (Fig. 5/2).

Man's face to woman's back; rear entry: There are several variations of this position. The man may lie behind the woman, his hands around her to caress her breasts or clitoris. She lies in front of him, her legs bent at the hips, her body slightly curved away from his. The man's penis is inserted into the vagina from the rear, and once inside she presses her thighs together and pushes backwards so that her buttocks make a firm

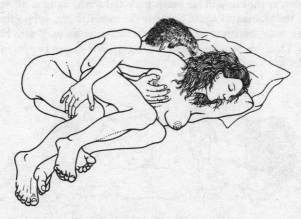

Fig. 5/3   Coital position. Rear entry.

contact against his lower abdomen and scrotum. Alternatively, she may lie on her stomach with her pelvis raised and her legs apart. The man lies on top of her, entering her vagina from the rear. Or she may kneel on hands and knees, her head and breasts touching the bed, the man kneeling behind her. In another variation, the man sits on the edge of a chair, or the bed, and the woman with her back to him, sits upon his penis and as it slips into her vagina, eases herself on to his lap.

The advantages of these positions are that the contact of the woman's buttocks on the man's abdomen, legs and scrotum may stimulate them both; he can readily caress her breasts or her clitoris; and the couple can rest on their sides during coitus. In late pregnancy this position is the most suitable one (Fig. 5/3).

Face to face, side by side: This position is, in fact, not exactly side by side, for penile entry would be almost impossible if it were. Usually the couple's legs are interlocked, and the man may lie largely on his back, the woman resting on his chest, or alternatively, the woman may lie largely on her back, one thigh beneath him (Fig. 5/4).

Sitting positions: The man sits on a chair, or the edge of a bed, and the woman sits astride his lap, his penis within her vagina, his arms around her body, and hers around his. Alternatively, the woman can lie on her back, the man squatting between her thighs, her legs clasped around his hips, his penis in her vagina. He can then make thrusting motions, or she can pull her pelvis back and forth. Another alternative is for the woman to squat between the man's thighs, supporting her weight on his outstretched arms, while he lies on his back with his legs apart. Once his penis is inside her vagina, she moves her pelvis in a circular fashion (Fig. 5/5).

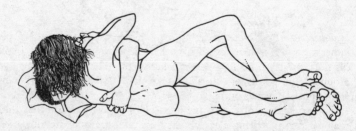

FIG. 5/4   Coital position. Face to face, side by side.

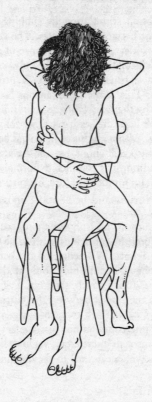

FIG. 5/5   Coital position. Sitting position.

Standing position: By bending his legs, the man can introduce his penis either facing the woman, or from the rear. She may put her hands around his neck and clasp his hips between her thighs. The couple may move around during coitus, or coitus may take place in surroundings different from normal, such as during a shower.

The advantages of the sitting and standing positions are that they may be more exciting because they are unusual and are not used routinely.

Extravaginal sexual stimulation

The man may obtain stimulation by rubbing his penis between the woman's thighs, or between her breasts. The advantage of these positions, apart from variety, is that the chance of conception occurring is remote, although ejaculation outside the vulva may lead to conception.

One 'notorious' extravaginal position is often followed by a deep emotional release. This is the simultaneous caressing of the woman's clitoris and vulva by the man's tongue (*cunnilingus*), while she puts his penis in her mouth and caresses it with her tongue (*fellatio*) until they both have orgasms. Although this position has been condemned by some clergy, and is whispered about by adolescents as the sixty-nine or soixante-neuf position, it is completely normal, and a couple need feel no guilt if they obtain mutual pleasure, happiness, sexual relaxation and release from it.

For sexual intercourse to be truly satisfying, after one partner has had an orgasm, or before, the other may wish to be helped to reach orgasm by cunnilingus or fellatio. The entry of the penis into vagina, or caressing with the tongue, should only come at the end of a sequence of pleasuring activities (body touch, stroking, hugging, exploration, talking) which draws the bonds between the partners closer, surrounding them with feelings of warmth to each other, and joy in their mutual embraces. Sexual intercourse is not just a silent monotonous thrust of an urgent penis into an indifferent vagina. It is a complex, varied group of activities which can lead to the maximum sexual joy for both participants.

Aphrodisiacs

Since the dawn of time, erotic stimulants have been sought by men who felt that their sexual performance was waning, and given to women who failed to respond to sexual advances. The oldest existing medical textbook, an undated Egyptian scroll from about 2000 BC, contains recipes for making 'erotic' potions. Shakespeare wrote extensively of aphrodisiacs. The great number of substances recommended as sexual stimulants indicates that none is of much value. Oysters are said to lead to amorous behaviour; rhinoceros horn powdered and drunk in wine is said to restore waning sexual function; while yohimbine, derived from the bark of an African tree, has long been used by the natives to increase their sexual powers. Cantharides, or Spanish Fly, which is an irritant of the urinary tract, also has an aphrodisiac reputation. All these beliefs are baseless, and none of the many foods, drugs or irritants recommended through the ages has any aphrodisiac property. Set apart because of its frequent consumption in Western society is alcohol, particularly champagne, which is credited as being a considerable erotic stimulant. Alcohol, it is true, causes dilation of the skin blood vessels and a feeling of warmth which extends to the genitals, and in small quantities it acts as a narcotic of the higher centres, producing a light-hearted approach and reducing the 'moral' block to sexual behaviour. In larger quantities, its narcotic effect reduces rather than stimulates sexual desire and performance.

In summary, there is no such thing as a true aphrodisiac, and no drug exists that the eager male could give to the resistant female which would render her unresisting and so full of sexual ardour that she would welcome seduction.

The new sexuality

Sexual research, in recent years, has established that many of the beliefs which surround sexuality are untrue, and today a better attitude towards sexuality is evident, especially among younger people. The research has shown, among other things, the following important findings:

- The 'double standard' of sexual behaviour has diminished, and today women can behave sexually much more freely. Some people regret this sexual 'permissiveness', but they are usually wrong. The change does not mean that most sexual relationships are a sequence of 'one-night stands' (which are unusual, except in certain groups) but that women, as well as men, now feel free to express their sexuality in any way they choose.
- Many more unmarried men and woman are living together, and most of these relationships, which may last for a longer or shorter period, are sharing, one-to-one relationships. This is something that those people who are anxious about today's sexual permissiveness and decadence fail to notice.
- Although some men and women may still feel uncomfortable about explaining their sexual and emotional needs to their partner, this inhibition is beginning to diminish.

- There is more open discussion about sex between men and women so that each becomes aware of the other's sexual desires and needs. This is good. Only when there is open discussion between lovers, will they become aware of each other's sexual desires and needs.

There are several other facets of sexuality which I believe should be emphasized. Many women have known about them, but male-dominated society has largely rejected them until recently. They include the following:

- Women have no less enthusiasm for sex, no less enjoyment of sex and no less sexual drive than men.
- A woman's sexual response is not intrinsically different from that of a man, but many women are slower to reach full sexual arousal than men, probably because of the sexual attitudes they learned during childhood.
- Women today feel comfortable and are able to tell men when they want sex. They are able to say 'yes' without shame, and 'no' without guilt when a man suggests that he wants sex. If he says, 'Unless you have sex with me, you don't love me,' it means that the man doesn't love the woman but wants to use her body. A woman need no longer be anxious that she may lose the man's love if she refuses his request and should be able to talk with the man about her decision.
- Women should be encouraged to expect that their relationship with a man is one in which mutual respect for the woman as a person replaces the older expectation that a woman should be dependent financially, emotionally and socially upon him. It is a relationship in which the mutual respect extends to each person's sexuality.

These changes should create an atmosphere in which sexuality is more open, more honest and more fulfilling, and the relationship between the two people should be more rewarding. The changes will neither increase, nor diminish, the number of people who obtain sexual enjoyment in a series of 'one-night stands' or who have relationships with several partners simultaneously, not serially. Provided all the partners accept and enjoy this convention, no psychological damage results, but two physical problems may arise.

The first is that each of the multiple partners has a greater chance of contracting a sexually transmitted disease, usually non-gonococcal genital infection or gonorrhoea (see p. 359) or even AIDS from another partner than would occur in a one-to-one sexual relationship (see

p. 362). The second consequence, which also applies to a one-to-one relationship, is that a woman runs the risk of becoming pregnant unless she or her partner take contraceptive precautions. Unfortunately, some women and men do not use birth control measures, and unwanted and unwelcome pregnancies continue to occur. With the change in society's attitude to single mothers, the problems of out of wedlock pregnancy have decreased, but sufficient disapproval and discrimination persists towards single parents to make the care of the child a burden to many unmarried mothers. Only if society provides sufficient financial and emotional support will the burden be reduced, and single parents be able to raise their children as satisfactorily as married parents.

Even so, an unexpected pregnancy can cause great stresses in a relationship, which may be so severe that the relationship is jeopardized. Today, with effective birth control measures (see Chapter 7) unwanted pregnancy should occur only rarely, provided adolescents and adults of both sexes have been informed about contraception and, if sexually active, have access to contraceptives. This means that all nations must implement the declaration their leaders collectively agreed to in 1974, at a United Nations conference in Bucharest. They agreed that 'all couples and individuals have the basic rights to decide freely and responsibly the number and spacing of their children and have the education and information to do so.'

The responsibility for avoiding an unwanted pregnancy is that of both partners. Unfortunately, at present, many women believe the man when he says he 'will be careful'. This is not enough. Contraception must be a mutual responsibility. If a woman is uncertain that her partner will use a condom, she must protect herself from becoming pregnant. A more permissive attitude to sex does not mean abandoning all sense of sexual responsibility.

Sexual responsibility should be a part of a new sexuality. If religious prohibitions and traditional sexual attitudes to premarital sex are increasingly abandoned, they must be replaced by the much more difficult concept of personal sexual responsibility. The code by which people live together is something only they can decide for themselves, but it should surely be based on emotional harmony, which includes sexual harmony. There is no place for emotional and sexual exploitation.

People who desire a return to traditional values of sexuality, that is sexual exploitation of women by men and the double standard, appear to believe that the new sexuality will lead to greater sexual self-indulgence, to less sexual responsibility, to the disappearance of marriage and family life and to the rejection of the 'deeper, basic values of society'. They ignore the fact that many young people who are trying to find new sexual values also reject other values which our society accepts as normal: deceit in government and business, greed for wealth and possessions, unequal opportunities for women, self-seeking by individuals and dishonesty by many individuals and companies.

Hopefully, these new sexual values will mean a sharing relationship with another person, in which the needs and desires of each are accepted. People accepting these values may not reject marriage, as over 90 per cent of people marry; nor will they reject the family as a social unit. But they may question whether the present family of 'legally' married father and mother and two children, living in relative isolation, is the best social unit, and ask whether other types of family may not produce better adjusted, happier, more 'sharing' people.

The marriage partnership

It is often asked, 'if women became sexually liberated and if society accepts the new sexual values, will marriage survive?' The evidence is that it will; but no one really knows why, in our society, two people fall in love with each other and marry.

In many societies, love is not a factor in marriage. In India for example, many marriages are arranged by the family, who select a suitable girl from one of several villages which traditionally supply brides to the village of the groom. The groom does not see his bride before the marriage. The evidence is that these marriages work fairly well; each partner knowing his or her duties and responsibilities, and the sexual aspect being limited. But in our society, the decision is made by the man and the woman that they will live together, will procreate and bring up children, will support each other, and will merge their personalities to some extent. This is not an inconsiderable undertaking, when one considers the different and unique background, training, experience, loves, hates, attitudes and personality structure of each partner. Studies have been made which show that, in fact, the choice of a mate is limited. The 'pool' of eligible males from which women select partners is usually determined by the race, the social class, the age, the level of education, the place of residence and also by religion. It is true that a few couples step over the expected boundaries and successfully marry outside their 'class' or 'race', but even in multi-racial societies, such as Malaysia and Fiji, inter-racial marriages are unusual.

As well as the 'social factor', there is a second, less understood factor which has been called the 'complementary need factor'. This factor is much more specific for each individual, and operates usually without their knowing it in their choice of a person with whom 'to fall in love'. A woman who needs to 'mother' another person may choose a man who has an obvious problem, and she gratifies her 'need' for mothering by looking after him and helping him to overcome his problem. An aggressive, demanding man may select a timid, passive woman, on whom he can vent his need for aggression, without receiving a rebuff. These are extreme examples, as many marriages are contracted for emotional rather than rational reasons. In these marriages, it has been suggested that the 'complementary need factor' may operate. The strongly-sexed male may be attracted to a girl who refuses his sexual advances because her upbringing has led her to believe that premarital sex is prohibited, and his main reason for seeking the marriage may be that she refuses to permit sexual intercourse. Meanwhile he has had sexual intercourse with other women, but because his upbringing has made him value virginity, he would not think of marrying one of them, although she might make him a more suitable partner.

In our society, sexual compatibility is an important factor in keeping a marriage stable but, of course, it is only one of many factors. If one of the partners to a marriage has been taught to believe that sexual intercourse is something shameful and dirty, and that for a woman sexual intercourse is something to be passively endured, rather than an activity for the mutual pleasure of the couple, problems will arise.

Clearly, incompatibility will not vanish even if both the partners have received some education in sexual matters, but the problems will be reduced. It would be wrong to suggest that all marital problems are the consequence of sexual incompatibility. In some cases, the couple may have a well-functioning sexual relationship, but may be unable to talk to each other about conflicts in other areas of the relationship, particularly each partner's emotional needs. The ability to communicate openly extends to all aspects of the marriage, not only the sexual aspects.

The behaviour of each partner in other areas of the marriage may also affect the relationship. For example, a knowledge of sexuality will not help the relationship if one partner is an alcoholic or a philanderer. Nor will it keep the marriage stable if the male is brutal, emotionally disturbed or completely selfish. But then any attempt by one individual to bend or damage the personality of another is a sin, if not a legal one, certainly one against humanity, particularly in a relationship where the two personalities are in intimate contact over a long time. Since the sexual side of personality is an important one, perhaps this is the reason why sexual compatibility plays such an important part in a stable marriage. It gives even greater emphasis to the belief that 'marriage should be made harder to obtain and divorce easier'.

Legalized marriage remains the most favoured institution for couples in most nations, despite the concern from some religious groups that so-called 'sexual permissiveness' will lead to the demise of the family.

Sexual problems

It is impossible to calculate the frequency of sexual problems which may mar, or destroy a relationship as, until recently, people were ashamed to seek help.

In men and women four sexual problems occur. In men the problems are (1) inhibited sexual desire (or drive), (2) premature ejaculation, (3) retarded ejaculation, and (4) erectile failure. A man who has an inhibited sexual desire is unable to become sexually aroused despite sexual teasing by his partner or by sexual fantasizing, and consequently cannot perform sexually, as he cannot obtain an erection. A man who has premature ejaculation becomes sexually aroused and obtains an erection, but ejaculates either before or very soon after he inserts his penis into his partner's vagina. The speed with which this occurs may prevent the woman obtaining sexual pleasure. A man who has retarded ejaculation is able to engage in sexual intercourse but fails to reach orgasm and ejaculate in spite of prolonged penile thrusting in the woman's vagina or prolonged masturbation. A man who has erectile failure usually is sexually aroused (although he may suppress this because of his fear of failure) but is unable to achieve an erection of his penis, so that he cannot engage in sexual intercourse. This may make his partner sexually frustrated and may damage his image of himself as a virile man who, in our society, is expected to be able to satisfy women sexually.

While disease, drugs and alcoholism may cause these sexual problems in a few men, about half of the men who have premature ejaculation or erectile failure have psycho-sexual problems, which usually can be resolved with the help of their partner and, perhaps, a counsellor.

In women four sexual problems also occur. The first is *inhibited sexual desire*. A woman who has inhibited sexual desire may not wish for, or enjoy, sex, but she may permit her partner to have sexual intercourse with her out of a sense of duty. Other women with this sexual problem are so upset by the idea of sexual intercourse that they refuse to have sex or make excuses to avoid having sex. The second problem is that *sexual intercourse is painful* so that it is either abandoned or else causes such a severe upset that it is never pleasurable. This problem is called *dyspareunia*, which means painful coitus. When the woman finds it too painful to let the man put his penis in her vagina and resists by tightening the muscles surrounding her vaginal entrance, the condition is called *vaginismus*.

The third problem is that although the woman has a normal sexual desire, at least in fantasy and in dreams, in reality she fails to be 'turned on' by her partner during sexual pleasuring. Because of this her vagina fails to become lubricated and wet, and the soft swellings at its entrance fail to develop. When sexual intercourse takes place she obtains little or no erotic pleasure, although she may enjoy caring for her partner in other ways The problem is called *lowered libido*.

The fourth sexual problem is that the woman is unable to reach orgasm. In other words she has '*orgastic dysfuntion*'. This term needs to be interpreted carefully. Some sex therapists believe that all women who fail to have orgasms during sexual intercourse have orgastic dysfunction. This is too restrictive. A woman has not got orgastic dysfunction if she usually has an orgasm during love-making, whether she reaches an orgasm by masturbating, while her lover is thrusting in her vagina, or by being stimulated by her lover before or after the lover has had an orgasm. Nor does a woman who has orgasms by masturbating when she is alone have orgastic dysfunction, even if she does not have orgasms when she is with her lover. None of these women is sick, nor are they 'frigid'.

Only women who never reach an orgasm, whatever the stimulation, have orgastic dysfunction. It is important for everyone to remember this. It is also important to remember that many women obtain a great deal of pleasure and emotional warmth from the closeness and intimacy of sexual intercourse even though they do not have an orgasm. Magazine articles which stress the need for a woman to become a real woman by having orgasms do a disservice. What should be stressed, instead, is that those women who obtain emotional closeness and pleasure during sexual intercourse will obtain even more pleasure if they are helped to reach an orgasm by their lover.

If you can have an orgasm, by whatever method you reach it, you are normal. If you do not have an orgasm during sexual intercourse, but reach an orgasm when your partner stimulates you, or by masturbation, you are normal. And the orgasm reached during sexual intercourse is no 'better' or more 'normal' than that reached in any other way.

But if you are unable to achieve an orgasm with your lover or are too ashamed to reach an orgasm by masturbating, and you are worried about this, you can be helped. Women with one or more of these sexual problems have been called 'frigid'. This term should be abandoned. It implies that the woman, because of some congenital condition, will never be able to respond fully sexually. This is untrue. With counselling and with the help of a lover, most women can become aroused sexually and nearly all can reach an orgasm. There is a difference in the speed of the change: women who are unable to become aroused sexually are harder to help than women who are aroused but who fail to reach an orgasm.

There are several reasons why some women have sexual problems, and they differ in different circumstances. The causes of women's sexual problems are very similar to those which cause sexual problems in men. They include: marital disharmony, or a poor relationship with the woman's partner; emotional stress due to environmental factors; ignorance about sexual matters, or guilt and shame about sexuality; illness, including psychological illness, such as depression and the effect of drugs used to treat illness.

INADEQUATE RELATIONSHIPS: If one of the couple feels hostility towards the other, and is unable to talk openly about the problem, marital disharmony may result, with a resulting reduction in sexual desire and arousal. Another cause of sexual dysfunction occurs if the couple are unable to talk to each other openly about their sexual needs and desires. For example, only a woman can tell her partner what turns her on sexually; he (or she) cannot know instinctively, and each woman has her own individual response.

Unless the partners can talk with each other (the fashionable word is 'communicate'), the sexual problem may become magnified. If the man has a lack of understanding of the woman's sexual needs, and a poor technique in helping her become aroused, the result may lead to antagonism, and a reduction of their mutual sexuality. Depending on the relationship, the woman may further inhibit her sexual response, or may reluctantly accept the man's sexual advances, although she gets little or no pleasure from them.

IGNORANCE: Faulty childhood upbringing by 'strict', sexually inhibited, parents who condition the girl to believe in the double standard of sexuality, to submit to her partner's 'demands' passively, and to expect to receive no sexual pleasure, can lead to a reduced sexual drive, and foster the belief that sex is a duty to be paid to a demanding, sexually aggressive man, rather than a mutually enjoyed pleasure.

Many women believe in sexual myths such as:

• A woman should always be available for sex with her husband whether she wants sex or not.

• Simultaneous orgasm is necessary for true sexual fulfilment.

• A man knows how to arouse a woman sexually and if you fail to be aroused it is your fault.

In recent years women's magazines have regularly printed articles on sexual matters, many purporting to teach women how to have better sex. The articles and the many books available may be damaging rather than helpful. They may make a woman feel sexually inadequate if she doesn't succeed in achieving the sexual pleasure the articles and books say she should achieve.

GUILT AND SHAME: Some parents may condition their daughters to believe that sex is a shameful activity in which a person 'indulges'. In these families, sex may never be discussed openly and such information (or more accurately, misinformation) as is obtained, is from the whispered confidences of girls of the daughter's own age. If the parents consider the human body, apart from the exposed face, arms and legs, to be indecent and punish the girl when she asks about it, or if they do not respond sensibly to the child's natural curiosity about sex and human reproduction, the child is likely to believe that sexual activity is indecent, shameful and something to be ignored as far as possible. These attitudes may influence her enjoyment of sex in later years.

The opposite attitude towards sex can also occasion shame. A 'sophisticated' woman who reads books about sex and who openly discusses sexual matters may also have a deficient sexual drive. In Western society success is lauded, and if in sexual relations success means reaching an orgasm during each episode of sexual intercourse, success may elude many women. This is not because they are inadequate for, as I have stressed, sexual desire and the ability to achieve an

75

orgasm vary very considerably over the years. But because a woman fails to achieve sexual success by having orgasms, she may become ashamed at what she believes is her sexual inadequacy. This shame can lead to a reduction in her sexual desire, as a safeguard against 'failure'.

She has become anxious about her ability to respond sexually, what the Americans call 'performance anxiety'. To avoid increasing the anxiety she suppresses her sexual arousal (in other words, her libido is reduced), or inhibits her sexual response (in other words, fails to reach orgasm).

During sexual intercourse, a woman can increase her sexual awareness by fantasizing about sexually-arousing stimuli. But if she keeps thinking how terrible it will be, and how inadequate she is if she does not have an orgasm, she may reduce her sexual desire by her over-determination to be a 'normal' woman. This feeling of inadequacy is increased by the cinema and by literature. So many films stress by implication, and so many books indicate explicitly, that when a woman has an orgasm, bells ring, lights flash, music falls from the air and the planets stop in their courses, she may believe she should experience all these explosive sensations. If she has an orgasm without fireworks or comets, she may believe that she is sexually deficient, although with it, a warm delightful sensation sweeps over her. The conflict created by this false belief may cause her subconsciously to reduce her sexual desires, so that she may avoid the pain and shame of failure.

Her sense of sexual 'failure' may be compounded by the knowledge that she can reach an orgasm if her lover stimulates her erotically, or if she masturbates. Many women have been brought up to believe that masturbation or stimulation is shameful. This myth is also believed by many men. The truth is that an orgasm is an orgasm however it is produced.

ILL HEALTH AND FATIGUE: A number of sexual problems are due to physical or mental illness, including depression, although ill health is a less common cause of sexual dysfunction than are the other causes which have been discussed. When help is sought concerning a sexual problem, the doctor will wish first to make sure that no physical or mental illness is present, and will wish to enquire if the woman has been prescribed any drugs which may reduce sexual responsiveness.

A fairly common factor, associated with a reduced sexual response, is fatigue. Fatigue is associated with a reduced sexual drive and sexual capacity in many people and, in our society, women may become more fatigued than men. Because women are subjected to so much physical and emotional pressure, by the demands of rearing children, maintaining a house, often simultaneously working at a job, and by demands for companionship and socializing, they may be too exhausted to respond sexually.

WHAT CAN BE DONE? If the woman has dyspareunia there may be a local cause, and a doctor would be able to make sure that she does not have candidosis or endometriosis, which could make sexual intercourse painful.

In most cases of dyspareunia, and in all cases of vaginismus, the problem is a psychological one which may be aggravated by an unaware lover. Many women still believe that intercourse is painful or impossible because they are 'small made' – meaning that their vagina is too small or the man's penis too large. Their lover can reinforce the belief if he fails to stimulate the woman before he tries to insert his penis into her vagina, so that it is insufficiently lubricated. Many women are ignorant about their genital anatomy. They have no idea where their clitoris is, nor how the labia surround their vagina. Many women have never looked at their vulva in a mirror so that they could see what it looks like. These beliefs and failures produce the fear that intercourse will be painful and may damage the woman, and consequently it is painful.

But with counselling, understanding and the lover's help, every woman who has vaginismus can be cured, but only if she takes the first step to obtain help from a concerned, helpful counsellor. Unfortunately, doctors have as many sexual hang-ups as their patients, and the couple have to find a doctor who has been trained to manage sexual problems. Some doctors still use surgery to 'widen' a narrow vaginal entrance. In very rare circumstances this operation may be needed, but they are so rare that if a doctor suggests surgery the woman should at once obtain a second opinion.

The solution to the problems of lack of sexual arousal (lowered libido) and the failure to have orgasms (orgasmic dysfunction) is rather more complicated.

If the couple do not relate adequately emotionally they may also not be able to relate sexually. If the woman is uncertain about her relationship and uncomfortable about her sexual desires, and has, as a partner, a lover who is sexually inhibited, uninformed and emotionally 'uptight', neither will be able to communicate with the other about their sexual needs. Lacking insight, the lover is unable to perceive that the woman has a problem and she is unable to talk about it.

The lover knows when he is sexually excited and how to reach an orgasm, which he often does quickly; he forgets that he should be involved in helping his partner to become sexually excited, and ignores the fact that it may take her longer than him to reach the pre-orgastic stage of sexual arousal, so that it is all over for him before she is ready. Because of their inhibitions in communicating their sexual needs, the woman is unable to ask her man to help her reach an orgasm by stimulating her, and he is too inhibited or too ignorant to take the initiative. Masters and Johnson have pointed out that in the resolution of a sexual problem, there is usually no uninvolved partner. A woman's sexual problem will only be resolved if her partner is prepared to help willingly and lovingly.

With his co-operation and with informed guidance from a counsellor who may be a family doctor, a psychologist, a gynaecologist or a psychiatrist, cure is likely. The counsellor first makes sure that the woman has no disease which may reduce her sexual desire. The next step is to find out what excites the woman sexually and conversely what 'turns her off' sexually, so that she can become sexually self aware, and so that her partner can become aware of her sexual needs. The counsellor next tries to help the couple obtain a relaxing, erotically stimulating environment in which they can learn to pleasure each other sexually, giving pleasure to get pleasure. In this relaxed environment, where there is no pressure to perform sexually, the woman's sexual desires are usually aroused. At first the arousal may be small but with continued pleasuring it increases. Only when she is really aroused do the couple try having sexual intercourse.

In spite of this generalization some women are content to give sexual pleasure to their partner, although they are not sexually aroused by him, either during pleasuring or during sexual intercourse. If the woman is happy with this and her partner is also sexually fulfilled she should not feel that she is less feminine than other women who respond fully to sexual stimulation.

If the woman's sexual problem is the failure to have orgasms, the couple use the same pleasuring techniques, but go through the learning stages more quickly. Often the man has to learn techniques of stimulating the woman erotically so that she reaches an orgasm. It is important that she tells him what gives her sexual satisfaction, rather than permitting him to do what he thinks will give her satisfaction. She is the director and the authority about what most stimulates her. When the problem is orgasic dysfunction, some women may find it easier to begin by masturbating when alone, using fantasy as an erotic stimulus, rather than to be stimulated erotically by a partner. If these methods fail to help the woman to reach a climax, the doctor may suggest that she uses a vibrator, which a woman can use to stimulate herself erotically so that she reaches an orgasm.

Once a woman has achieved one orgasm, by whatever method, she is well on the way to being regularly orgasmic. With the help of a co-operative, gentle, sympathetic partner, most women who have failed to have an orgasm and a large number who could not be aroused sexually find their sexual response heightened and reach an orgasm regularly.

A few doctors continue to treat women's sexual problems, particularly lack of sexual desire and arousal, by giving the patient injections or tablets of the male hormone, testosterone. In carefully designed research studies it has been demonstrated that testosterone provides no benefit. It should not be prescribed.

Homosexuality (lesbianism)

Over 90 per cent of women find companionship, a stable relationship and sexual fulfilment with a member of the complementary sex. Note that I have called men the complementary sex – not the opposite sex. This is what men are to women, and women to men – the sex of each complements that of the other partner. About 5 per cent of women, perhaps more, are bisexual; that is at some time, or for several periods of their lives, they choose to cease to have a sexual relationship with a man and form a relationship with a woman. In both kinds of relationship they give and receive sexual pleasure, so that they obtain emotional contentment from both. Bisexual women say that they relate differently to a male lover and to a female lover. Sexual relationships with a man may be conditioned by the man's cultural belief that he must be the initiator, that he is the sexual expert and that his sexual needs are paramount. The woman may be conditioned to be passive, to aim to 'please' the man sexually, to adjust her response to his and to hope, but not expect, that he will help her reach her sexual fulfilment including an orgasm. By contrast, bisexual women say that when their lover is a woman, the mutual pleasuring is slower, more innovative and lasts longer. They have a total body response rather than a genital one, and feel a warmer, deeper, reaction to their lover, because each is more sensitive to the other's need. The information is fragmentary at present, but in the next few years, more may be discovered and the social constraints towards bisexuality may diminish.

About 5 per cent of women have no sexual interest in men, although they may have friends who are men, and their sexual interests, their need for companionship, are met by alliance with another woman. These women are homosexuals: their sexual desires are directed to members of their own sex. They are also called lesbians, because a group of homosexual women, prominent among whom was the poetess Sappho, lived on the island of Lesbos in the time of the ancient Greek civilization. This civilization, lauded as one of the peak periods of human creativeness, incidentally was relatively permissive in regard to sex.

Until recently it was thought that a homosexual tendency was inborn, in other words, it was there before birth. Although it is true that there are shades of femininity and masculinity in every person, it is now known that homosexual attitudes are *acquired* during the child's upbringing. It was also thought at one time that feminine men and masculine women were so because the man manufactured too much female sex hormone, and the woman too much male hormone. It is true that women do manufacture some male hormones in a gland called the adrenal, but the quantity is small, and there is no difference in the amount of hormone secreted by homosexual or heterosexual women. A similar consideration applies to men, and the much-derided 'pansy', 'fairy' or 'queer', although different in character, has the same amount of male sex hormone (androgen) circulating in his blood as a bovine football hero. Very rarely a woman may develop a tumour which manufactures androgen, and as the concentration of androgen increases in her blood, she becomes physically less feminine: hair appears on her body and face, her breasts become smaller, her clitoris enlarges, but her feminine attitudes do not change.

Small children have no particular thought about sex – except perhaps to note that little girls do not have a penis – and until parental attitudes direct them into one sexual role or another, they are content, each seeing the other merely as a playmate. However, the cultural attitudes of our society towards sexual differences are soon imposed on the child. A girl is taught to be quiet, play with dolls, help mother, wear 'pretty dresses', be demure; a boy is expected to be untidy, play 'rough' games, like toys which are destructive, to be 'manly' and to imitate father. Most societies recognize that a distinction between the sexes is needed for survival and each sex is trained to believe that certain activities are predominantly theirs – housework and cooking are for girls; car-cleaning, wood-cutting, painting are boys' work. Ultimately, then, the sexual inclinations of the child are determined by the attitudes of its parents, and some parents unwittingly encourage homosexuality in their children. These parents would be shocked to learn that this is what they have done, for they are often more rigid in their attitudes, more puritanical towards sex, and more derogatory about homo-sexuality than average. A brutal father may make his son fearful of men and drawn to his oppressed, humiliated mother, so that he identifies himself with her, and in adult life becomes a passive, 'female type' homosexual. Oddly enough, opposite parental attitudes can encourage homosexuality. The mother who perpetually pampers her son, who never lets him out of her sight, who forbids his playing with 'common, dirty' companions, who surrounds him with 'smother love', may turn him towards homosexuality. This is even more marked when the sex of the child is in some doubt at birth. Since most of these children look like girls, they are brought up as girls, and find that they are quite happy in the female role. Later it may be found that the 'girl' was in fact gentically a male – she had the Y chromosome in all her body cells – but by this time it is almost impossible for her to exchange roles, and unwise for her to be forced to do so unless she wishes it herself.

As far as girls are concenred, it appears that the mother is the dominant parent in the child's sexual development, although a poor relationship with the father is an important factor. The mother who 'wanted a boy but got a girl' may consciously or unconsciously impose her disappointed desire on her daughter, so that in life she has many masculine attitudes. This does not mean that she will become homo-sexual, but she may. Similarly a mother who has an unhappy relation-ship with her husband, may influence her daughter to hate men, and later to seek affection and companionship only with women.

In these ways homosexuals are created. Of course, only some child-ren whose backgrounds resemble the ones described become homosexual. Most are heterosexual, although their sexuality may be impaired or damaged, so that they find it difficult to achieve a happy relationship with their chosen partner.

Ultimately it is the sensible attitude of the mother to the upbringing of her child which counts. But, as always, the behaviour of both parents towards each other and towards the child influence the way she will develop.

In the normal sexual development of a child, psychologists consider that there is a period when homosexual alliances are normal. This period is usually of limited duration during early adolescence, and is marked by a special closeness for a friend of her own sex. For a period, life away from the chosen one is intolerable, the clothes they wear must be the same, they must do the same things, they are miserable when separated. The intense homosexual friendship wanes as the girl grows older and forms heterosexual companionships. Often it is replaced by a more emotionally stable friendship, which persists throughout life. In some 10 per cent of cases of adolescent homosexual friendship, the sexuality of the girls is stronger than usual, and they mutually masturbate by stimulating each other's clitoris. There need be no parental anxiety about this, as mutual masturbation is without any consequences, and certainly does not predispose to homosexuality in adult life. Another form of the adolescent homosexual phase is the development of a 'crush' or 'pash' for an older person. Again this is a normal phase, and may be less traumatic to the child, and to her parents, than the heterosexual 'crush' on the latest 'pop' or TV star which replaces or follows it. Hero-worship is a normal development in which the child, beginning to be independent, sees in the hero a substitute, stronger and more romantic than either a dominating or a cold indifferent parent. By the age of 15, the homosexual phase has waned in most girls. They are now more interested in boys, their friendship for other girls lingering on, but with much less intensity. A few remain homosexual.

In our society, female homosexuals are oppressed far less than male homosexuals. There are several reasons for this. Homosexuality in the male is thought more of a danger to a male dominated society, where 'men are strong and dominant' and women 'weak and submissive', than is lesbianism. In our culture, women are permitted to show greater physical intimacy between each other than men: girls habitually hug and kiss; if men do this, it is considered improper. For these reasons, female homosexuals may live together in complete intimacy, rarely incurring the disapproval of the community. Male homosexuals living together are sometimes sneered at and attacked. It is true that male homosexuals appear to be less able to form stable associations with each other, and tend to change partners or seek new sexual contacts more frequently than female homosexuals, who are generally monogamous with one partner. This may give some point to society's condemnation of male homosexuals, even if most of it is due to ignorance, prejudice and perhaps to unsolved sexual problems among those who condemn.

Most female homosexuals form happy, stable relationships and lead full, contented lives. A few homosexual women have emotional problems, but these only differ in degree from the emotional problems of heterosexual women.

The increased threat to a lesbian's emotional health is due to society's condemnation of homosexuality, which increases her insecurity.

It is intolerable that a civilized society should single out a group of people for disapproval, aggravating their problems. The only difference between a homosexual and a heterosexual woman is her erotic preference.

CHAPTER 6

The Infertile Marriage

It is a strange thing that in a world where one of the main problems facing mankind is the 'population explosion', or the birth each year of too many children, a fairly large group of women are seeking desperately to become pregnant. In times past barrenness was always blamed on the woman, but today it is known that in many cases the reason for the childlessness lies with the man.

If a couple are normally fertile, and have sexual intercourse reasonably regularly, a pregnancy will result within one year in 90 per cent of cases. For this reason, a couple is considered to be infertile after this time, and may require investigations, tests and treatment if they wish to have a child. With treatment about 45 per cent of the infertile couples will achieve their desire – a pregnancy, resulting in the birth of a healthy child. The majority of women becoming pregnant do so within one year of the investigations and treatment, but pregnancies occur up to 10 years after the investigations have been completed. In recent years the numbers of tests, investigations and suggested treatments have increased very considerably, but the success rate after the investigations has remained stubbornly at the same 45 per cent.

This is not to say that an infertile couple should not be investigated. It is well worth while, but neither the enthusiasm of the doctors, nor the couple's desire to clutch at every straw should lead them on the round of visits to many doctors in many places to receive a variety of treatment to achieve nothing.

Careful investigation of the causes of infertiity has shown that in about 35 per cent of cases the woman has a fertility problem and in the same proportion the problem lies with the man. In the remaining 30 per cent of cases factors which affect them both are present.

It is usual for the woman to consult the doctor first when pregnancy fails to occur. This is correct and proper, for it is she who will carry the growing baby in her uterus for the 40 weeks of pregnancy. At this first visit the doctor enquires about the past operations and illnesses she may have had, about her present health, and about her menstrual history. He will want to know when menstruation first started, of its duration, the interval between periods, and if the periods were painful. Also he will enquire about the couple's sexual habits. The patient should not be embarrassed at this, for it is essential for the doctor to know the frequency of sexual intercourse, and whether the woman felt it to be satisfactory. It is then usual for him to examine the woman thoroughly, first to make sure she has no disorder which would make pregnancy hazardous to her, and second so that he may perform a pelvic examination to make sure that her genital organs are normal, as far as he can tell from this examination. In several surveys of infertile couples, it was found that in 1 per cent sexual intercourse had not taken place properly, and the women was still a virgin. It was hardly surprising that pregnancy had not resulted!

The doctor should outline what he intends to do. He will explain that investigation of infertility usually takes several visits, and that as the problem concerns the husband as much as the wife he would like to see him as well as her at the next visit.

Infertility factors

The factors which may lead to infertility are rather complex, but can be understood if a little thought is applied. The male seeds, or spermatozoa, have to be ejaculated into the upper vagina. They then wriggle their way through the cervix, swimming up between the seaweed-like strands of mucus which stretch downwards from the cells which line the cervical canal. They have to negotiate the cavity of the uterus, and by the time they have done this, of the millions ejaculated, only hundreds remain active. They then have to get through the narrow opening joining the cavity of the uterus and the hollow tube of the oviduct. Only a few dozen spermatozoa succeed in doing this. They then swim along the oviduct, against the current as it were, to reach the outer portion. If this occurs just at the time when the ovum has been expelled from the ovary, and if the ovum has been taken up by the fine finger-like projections at the end of the oviduct, conception may occur. If it does, the fertilized egg has to pass down the oviduct again, spending three days in the process, during which time it has divided and the one original cell is now a collection of cells, still within the shell of the *zona pellucida*. The fertilized egg reaches the cavity of the uterus three days or so after conception, and then by shedding the zona pellucida, implants itself into the soft, juicy lining of the uterine cavity. If all goes well, it now grows and becomes a baby; if all does not go well, an abortion occurs, which may or may not be noticed by the woman. It has been calculated that where no bar to conception is present and where every chance of becoming pregnant has been taken, in any one month of 100 fertile women, 60 will become pregnant and 40 will not. Of the 60 who do become pregnant, 25 deliver a live baby and 35 abort, but in 25 the abortion is undetected as it happens so early.

Considering the long journey made by the sperm to fertilize the egg, and the long journey made by the fertilized egg to reach the uterine cavity and implant itself there, it is surprising how readily pregnancy occurs. This description of how fertilization takes place enables a list of factors which prevent fertility to be made.

The male factor

The man may fail to manufacture any spermatozoa, or because of illness which has damaged the tube (the *vas deferens*) linking his testicles to the collecting areas (*seminal vesicles*) in his prostate gland, the spermatozoa may fail to reach the collecting areas (Fig. 6/1). The spermatozoa may be few in number or weak in activity, so that they have not the strength to swim up the genital tract of the woman. Finally, the man may not be able to ejaculate, or even to practise sexual intercourse properly. Because of these possibilities, the doctor enquires from him about any illness he may have had, particularly mumps which may have damaged the testicles, and gonorrhoea which may have damaged the vas deferens. He will also ask about his smoking and drinking habits, for excessive smoking and too much alcohol both reduce sperm production and reduce the frequency of coitus. He will require to know his occupation, for some jobs reduce sperm production; and about his sexual habits. He will perhaps require to examine the man, although this can be avoided if the man is embarrassed provided that the doctor is supplied with a specimen of his semen. This can be obtained if the man goes to the laboratory and masturbates, but many men find this inhibiting. The other ways are for the couple to masturbate or to have sexual intercourse. If they choose the latter, just before ejaculation the man withdraws his penis from the woman's vagina, and ejaculates into a dry, wide-mouthed jar placed beside the bed. His specimen is

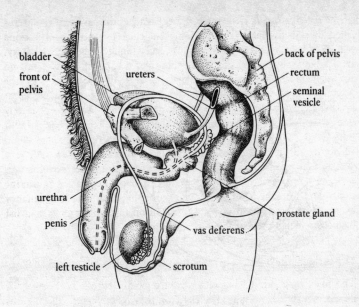

bladder

front of
pelvis

ureters

back of pelvis

rectum

seminal
vesicle

urethra

penis

left testicle

scrotum

vas deferens

prostate gland

FIG. 6/1   The male genital tract.

then brought to the laboratory by the woman, if this is more convenient. She should note the time the specimen was produced and bring it to the laboratory within two hours. Another method is not so satisfactory, but is preferred by some patients and some doctors. In this method, the couple have sexual intercourse normally. Six hours later the woman goes to the doctor, who introduces a speculum into her vagina and takes a sample of the semen which is in her cervix (Fig. 6/2). This method, called the 'postcoital' test, has one particular advantage, it *proves* that normal coitus takes place and that the man ejaculates into the woman's vagina; but it is impossible to determine the quality of his semen from this method.

The main purpose of all the methods I have mentioned is to determine the quality as well as the quantity of the sperms in the seminal fluid. If the test shows that the man's sperm has a poor quality, the test is repeated at least twice, sometimes after giving antibiotics, before any final decision about its quality can be made. If no sperms are found in any of the tests, or if the count is very low, a blood sample is taken

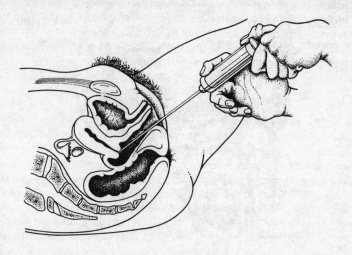

FIG. 6/2   The postcoital test.

and the level of FSH (see p. 27) is measured. If this is high, no treatment is available. The man's sperm production is irrevocably damaged. But if his FSH level is normal or low, there is some hope, but only if some spermatozoa are found in the tests. If no spermatozoa are found, no treatment is possible. The man is sterile.

A man who has a low sperm count and a normal FSH level, may be able to improve the quantity and quality of his spermatozoa by certain treatments. The man may have varicose veins around his vas deferens, for example. It has been found that the surgical treatment of these varicose veins is sometimes effective in producing a better quality semen. If the man has no varicose veins, changes in living habits, in tobacco and alcohol consumption may help. Many vitamins, drugs and hormones have been suggested in the hope of improving the sperm count. Nearly all have proved expensive and without effect. Recently, the use of a particular drug given to men, whose sperm count is more than 5 million per millilitre and whose FSH level is normal, has been shown to produce some improvement but the work is still preliminary and more research is needed.

Because it is so easy to check the male factor by examining the semen, this is usually one of the first tests made when infertility is investigated. Indeed, logically, a semen analysis should be made before any complicated tests are made on the woman. For example, if the man were found to be sterile, it would be pointless and heartless to perform tests on the woman.

The ovulation factor

Quite obviously if the woman fails to produce an egg, pregnancy cannot occur. Although in the years before the age of 18 and after 38 ovulation occurs less regularly, between these years most women ovulate each month. In the past an infertile woman was usually asked to check if she was ovulating by taking and charting her temperature each morning before getting out of bed or drinking anything. The method is not very accurate and today most doctors determine if ovulation has occurred by measuring the level of the hormone progesterone in a blood sample taken in the week before menstruation. If lack of ovulation is confirmed over several months, one of the 'ovulating drugs' may be prescribed, provided no other reason for the couple's infertility has been found. The use of the 'ovulating drugs' is fairly complicated, and most doctors insist that they are only given by specialist gynaecologists who have access to special laboratories, so that the exact dose required for the particular patient may be determined.

The oviductal factor

The sperm has to pass upwards along the oviduct to reach the egg, and the fertilized egg has to pass downwards along the oviduct to reach the uterine cavity. If the oviduct is blocked, these essential events cannot happen. The next step in the investigation, after the man has been found to be normal, and the woman to be ovulating, is to determine if the oviducts are clear. The most informative way of finding out is to ask the woman to come to an x-ray department which has an image-intensification unit. This apparatus enables the doctor to obtain the most information with the least discomfort to the woman. No anaesthetic is needed for this investigation.

In the x-ray department, the doctor inserts a speculum into the woman's vagina and puts a narrow tube into her cervix; this tube is connected to a syringe which is filled with a substance opaque to x-rays. The doctor injects the watery substance slowly so that it fills the uterus and then passes along the oviducts. He watches what he is doing on the television screen of the image-intensification apparatus. The woman can also watch what is happening and a sensitive doctor can explain to the woman what he sees.

The test will show if the oviducts are normal and unobstructed so that sperms can wriggle along them to reach the ovum. If the test suggests that the oviducts are blocked somewhere along their course obviously the chance of pregnancy is reduced. All tests have errors so that if the test appears to be abnormal it is repeated one or two months later. The test is called a hysterosalpingogram. The alternative method of finding out if the Fallopian tubes are patent, is for the doctor to use a laparoscope. This instrument, which is like a narrow telescope, is introduced into the abdominal cavity through a tiny cut in the lower part of the umbilicus, after filling the abdomen with carbon dioxide gas. The doctor looks through the laparoscope and can see all the pelvic organs. If a dye is injected into the uterus through the cervix as is done for a hysterosalpingogram, and the tubes are patent, the doctor will see the dye dripping from the outer ends of the tubes. One problem is that, unlike the hysterosalpingogram, the woman has to have a general anaesthetic, and may have pain in the abdomen for 24–48 hours.

Surgery in infertility

If tests show that the woman's oviducts are blocked, surgery is possible. Because the oviducts are so narrow and delicate, the surgery should be undertaken by a gynaecologist who has made a special study of infertility surgery and is skilled at micro-surgery. Even in these circumstances only one woman in every five operated upon becomes pregnant later and delivers a live, healthy baby.

In vitro fertilization ('test-tube baby')

If a woman's oviducts are so damaged that surgery is unlikely to be successful, the new technique of in vitro fertilization (IVF) may offer hope in the future. The first in vitro fertilizations took place in 1978 in Britain, and further successes have been obtained in many countries since 1979. By 1989, over 10 000 healthy babies had been born to women who had had an ovum fertilized in vitro. But it must be remembered that following one IVF only about 15 per cent of the women give birth to a live baby. If IVF is repeated two or more times on the same women, the 'success' rate increases to about 20 per cent.

The technique is complex. Hormone studies are made daily to identify the time of ovulation and ultrasound is used to see if the follicle is growing properly. When the tests show that ovulation is about to occur, the egg is recovered from the ovary using a meticulously gentle technique. This is done by inserting an ultrasound instrument, the size of a thick sausage into the vagina and making a real time picture (like a video) of the ovaries. A needle is guided along a groove on the side of the ultrasound probe and watched on a TV screen as it is pushed through the vagina into the ovary. Eggs are sucked out of follicles under vision.

The egg (ovum) is placed in a small test-tube containing a nutrient broth, and the father's fresh sperm are added immediately. If fertilization occurs, the division of the fertilized egg is watched closely and when it has divided three or four times (to make between 8 and 16 cells in a bunch like a mulberry) it is removed from the test-tube in which it has been growing. It is then delicately introduced into the woman's uterus through a narrow tube. Inside the uterus it 'floats' freely, and hopefully attaches itself naturally to the lining of the uterus, to develop into a baby.

Developments in the technique of IVF are occurring each year, and an increased success rate is occurring. In vitro fertilization is used if the woman has blocked Fallopian tubes, in some cases where the quality of the man's sperm is poor and in some cases where the cause of the couple's infertility cannot be explained. For these couples another form of artificial fertilization is often used. This is called GIFT – which means gamete intra fallopian transfer. In this technique, eggs are obtained from the woman's ovaries and sperms are added in a test tube. Immediately after the addition the mixture is introduced into the outer end of a Fallopian tube under vision using a laparoscope. GIFT is followed by a higher 'take home' baby rate than IVF, and is the preferred treatment if the woman has undamaged Fallopian tubes.

Because of the considerable ethical problems associated with IVF the procedure is only licensed to be performed in certain centres and is controlled.

Other tests

Certain other tests are frequently made although their practical value is doubtful. As I have mentioned, some doctors believe that the mucus secreted by the cervical glands is sometimes 'hostile' to spermatozoa. If this really does occur, then obviously pregnancy is less likely. To test this, the doctor takes a specimen of the mucus at ovulation time, as this is the only time when the spermatozoa can wriggle easily through the strands of mucus. He places the mucus on a glass slide and adds some of the husband's spermatozoa so that the two touch. He then measures how many spermatozoa penetrate into the mucus and how far. For convenience, he can do this test at the same time as he does the 'postcoital' test using the spermatozoa which are still in the vagina. If few spermatozoa penetrate the mucus he says that the mucus is 'hostile' and suggests treatment. The reservation I have about the test is that many couples who have been found to have poor sperm penetration of the mucus get pregnant with no treatment at all. This suggests that the treatment has little real value.

Recently, tests have been made to see if a woman has made antibodies to the man's spermatozoa which either make them immobile or cause them to clump. In either case they would not be able to make the journey through the uterus and oviducts. While studies have shown that more infertile couples have sperm antibodies than are found in fertile couples, it is not clear if they are of any real significance in preventing pregnancy and there is no effective treatment if they are found.

Donor insemination

It may be that the only reason for the barrenness of the couple is that the husband is sterile. In these circumstances, some couples decide that they would prefer to let the wife bear the child of an unknown donor, rather than adopting a child or doing nothing at all. The procedure is called DI (insemination of a donor's semen). In recent years fewer babies have become available for adoption and the waiting time has increased, often lasting for 5 years. For this reason DI is becoming increasingly popular. The physical characteristics of the husband are matched as closely as possible to the unknown donor. He is never seen, or known, by the couple, nor does he know to whom his donated semen has been given. The semen may be freshly obtained, which means that the donor has to masturbate and ejaculate within an hour before the insemination is to take place, or it may be frozen. In this case the donor supplies his semen which is then drawn into plastic straws and frozen in liquid nitrogen. It can be kept frozen until it is required.

At about ovulation time, which the woman detects by checking her temperature chart, or by observing the cervical mucus, the woman goes to the DI clinic or to the doctor's surgery. The fresh semen or a straw of defrosted semen is injected gently into her cervix and upper vagina. The procedure is repeated on the next day. On average two or three inseminations a month are required for three to six months before pregnancy occurs.

During the period, between 50 and 65 per cent of women will become pregnant, and most will give birth to a live baby. This child is brought up as the natural child of the father.

Infertility investigations take time and pose problems. Because of this, the couple must co-operate fully and should seek a doctor who has an interest in infertility, who is sympathetic to the patients, and who is careful never to do too much to little purpose. Although 45 per cent of couples will achieve a pregnancy, it is kinder to tell some of the others that pregnancy is impossible, and to suggest adoption while they are still relatively young. An adopted child can give as much joy to a family as a natural child.

CHAPTER 7

Birth Control and Family Planning

Of the many interlinked problems facing humanity in the last quarter of this turbulent century, that of the rapid rate of population growth is a major one. Because of the reduction in the deaths of infants and children due to better sanitation and the control of diseases, increasing numbers survive to reach their reproductive years and, being human, they reproduce. The scale of population growth is immense. In 1786, the population of the world was about 1000 million. In 1886, 100 years later, it had risen to 1500 million. In 1986, it reached 4800 million and by 2000, it is likely to reach 6500 million, unless global disaster occurs before that time (Fig. 7/1). All these people need to be able to eat adequately, to receive some education, to find some form of employment and to have some enjoyment of life.

In the rich, developed nations of the world, the population growth rate has diminished as women (and men) have chosen to have fewer children and, by using birth control methods, have been able to have smaller families. By contrast, in most of the poor, hungry developing nations, the birth rate remains high, and only a few couples limit the size of the family. This is because children are seen as valuable in societies in which social welfare measures are few and provision for old age almost impossible because of poverty. Children are also esteemed as they demonstrate the masculinity of the man, and are useful extra hands in rural communities. But even in these nations, surveys show that women want fewer children than they actually have, so that the desire to limit the size of the family is present. There is also the realization that if children are 'spaced' so that an interval of between two and three years separates each birth, the health and welfare of each child, as well as that of the mother, benefits.

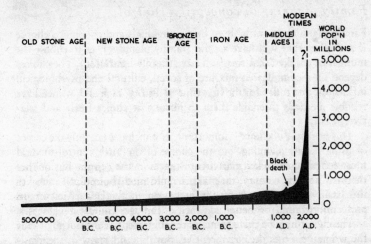

FIG. 7/1   The growth of the world's population.

In all nations, for one reason or another, women are beginning to realize that they need no longer be condemned to a life of constant childbearing and child-rearing, but are increasingly able to choose how many children, or how few children, they want to have.

The choice of method may be to prolong breast-feeding, which considerably reduces the chance of another pregnancy, or to use contraceptives which effectively prevent a new pregnancy occurring, or to have an abortion which ends a new pregnancy. Obviously, it is better to prevent a pregnancy than to terminate it – better on medical and social grounds. Yet, induced abortion is still the most usual way by which women limit the size of their family, although the use of modern efficient contraceptives is replacing it. However, even in the most sophisticated societies, induced abortion remains as an important method of birth control for women who have an unintended pregnancy, either because they do not use a contraceptive or do not follow the directions for use. A study in Britain in 1989 showed that a third of the women studied said that their pregnancy had been unintended. Some continued with the pregnancy whilst others sought an abortion. For this reason I will discuss abortion later in this chapter.

95

Family planning or conception control

Family planning is available to help individuals and couples to choose if and when they will have a child (family planning), or to choose the number of children that they will have (family limitation). The choices depend on a complicated mixture of social, cultural and psychological influences; and today for the first time in history, men and women have reliable methods to enable them to make that choice freely and relatively easily.

This principle of choice is important, as it includes not only the choice of using family planning, but the choice of the birth control method most suited to the particular circumstances of the couple. But neither the man nor the woman can make an informed choice until each has the basic knowledge of the different methods, their efficiency in protection against pregnancy and their advantages and disadvantages.

The choice may be that the man uses contraceptive measures; or that the woman chooses the contraceptive. Both should know of the available methods so that the decision is made carefully. The choice is helped if each partner has an idea of how efficient the method chosen is in preventing an unwanted pregnancy. A measure of contraceptive efficiency which is used by many people is the Pregnancy Index or the Pearl Index (from the name of the man who first used it). The Pregnancy Index, is calculated in the following way.

$$\frac{\text{The number of pregnancies} \times 1200}{\text{Total months of exposure to pregnancy}}$$

The result is expressed as the number of pregnancies per 1200 months of exposure, or preferably as the number of pregnancies per hundred 'woman-years'. This shows how many of every 100 women making use of the particular method chosen are likely to become pregnant if the method is used for one year.

Contraceptives for men

The choices available to a man are for him to use a temporary method, so that he remains fertile; or a permanent method so that he becomes sterile. Compared with the contraceptives available to women, those available to men are limited. This is not due to lack of research but to the fact that sperm production in man is infinitely greater than the production of ova in women, and methods of hormonal or chemical suppression of sperm development are consequently much more difficult to discover. It will be some time before a male contraceptive pill or injection is available which is both effective and acceptable.

At present, two temporary contraceptive measures are available to men. These are coitus interruptus (withdrawal) and the use of the condom. One excellent permanent method is currently available. This is vasectomy.

COITUS INTERRUPTUS (WITHDRAWAL): For many years withdrawal of the penis from the vagina just before ejaculation has been used to avoid pregnancy. In several investigations, made in the days before the Pill became available, it was found to be the most usual method adopted. It relies, of course, on the ability of the man to recognize the sensations which occur in his genitals just before ejaculation, and for him rapidly to withdraw his penis from the vagina and ejaculate outside. This requires great self-control, as the man will often want to keep his penis in the woman's vagina for as long as possible to obtain the greatest amount of pleasure. As the first spurt of semen, which contains the most spermatozoa, may either be ejaculated during withdrawal or may spurt into the vaginal entrance, the risk of pregnancy is high, and the pregnancy index is 25 per 100 woman years.

Coitus interruptus is said to lead to pelvic discomfort in a woman, who is stimulated but not relieved (unless she reaches a climax first), and in the man who has to withdraw at a moment when he would penetrate more deeply. Over long periods it was said to cause mental disorders. There is no evidence that coitus interruptus leads to either of these conditions, or indeed to any disease at all, but it may not be a very satisfying method for either sexual partner. Better methods are available. If a couple have used coitus interruptus successfully for years and it suits their particular sexual needs, no pressure should be put on them to change, but they might wish to know of other more reliable methods now available.

THE CONDOM: If the male covers his penis with a sheath, which is so thin that it is not noticed by either sexual partner, but so strong that neither the movement of the penis in the vagina, nor the ejaculation of semen tears it, pregnancy will be prevented as no spermatozoa will be deposited near the cervix. The sheath (or condom), which today is made of fine latex rubber, has been used since Roman times (Fig. 7/2). In the past century its use has been widespread, and although primarily

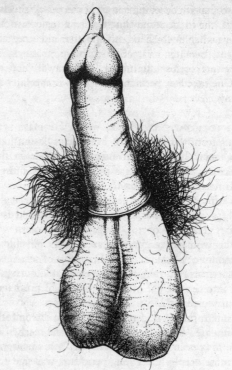

FIG. 7/2   The condom drawn on to the erect penis.

used to prevent conception, the condom was issued to soldiers who were going to fornicate with prostitutes as a method of reducing the chances of catching venereal disease. If the penis was 'protected' by the condom, the germs which lived in the genital tract of many prostitutes were unable to get into the delicate tissue of the opening of the 'eye' in the glans of the penis, or to invade the glans itself. In this way the spread of gonorrhoea and syphilis was to some extent prevented.

The disadvantages of the condom, or French letter, as a method of contraception are that the male must put it on, usually waiting until he has an erection of his penis. When he puts it on he must make sure that no bubble of air remains in the tip and that the condom is fully unrolled, so that it covers the length of the penis. Unless he takes these two actions, the condom may burst when he ejaculates, or it may come off his penis when he loses his erection after orgasm. If his penis is still in the woman's vagina this could let the sperm escape. Because of the need to put on a condom carefully the man may decide 'to take a chance'. This disadvantage can be avoided if the woman puts the condom on to the man's erect penis during love-play.

In the past few years because of AIDS and the increase in the number of women who have developed pelvic inflammatory disease or wart virus infection, the use of the condom is being encouraged. In fact it can be stated that if a woman enters a sexual relationship with a man, she should insist that he uses a condom until she is certain that he has not been infected with wart virus, chlamydia or any other sexually transmitted disease.

This is easy to state but experience shows that it is not so easy to achieve, particularly by sexually active teenagers.

The advantages of the condom are several. First, modern condoms are prelubricated by adding silicone and are individually packed in hermetically sealed aluminium foil sachets which enables them to be kept for a long period. The quality of the condom and its prelubrication make it easy to put it on to the man's penis by unrolling it. Provided the man makes sure that no bubble of air is left in the closed end, it is very efficient. Air, together with the ejaculated semen, can lead to the condom's bursting. Because of this slight risk, many doctors recommend that the woman puts some spermicidal cream in her vagina if the man uses a condom. Second, the condom is probably the suitable contraceptive if sexual intercourse takes place infrequently and unpredictably. In such circumstances a man may choose always to carry a condom in his wallet, and a woman may either have a condom or a vaginal diaphragm available should erotic stimulation lead to sexual intercourse and the man does not have a condom available. Third, there are no side-effects, because no hormones or chemicals are used, and the condom protects by acting as a mechanical barrier, preventing the spermatozoa reaching the cervix. Fourth, the condom reduces the chance of transmitting a sexually transmitted disease, especially non-gonococcal infections such as chlamydia (see p. 359) and genital wart virus (p. 358).

The assumed disadvantage that the condom reduces sexual pleasure is untrue. Modern condoms are usually unnoticeable to either partner, and a reduction in sexual pleasure is not so much due to the physical presence of the condom, as to psychological 'hang-ups' about its use.

A more real disadvantage is that the condom may slip off the man's penis when it becomes small after ejaculation, or may burst. If either of these events occurs and sperm escapes into the woman's vagina, pregnancy may result if intercourse took place at about the time of ovulation (page 14). Some doctors provide women, whose partner uses a condom (or if she chooses to use a diaphragm), with the morning-after pill (see page 116) to take should such an eventuality occur.

Because of its cheapness, its reliability, its ease of purchase and of use, the condom continues to be a popular method of birth control in all nations. Its reliability in protecting the woman against an unwanted pregnancy is more difficult to estimate and depends on the motivation of the couple always to use a condom during sexual intercourse. Among highly motivated couples a pregnancy rate of less than 2 per 100 woman-years is reported, but most reports show a pregnancy rate of about 5 per 100 woman-years.

VASECTOMY: Increasing numbers of men are becoming interested in vasectomy as the operation provides an easy, relatively painless method of making a man sterile without interfering with the couple's sexual enjoyment. Vasectomy must be clearly differentiated from castration, in which the man's testicles are removed surgically. Vasectomy merely prevents the sperm from being ejaculated. The testicles remain and function normally so that a man who has had a vasectomy is no less

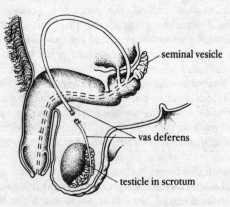

FIG. 7/3   Ligation of the vas deferens.

masculine, nor does he have any fewer sexual desires. He is able to perform and enjoy sex as much as, or more than, a man who has not had the operation.

The operation is relatively simple. The principle is to cut a small segment out of the vas deferens, the narrow tube which carries the spermatozoa from the testicles, where they are made, to the area of the prostate gland where they mature (Fig. 7/3). If you gently palpate a man's scrotum, at the level where it joins his body, by putting your thumb in front and your index finger behind, you will feel a cordlike tube as you roll the folds of skin between your thumb and index finger. This is the vas. There is a vas from each testicle, so you will feel one on each side.

The operation is made through a tiny cut into the skin, and can be done under local anaesthesia or using a general anaesthetic if the man prefers it. Each vas is identified and a small segment is cut out, after which the cut in the skin is closed. The operation takes about 15 minutes, and throughout the world about 10 million operations are done each year. Chinese doctors have simplified the operation even further, and have developed a 'no-scalpel' technique, which requires no stitch and takes less than 8 minutes.

Sexual intercourse can be resumed as soon as the man wishes, but the couple must continue using some form of contraception until the man has had about 12 ejaculations. This is because he has to ejaculate all the spermatozoa which have been stored in his prostate gland. Once

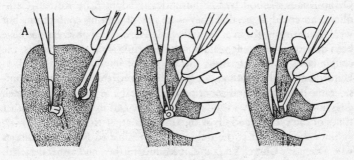

Fig. 7/4 In a no-scalpel vasectomy the vas (dotted line) is grasped by special ring forceps and the skin and the vas sheath are pierced by sharp-tipped dissecting forceps (A). The forceps then stretch an opening (B) and the vas is lifed out (C).

all these sperms have been ejaculated, the man is sterile, although he continues to ejaculate fluid which is made in the prostate gland so that neither he nor his partner notice any difference in their sexual pleasure.

What happens to the spermatozoa which are produced in the testicles but cannot escape because of the cut vas? They cease to be produced after a short time, so there need be no anxiety about the testicles becoming bloated with sperms!

The effect of the operation on the sexual pleasure of a couple has been investigated sufficiently to establish that over 70 per cent of men find that after vasectomy their sex life is improved, and only 2 per cent find it to be worse. The remainder said there was no change.

Methods requiring co-operation

PERIODIC ABSTINENCE (THE SAFE PERIOD): In a woman with a normal menstrual cycle, ovulation will occur approximately 14 days before the anticipated menstrual period and the ovum can only survive for 2 days unless it is fertilized. After intercourse, the ejaculated spermatozoa survive, and are able to fertilize the ovum, for 4 days at the most. From these facts you can deduce that if coitus is avoided from 4 days before to 4 days after ovulation pregnancy should not occur. Coitus should therefore be restricted to the days of menstruation, to the 4-6 post-menstrual days and the 10 pre-menstrual days. The physiological concepts of ovulation were independently observed in 1929 by Dr Knaus in Austria, and Dr Ogino in Japan. The so-called Ogino-Knaus method was enthusiastically adopted by Roman Catholics who could argue that they were not preventing conception, but were regulating births in a 'natural way'. The original observations have been developed in recent years but the principle is the same: that is, the couple have to restrict coitus to the time of physiological infertility. Unfortunately the method, despite the improvements, requires considerable motivation and is not particularly safe, as the average women does not have an exactly regular cycle, and ovulation may occur at other times of the cycle, especially if the emotions are stirred.

Since the method is the only one permissible to Roman Catholics who accept the Church's dictates, it requires further, and rather detailed, consideration in its three techniques of periodic abstinence: the 'calendar method', the 'temperature method' and the 'mucus method'.

The calendar method: If a woman is prepared to use a calendar, and over a period of 6 menstrual cycles to record the duration of each cycle, she can determine her own safe period by calculating the date of ovulation in each cycle, and then subtracting 3 days from that day in the shortest cycle and adding 3 days in the longest cycle. Coitus should be avoided during the danger period. If a woman has a cycle of less than 20 days, or if the duration of her cycle varies by more than 10 days, she will only be able to have 'safe' sexual intercourse at infrequent intervals and sexual frustration is likely to occur. A careful study in Washington DC of 30 000 cycles in 2316 women showed that only 30 per cent of them would qualify for the calendar rhythm method on the basis of a cycle range of 8 days or less. The cycle range varied with age, the smallest variation being in the age group 30 to 34, when 40 per cent had a cycle with a range of 8 days or less. However, if the couple are prepared to accept that coitus takes place in accordance with the calendar, not with desire, then the method is reasonably successful.

The temperature method: This is a more accurate method of pinpointing ovulation. It is based on the physiological observation that when ovulation has occurred the body temperature rises slightly. To detect this temperature rise a woman has to be sufficiently motivated to take her rectal, or vaginal, temperature each morning on waking and before she gets out of bed (which may be difficult for a woman with a young family), or has any food or drink. From the daily reading she makes a chart, and can have coitus safely 3 days after the temperature rise has occurred. The problems are that not all cycles show 'ideal' temperature rises and if the woman has a cold, flu or some other infection, the method cannot be used. It also requires considerable motivation to remember to take the temperature each day.

The mucus method (or ovulation method): The woman learns to examine her vaginal orifice for the presence of mucus. Immediately after a menstrual period the vaginal orifice feels dry, but as ovulation time approaches mucus can be detected. Initially, it is cloudy and sticky, but as the level of oestrogen rises, the cells of the neck of the womb (the cervix) are stimulated to secrete more mucus and its character changes. It becomes clearer, strands stretch without breaking and it 'feels slippery'. The peak of the clear mucus is reached on the day of ovulation, after which the mucus becomes cloudy again. The physiological concept of this sequence is correct, but the detection of mucus at the vulva requires considerable motivation, and perhaps the eye (and finger) of

103

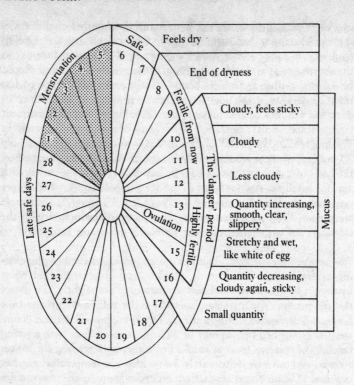

FIG. 7/5   Periodic abstinence: the mucus (ovulation) method.

faith. As well as this, vaginal secretions, either physiological or pathological, can confuse the issue. The motivated woman is given a chart and enters her findings each day using differently coloured stickers for different types of mucus. Coitus is 'safe' when there is no mucus, and more than 3 days after the last day of the clear mucus (Fig. 7/5). Between these times coitus should be avoided. Couples who have been trained in the method and conscientiously adhere to it, have a low failure rate, but most couples are not so motivated and the failure rate is between 15 and 25 per 100 woman-years, which is about the same rate as that of the other 'safe-period' methods. The problem is one of motivation. If the couple avoid coitus whenever there is any mucus, the woman will avoid pregnancy; she may also have to avoid coitus for most days of the month, which can be frustrating to both sexual partners. However, when a couple choose one of the 'natural' methods of birth control, they only have to avoid sexual intercourse on the 'dangerous days'. They can still enjoy cuddling, kissing and body contact and if aroused sexually, can be helped to orgasm by oral or digital stimulation of the woman's clitoris area and the man's penis.

Contraceptives for women

DOUCHING: Many women believe that if they douche immediately after coitus, they will prevent pregnancy occurring. There is no truth in this belief, as the spermatozoa enter the cervix almost immediately after ejaculation. The douche only washes the vagina, and clears the semen left there. As the woman has to go and douche immediately after the man has ejaculated, she may not have an orgasm herself and the need to leave may interfere with their mutual pleasure considerably. Douching is not a method of contraception, and has other disadvantages (see p. 370).

VAGINAL JELLIES OR CREAMS: These are preparations containing chemicals which will kill spermatozoa if the sperms are in contact with the chemical for sufficient time. Used alone, the jelly or cream (which may foam) is introduced high into the vagina with a tube and plunger, just prior to coitus. It is a poor method of contraception, about 35 women in every 100 using it for a year become pregnant. Spermicidal jellies and creams are also used in conjunction with vaginal diaphragms, or when the man uses a condom, which may increase their protective value against an unwanted pregnancy.

THE VAGINAL DIAPHRAGM: As its name implies, the vaginal diaphragm, or Dutch cap, consists of a thin rubber dome which has a coiled or flat metal spring in the rim. The diaphragms are made in various sizes, and the woman must be examined vaginally and given the size most suitable for her vagina. Most women smear spermicidal jelly in the dome and around the rim of the diaphragm although the use of a spermicidal jelly may not be necessary. Usually she squats, or stands with one foot on a chair, to introduce the cap, and inserts it into her vagina in an upward and backward direction. Inside the vagina, it regains its shape and fits snugly across the vagina covering the cervix (Fig. 7/6). After childbirth, the capacity of the vagina may increase to

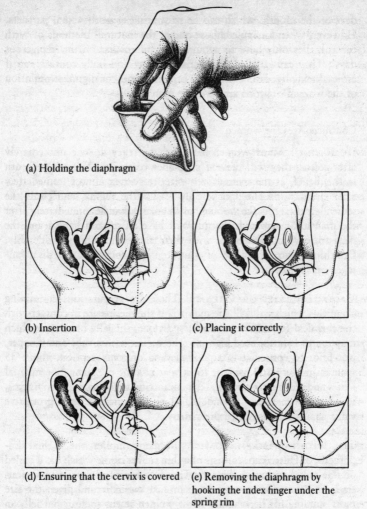

(a) Holding the diaphragm

(b) Insertion

(c) Placing it correctly

(d) Ensuring that the cervix is covered

(e) Removing the diaphragm by hooking the index finger under the spring rim

FIG. 7/6   The technique used in inserting the diaphragm.

some extent and the woman should be refitted if she intends to continue to use the diaphragm as a contraceptive method.

The advantage of the diaphragm is that it is completely without side-effects (although a few spermicidal creams may cause a mild vaginal irritation, which disappears when the cream is changed).

The psychological problem to a sexually aroused couple of the woman having to go away to put in her diaphragm is obvious. The alternative is for the woman to put the diaphragm into her vagina at a convenient time each day, or if she prefers during love play helped by her partner. Once inserted she can leave the diaphragm in her vagina for 24 hours. However it should be left in place for 6 hours after the last time she has sexual intercourse. When she removes the diaphragm she should wash it and either replace it in her vagina or dry it and store it depending on her desires and circumstances.

If a woman chooses this method of birth control she needs to be seen by a doctor so that the size of the diaphragm most suited to her can be chosen and so that she can learn how to introduce it into her vagina and how to remove it. If she chooses to use a spermicidal cream in conjunction with the diaphragm, she learns to place a large blob in the centre of its upper surface and additional cream around the rim. This also makes its introduction easier. She learns how to be sure that the diaphragm is in place, and to know this she must feel her cervix through the rubber. A woman generally needs to have some knowledge of her anatomy, many quite incorrectly believing that the vagina runs vertically upwards rather than upwards and backwards, and she should practise introducing and removing the diaphragm at home (Fig. 7/6). If she can, she should revisit her doctor a few days later, wearing the diaphragm, so that she can be reassured that her technique is good, and so that her additional questions can be answered.

It will be realized that the complexity of fitting the diaphragm, the necessity for the patient to have skills for its insertion, and the need for her to be so motivated that she makes sure it is in place every time she expects coitus, has limited its popularity. The pregnancy rate is less than 2 per 100 woman-years when a motivated couple use the method but for all couples the rate is about 4 per 100 woman-years.

The place of the diaphragm as a method of birth control should not be minimized, as it has no side-effects, is probably protective against cervical cancer, and if maintained properly can be used for one to two years before being changed. In the past few years, the popularity of the vaginal diaphragm as a contraceptive method has increased, and more women are using this method.

As well as the vaginal diaphragm, many family planning clinics and doctors have other forms of 'barrier' caps available. These tend to be smaller and fit over the cervix. They are rather more difficult to place correctly but some women may prefer to take the extra trouble and choose the smaller device.

HORMONAL CONTRACEPTIVES: To most women, hormonal contraceptives mean the Pill. Since it was first used in 1955, the number of women taking the Pill at any one time has increased to over 65 million. Nor is the Pill used today the same as that used more than 20 years ago. Today's Pill contains less oestrogen and less progestogen than the original Pill and so is a much safer product. And although the Pill is a method of contraception most favoured by women, the two hormones may be used singly, or together, given my mouth or by injection to suit the needs of different women.

The two hormones which are used in the Pill are laboratory-made substitutes of the two female sex hormones, oestrogen and pro-gesterone, which we discussed in Chapter 4. The hormones give a women her feminine contours, they prepare her uterus each month to receive a fertilized egg and they encourage it to develop into a child.

You may remember (if you don't you can find out again by reading Chapter 4) that ovulation is controlled by a special area of the brain – the hypothalamus. From cells in this area, hormones travel to the pituitary gland, at the base of the brain, and stimulate it to release a hormone, called follicle-stimulating hormone, into the blood. This, in turn, stimulates between 12 and 20 egg cells (or follicles) in the ovary to grow. As they grow they produce oestrogen. The oestrogen levels rise and 'feedback' to the hypothalamus. This has the effect of reducing the amount of follicle-stimulating hormone released, and of causing the release of a second hormone, the luteinizing hormone. The sudden surge of this hormone in the blood causes an egg, and usually only one egg, to escape from one of the growing follicles. The egg is expelled and the follicle, which looks like a tiny thick-walled balloon, collapses. It quickly undergoes conversion into a yellow-coloured structure which produces not only oestrogen, but also progesterone. If pregnancy occurs the yellow-coloured structure continues to live, but if pregnancy does not occur it ceases to produce hormones after a life of about 12 days. When this happens, menstruation starts.

The hormonal contraceptives upset this sequence. There are two main types. In the first, both oestrogen-substitute and progesterone-substitute are given from soon after menstruation. At the dose chosen, the hormones 'feedback' to the hypothalamus and prevent the release of the follicle-stimulating and of the luteinizing hormones, so that ovulation is prevented. In addition, they alter the lining of the uterus so that it is not receptive to a fertilized egg, and they alter the secretions of the cervix so that they become thick and sticky. This prevents most spermatozoa from travelling upwards from the vagina and entering the cavity of the uterus. The 'combined' hormonal contraceptives protect a woman against an unwanted pregnancy in these three ways. But if a woman takes the Pill by mouth, she must remember to take a pill every day as the hormones are rapidly inactivated in her body, and the level may fall too low for the protection to occur, should she miss more than two days. The Pill is taken each day for 21 days and then stopped for 7 days, but in most formulations sugar pills are given for the 7 days so that the woman takes a pill every day.

The second type of hormonal contraceptive avoids the use of oestrogen, and contains only the progesterone-substitute, which is called progestogen. The progestogen hormonal contraceptives do not prevent ovulation consistently, but do alter the secretions of the cervix so that sperms have difficulty in wriggling through. The hormone also alters the lining of the uterus so that the egg, if fertilized, is unable to implant itself. The progestogen hormone can be taken by mouth each day, or can be given by injection at one-monthly, three-monthly or six monthly intervals.

The 'injectables' are increasing in popularity. A single injection, every three months, is felt by some women to be more convenient than having to remember to take the Pill each day, and since the injectables do not contain oestrogen many of the side-effects of the Pill (which are due to oestrogen) do not occur. Against these two advantages are the disadvantages. In the first six months, about one woman in four has quite irregular and unpredictable episodes of bleeding, and one woman in six ceases to menstruate. After six months an increasing number of women (up to 30 per cent) cease menstruation. Medically, there is no need for a woman to menstruate at all, unless she wants to have children when menstruation usually indicates that ovulation has occurred. Absence of menstruation does not damage a woman's health, and many women may prefer not to menstruate, although some will worry that a pregnancy has occurred. The other disadvantage (which is only temporary) is that if a woman stops having injectables because she wants to become pregnant, fertility is usually delayed (in other words ovulation and menstruation fail to occur) for 9 to 12 months.

As I mentioned, the progestogen can also be taken by mouth, each day. The advantage of this type of hormonal contraceptive, which has been called the 'mini-pill' is that it increases the flow of milk in some lactating women. Unfortunately, the progestogen mini-pill disturbs the menstrual cycle in a number of women, so that it is not so convenient or acceptable as the combined pill, and its main use is for women who are breast-feeding but want the added security that a new pregnancy will be avoided.

When a woman weighs up the advantages and disadvantages of the hormonal contraceptives, she has to know how efficient the various hormonal contraceptives are in protecting her against an unwanted pregnancy. The combined oral contraceptive, the Pill, is the safest and provided it is taken daily as recommended, gives nearly 100 per cent protection, a pregnancy rate of 0.3 per hundred woman-years occuring. The 'injectables' are associated with a pregnancy rate of about 0.25 per 100 woman-years; and the 'mini-pill' with a pregnancy rate of about 2 per 100 woman-years.

When given the choice, most women prefer, at least initially to use one of the combined oral contraceptives, rather than one of the other types. Because of concern about side-effects (which we will discuss later) the majority of formulations of the Pill now contain only a small amount of oestrogen (which is two or three times less than the amount contained in the original Pill). As well as this, the amount of progestogen has been reduced over the years and today's Pill contains considerably less than some years ago.

The lower-dose formulations probably should be the first choice for most women. Three kinds of lower-dose formulations are available. In the first the same dose of each of the two hormones is taken each day. This is *monophasic* formulation. In the second, the dose is varied once in the cycle (the *biphasic* formulation). In the third, the dose of each hormone is varied twice in each course, producing a *triphasic* formulation. The advantage of this formulation is that it contains the lowest total dose of oestrogen and progestogen. A disadvantage is that the woman must *remember to take the Pill at about the same time every day*, or she may become pregnant. A disadvantage of all of the low-dose formulations is that 'break-through bleeding' may occur.

It is important for a woman choosing the Pill to read the leaflet enclosed in the package for detailed advice about how to take the Pill she has chosen. If the woman chooses a 28 day pack (which contains 21 days of hormones and 7 days of a sugar or a sugar-and-iron Pill) she takes a Pill every day. If she chooses a 21 day pack she should start taking the Pill from the new pack after a 7 day pill-free interval. She should not relate the time of starting to her menstrual bleed.

The missed Pill

If you miss a pill:

Take it as soon as you remember, and the next one at your normal time. If you are 12 or more hours late with any Pill, especially the first in the packet, the pill may not work. As soon as you remember, continue normal Pill taking. However, you may not be protected for the next seven days and must either not have sex or use another method such as a condom. If these seven days run beyond the end of the packet, start the next packet at once when you have finished the present one. (If you are using everyday (ED) pills, miss out the seven inactive days.) Do not leave a gap between packets. This will mean you may not have a period until the end of two packets but this will do you no harm. Nor does it matter if you have some bleeding on days when you are taking the Pill.

It is particularly important to remember to take the Pill at the end of the Pill free period, or if a 28 day pack is used at the end of the sugar tablet section. Delay in taking the first hormonal Pill may allow ovulation to occur in that cycle. This is one of the causes of an unintended pregnancy occurring whilst taking the Pill.

To avoid these problems some doctors now suggest to women that they take monophasic Pill (such as Marvelon) every day for 3 months by using three packets one after the other. This reduces the chance of an unintended period occurring and means that the woman only has 4 periods a year.

Side effects of the Pill

The side-effects of the Pill prevent it from being the 'perfect' contraceptive and reduce it to being a very good contraceptive. Since contraception is such an emotional matter, the incidence and severity of the side-effects are influenced by gossip and by sensational articles in women's magazines, which are often rich in speculation if poor in scientific observations.

The side-effects most often reported are listed in Table 7/1. This table does not prove that a side-effect is due to the Pill as many of the complaints are found in women not taking the Pill. But if you believe that the Pill is causing a particular side-effect which distresses you, you should consult a doctor and if necessary change to another method of contraception.

Table 7/1.
The side-effects attributed to oral contraceptives (the Pill)

Acne	Some increase in some women who take the combined Pill. The use of a 'sequential' pill reduces the incidence of acne.
Blood pressure	About one woman in every 20 taking the Pill experiences a small rise in blood pressure. A few susceptible women, generally over the age of 35, get a rather greater rise in blood pressure. The newer low-dose Pill does not seem to affect the blood pressure as much as the older higher-dose Pills.
Depression, mood changes	No increase, except among women who were depressed before taking the Pill, or who feel guilty about taking the Pill. Some, but not all, women who have depression when taking the Pill find that it is relieved by taking tablets of pyridoxine (vitamin B6)
Headaches and migraine	In carefully controlled investigations, no increase has been found. However, if a woman taking the Pill develops severe migraine which is localized, she should consult a doctor.
Heart attacks and strokes	Women who are aged 35 or more, who are overweight, who smoke cigarettes and who choose the Pill have five times the chance of having a heart attack or a stroke than similar women using other kinds of contraception. The risk is low, no more than 8 in every 100 000 women each year, but women who are overweight, over 35 and smokers should either stop smoking or choose some other method of contraception. Recent research suggests that the main reason for the higher incidence of heart disease and strokes is cigarette smoking rather than oral contraceptives. If a low-dose pill is chosen the risk is reduced further.
Menstruation	Tends to be reduced in amount, and often the colour changes from red to dirty brown. This is unimportant and does not mean that toxic substances are collecting in the body. Menstruation occurs on a predictable date, but a few women have spotting of blood, or a small bleed, on an unexpected day. If this is repeated in another cycle, a doctor should be consulted.

Nausea and vomiting	Fairly common in the first and second cycles on the Pill, thereafter unusual.
Pain with periods	Women taking the Pill usually have painless periods; this is a beneficial side-effect of the Pill.
Sexuality	Despite a good deal of anecdotal information, sexuality, sexual desire and enjoyment are usually unchanged.
Thrombosis in veins	There is evidence from investigations in Britain, the USA and other countries that women taking hormonal contraceptives (especially if they contain oestrogens) are more likely to develop clots in deep leg veins (deep venous thrombosis) than women using other methods. The risk is not great, but is increased if you are overweight, and smoke.
Vaginal discharge	The vagina is normally kept moist by secretions from the cervix. Women taking the Pill may expect increased vaginal moisture, and some discharge. If this is not irritating it is of no consequence. If it is irritating, a doctor should be consulted at once, as you may have developed monilia, which is slightly more common among women on the Pill.
Weight gain	Most women, whether taking the Pill or not, gain a little weight from retaining fluid in the few days before menstruation. This disappears when menstruation starts. Some women taking the Pill gain weight after a few months of use. This may be due to the hormone, progestogen, or to an increased appetite when the fear of pregnancy is lifted. Weight gain is usually controlled by a proper diet.

This information should help you decide if you would prefer to use oral contraceptives to the other methods available. Perhaps it will help even more if some questions asked are answered.

Are there any women who should not use the Pill? Because of the reported side-effects, which in turn are due to complicated biochemical changes in the body, some women should not use the Pill. These include some women who have infrequent menstruation; women who previously had a clot in a deep vein or a pulmonary embolism; women who have liver disease; women who have severe migraine, especially if it localizes to a small area of the head; and women who have certain blood disorders. As well, some women with high blood pressure or women with severe diabetes would be wise to use another method of birth control as both conditions may worsen when taking the Pill.

Does a doctor have to prescribe the Pill? The answer is yes, at least in most countries. Before prescribing the Pill, the doctor should find out if a woman has any of the diseases just mentioned. He should take her blood pressure and check her urine for sugar. Since she is well, and seeking protection against pregnancy, he should offer her protection against breast or uterine cancer by palpating her breasts and taking a 'cervical smear' (see p. 375).

The problem is that many young women are deterred from obtaining the Pill because they have to go to a doctor, and so fail to obtain protection against pregnancy. If they become pregnant, they seek an abortion. Because of this and because many doctors fail to do the examinations I have mentioned, and because in young women the diseases mentioned are unusual, I believe that a young woman should be able to obtain the first supply of the Pill without having to go to a doctor, provided she has regular periods, but should be encouraged to go to a doctor to obtain a repeat prescription.

Does the Pill lead to promiscuity? Some people believe that a woman avoids intercourse, because of fear of pregnancy, and fear of venereal disease. The Pill has removed the first fear but has done nothing to reduce the risk of getting a sexually transmitted disease. It happens that a relaxation of the double standard of sexuality and so a more liberal attitude to women's sexuality has coincided with the availability of the Pill. There is no evidence that the Pill increases promiscuity, whatever may be written or said.

Should the Pill be stopped for a month or two each year? This idea originated from the belief that as the Pill suppresses ovulation, it was wise to give the ovaries a chance to function normally each year. It is nonsense and is dangerous because an unwanted pregnancy can occur unless some other efficient contraceptive method is chosen. A woman can take the Pill, without a break, for as long as she wants. But if she is told to stop taking the Pill she must make sure that she uses some other reliable contraceptive method.

If a woman takes the Pill before she is married, will it prevent her from having a baby when she marries? This is a particularly insidious, nasty myth. In Chapter 6, I pointed out that about 1 couple in 7 is unable to have a baby. It is true that after ceasing the Pill (and sometimes when taking the Pill) the periods do not always come on time. In the first month after ceasing to take the Pill, ovulation is often delayed for 2 or 3 weeks, but after this most women ovulate regularly. In a few women, ovulation and menstruation take longer to return, but by six months 99 out of every 100 ex-Pill takers ovulate regularly. In only 2 in every 1000 does lack of ovulation and lack of menstruation persist for more than one year. The women who develop post-Pill amenorrhoea are of all ages, have been taking the Pill for a short time or for a long time, and have had infrequent or normal periods before using the Pill. There is no way of detecting which women will menstruate immediately and in which women ovulation and menstration will be delayed. But should this happen, treatment is available which generally enables a woman to ovulate, should she want to become pregnant.

When can a woman start using the Pill? She can start using the Pill from the time she becomes sexually active and at risk of becoming pregnant provided her periods are regular. If her periods are irregular, some other method of contraception may be preferred.

When should a woman start contraceptives after childbirth? If she is not breast-feeding she should start within 4 weeks. If she is breast-feeding it is unlikely that ovulation will occur for about 20 weeks, although it sometimes does. For this reason, many women do not want to take the chance and decide to take hormonal contraceptives. The progestogen-only Pill is to be preferred as it stimulates, rather than reduces, milk flow, and can be started when leaving hospital after the birth of her child or at the postnatal check-up.

When should a woman cease using the Pill? It is not certain for how many years a woman past the age of 40 should use contraceptives in order to avoid any possibility of pregnancy. Ovulation occurs less frequently after the age of 40, and rarely after the age of 47. At the moment, then, it would seem wise for her to continue with contraception until the age of 50. If she is taking the Pill she will, of course, continue to bleed each month, and will not know when she has reached the natural menopause, or 'change of life'.

Because of the increased risk of deep vein thrombosis, pulmonary embolism and stroke in women over 35 who are overweight and are also heavy smokers, it has been suggested that such women should use other methods of contraception. This belief has been extended by some doctors to apply to all women over 35. I do not agree, particularly as the new low-dose Pill is available. The amount of oestrogen (30 micrograms) in this Pill is little more than the amount many women are recommended to take by doctors to avoid menopausal symptoms.

What is the morning-after pill? This is a method of preventing pregnancy in a woman who has had sexual intercourse at ovulation-time when neither she nor the man have used contraceptives. Two pills (each containing oestrogen 50 micrograms and levonorgestrel 250 micrograms) are taken and the dose is repeated 12 hours later. The first 2 pills must be taken no later than 72 hours after the coital experience. The morning-after pill has also been suggested for women who only have intercourse once a week or less frequently and in this instance a large dose of progestogen is taken *within 3 hours of each coital episode*.

The amount of oestrogen makes one woman in four nauseated and vomit, but the progestogen seems to have few side-effects. The protection against pregnancy is very high when oestrogens are used after a single coital episode, but when progestogens are taken after each episode, the pregnancy rate is about 3–5 per 100 woman-years.

Fear has been expressed that hormones used in this way may cause abnormalities in the fetus should pregnancy occur despite the drugs. There is no evidence of this, but if a woman requests an abortion it should be given to her.

A recent development is to take a single dose of RU486 (mifepristone), a drug used to induce abortion, in countries where mifepristone is available. Mifepristone causes less nausea and vomiting than the present morning-after pill, and is nearly 100 per cent successful in preventing a pregnancy.

If the woman doesn't like the idea of taking these drugs she can wait to see if her period comes on time. If it does not she can have a sensitive pregnancy test made. If this is positive she can seek help from a doctor who uses 'menstrual regulation' (see p. 129) or to seek an abortion.

What are the long-term effects of taking the Pill? The Pill has now been available and used for over 20 years. No long term side-effects have been found. It does not increase the risk of cancer of the breast or uterus. It does not lead to the birth of abnormal children to women who have taken it for some years. It does not increase the incidence of diabetes or liver damage.

Isn't the Pill dangerous? No. The dangers of oral contraceptives have been exaggerated. Newspapers, women's magazines and the media find that a scare headline sells more copies than an item about the value of the Pill. The truth is that the Pill is not perfect, but no other 'drug' has been subjected to so much careful investigation in the whole of history, and the safety:efficiency ratio of hormonal contraceptives is equal to or better than that of any other known drug.

The benefits of the Pill. The use of hormonal contraceptives does have real advantages. The obvious one is that they enable women to control their fertility with ease and, in general, with little upset. But the Pill confers other benefits. A woman taking oral contraceptives is unlikely to have dysmenorrhoea, her menstrual flow will be reduced (which in turn helps to prevent anaemia) and she is likely to have a reduced amount of premenstrual tension. In addition women taking the Pill have a lesser chance of developing ovarian cysts. Recent work suggests that a woman has a lesser chance of developing the lumpy condition of the breasts which is called by various names, usually benign mammary dysplasia. These benefits are usually not publicized, but they are real.

In the end, *you* have to choose whether or not you want to take hormonal contraceptives to prevent an unwanted pregnancy. You may prefer to use another method – a popular choice is to use an intrauterine device – an IUD.

The intrauterine contraceptive (The IUD)

The IUD is being chosen by some women who wish to avoid pregnancy. It has an advantage over the Pill, in that once it has been placed inside the uterus and has been accepted, the woman has not got to do anything else to protect herself. She does not have to remember to take the Pill each day. She can have sexual intercourse with reasonable safety and without worry.

There is nothing new about the IUD. Arab camel drivers in Biblical times used the method. They used to introduce a round stone, the size of a pea, into the uterus of their female camels, which then repulsed the advances of the male camels, and worked harder! In the 1920s, a German gynaecologist used a silver or gold device which he introduced into the womb. Unfortunately it caused many complications and was abandoned by most doctors as unsafe! A revival of interest in this form of contraception occurred after the discovery of polythene. Polythene

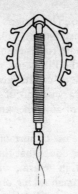

FIG. 7/7 The Multiload IUD

is a plastic which easily regains its shape after stretching, is not irritating to the tissues, and can be made free from germs quite easily. Because of the urgent need for some cheap form of contraceptive device, various shapes of polythene were devised to see if they would prevent pregnancy when inserted into the uterus of a woman. Of the bewildering and fanciful shapes which have been produced over the past two decades, only two remain. These are IUDs which have copper wire wound round their stem. One is shown in Fig 7/7. This permits a smaller IUD to be used, which effectively prevents pregnancy for 3–5 years.

No one yet knows how the IUDs work. The most recent evidence suggests that they cause a change in the environment inside the womb which makes its lining 'hostile' to the egg. It is known that the larger the device, the lower the pregnancy rate. Unfortunately, the larger the device, the more likely is the woman to have cramping pains and to have heavy periods, which are a considerable disadvantage. This was the reason for adding copper wire to the device. Inside the uterus the copper slowly ionizes, and this affects the lining of the uterus so that it rejects the egg. Copper has permitted scientists to make the device smaller, and consequently to reduce the side-effects while giving the same protection against pregnancy as with the larger devices (Fig. 7/8). The smaller device is also easier to introduce into the uterus of a woman who has never had children. There is one problem with the copper-containing IUDs. It is that as the copper slowly ionizes, the device becomes less efficient. At the moment, scientists think it should be

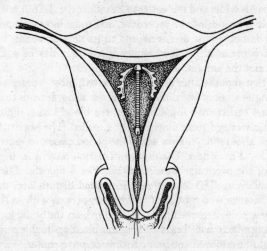

FIG. 7/8   An IUD in the uterus.

changed every 24–36 months, while the loop can stay in the uterus and give protection against pregnancy for as long as a woman wishes. The newer progesterone-containing IUD has to be changed each year.

Before the IUD is inserted it is important that the woman should talk with the health worker – doctor or nurse – so that she can learn about her genital anatomy and have the opportunity to ask questions. The health worker will examine her vaginally so that the size and position of the uterus can be determined. Once this has been done, the IUD is put into the womb painlessly and easily. Modern devices are prepacked in sterile packs and it is simplicity itself to introduce it into the woman's uterus. Usually she lies on her back with her legs apart. The health worker puts a small instrument into her vagina so that the cervix can be seen. It is cleaned with a gentle antiseptic, and then the introducer, preloaded with the IUD, is slowly pushed along the canal of the cervix so that its tip lies in the cavity of the uterus. The plunger is pushed, and the device is expelled to lie in the womb. There is no need for an anaesthetic, and the woman can go home immediately after.

The best time to put an IUD into the uterus is in the last days of menstruation; at a postnatal visit, which usually takes place six to eight weeks after childbirth; or just after an abortion. At these times the canal of the cervix is wider and it is easier to introduce the IUD. A few women feel a little faint during the procedure, and some have cramping pains for a few hours, as the uterus adjusts to its new occupant, but most have no trouble at all. A few women bleed for a day or so after the insertion, but the amount is slight.

In the first months after an IUD is inserted, most women report an increase in the amount and duration of menstruation. It tends to start one or two days earlier than usual. At first, the blood loss is slight, but it becomes heavier and some clots may be expelled. The heavier bleeding goes on for about 4 days, after which the period ceases, or spotting may continue for 2 or 3 days. Usually menstruation returns to the pattern normal for the particular woman within 3 or 4 months. The smaller copper-containing IUDs cause fewer menstrual disturbances than does the loop. Women who continue to have heavy periods with an IUD, find that the new progesterone-containing IUD reduces the blood loss. A few women continue to have heavy or irregular bleeding. If this persists, the IUD should be removed and another contraceptive chosen.

Apart from cramp-like pains experienced by some women when the IUD is inserted and some discomfort during menstruation when clots are expelled, pain is unusual. Should a woman have pain in her lower abdomen and this is associated with an increased discharge from her vagina and perhaps pain during intercourse, it may be a warning that she is developing a low-grade infection in her oviducts or in the other organs in her pelvis. In recent years there has been much concern about the relationship between IUD and pelvic inflammatory disease. Originally it was thought that the introduction of an IUD increased the risk of PID six-fold. It is now known that the risk is only increased if the woman has had a sexually transmitted disease in the past or has been infected without showing symptoms.

For this reason the IUD is not a good choice for a woman who has had several sexual partners or whose sexual partners have had several sexual partners. If the woman and her partner are faithful to each other the IUD may be a good choice.

The research has also shown that the greatest risk of PID occurs in the first 20 days after the IUD is inserted, and doctors are recommending that women who choose an IUD and have had several partners are given a course of antibiotics at the time of the insertion. A woman should seek medical help if she develops lower abdominal pain which persists, or if she gets pain during sexual intercourse when her partner's penis is deeply inside, or if she develops a heavy offensive vaginal discharge. If the doctor diagnoses pelvic infection the IUD will be removed and antibiotics given.

Two other problems should be mentioned. About 2 women in every 100 find that the presence of the IUD increases the contractions of the uterus so that the device is expelled. This usually takes place during menstruation but it can occur at other times. Of course, if the IUD is not in the uterus the woman is not protected against an unwanted pregnancy. This is one of the purposes of the nylon thread attached to the tail of the IUD. A woman should examine herself vaginally after each menstrual period to make sure the thread is there. If it is, all is well. She need not worry that the nylon will injure her sexual partner. The nylon is soft and there is no danger that it will spike his penis! In a very few women, the contractions of the uterus propel the IUD in a different direction – the IUD being pushed through the wall of the uterus to lie in the peritoneal cavity. This occurs in 1 insertion of every 1000 made. Once again, the nylon thread can no longer be felt when the woman examines herself. The woman should see her doctor so that he can decide if the device has been expelled or has been pushed through the uterine wall. The second problem is that an IUD should not be used by certain women. These include women who have had pelvic infection or an ectopic pregnancy in the past; women who have heavy menstrual periods and diabetic women.

As a method of contraception, the IUD is not as efficient as the Pill or the injectables. About 2 women in every 100 become pregnant while wearing an IUD and the rate seems to be the same whichever device is chosen. If pregnancy occurs the woman has two choices. She can ask to have an abortion, and her request should be granted without any difficulty, as in a few cases of pregnancy occurring with an IUD in the uterus, a spontaneous abortion (or miscarriage) occurs in the second quarter of pregnancy. Rather a high proportion of these abortions are accompanied by infection which may reduce the woman's chance of becoming pregnant later, when she wants to have a baby. Alternatively, she can continue with the pregnancy. She should visit her doctor as early as possible, after she knows that she is pregnant. The doctor will try to pull out the IUD without disturbing the pregnancy but if he fails the pregnancy may continue. But should signs of a 'threatened' spontaneous abortion arise (see p. 291), she should see the doctor again, and be checked for signs of infection.

Provided she does not abort she can be reassured that the IUD will not harm her baby in any way – there is no truth in the story that a copper-containing IUD causes abnormalities in the fetus.

Tubal ligation

Increasingly, couples who have completed their families are seeking permanent methods of birth control. In many cases the man chooses to have a vasectomy, as the operation is simple to do, relatively painless and highly efficient. In other cases the woman chooses to take the permanent measure. In her case the operation consists of cutting out a portion of the oviducts. These are the tubes which stretch from the upper corners of the uterus towards the ovaries. The egg, whether fertilized or not, passes along the oviduct. The sperms swim through the cavity of the uterus and along the oviduct where, when conditions are favourable, one of them fertilizes the egg. If a segment of the tube is clipped or is excised, and the cut ends tied, the sperms cannot reach the ovum and pregnancy will be prevented (Fig. 7/9).

This is the principle of the operation of tubal ligation. It is also called tubal sterilization, as the woman is permanently prevented from having children. Unfortunately, many women believe sterilization means castration, and confusion occurs. The ovaries are never removed in tubal ligation operations and after the operation continue to function normally, producing the hormones which help to make a woman a woman. Neither her femininity, nor her sexuality is diminished. Some women who contemplate having tubal ligation are anxious lest the eggs, released from the ovary each month, collect in the abdomen 'like frog spawn', as one of my patients said graphically. This fear is unfounded. At the most, only one egg is released each month, and it at once migrates into the oviduct where it is destroyed by other body cells.

Before deciding on the operation a woman should talk it over with her doctor, who will be able to answer all her questions. He will also need to examine her vaginally as certain conditions make tubal ligation inadvisable. These conditions include uterine 'fibroids', a marked prolapse, or a history of irregular menstruation which has not responded to hormones. If a woman has any of these conditions, and also wants permanent birth control, a hysterectomy is the preferable operation.

Nowadays, tubal sterilization is a relatively simple procedure requiring only a short stay in hospital. The operation is often done in the first days after childbirth, or it can be done apart from childbirth. In general (and there are obvious exceptions, for example after a third or

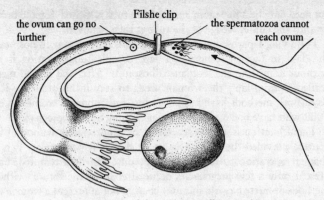

the ovum can go no further — Filshe clip — the spermatozoa cannot reach ovum

FIG. 7/9   Ligation of the oviducts (Fallopian tubes).

fourth caesarean section), tubal ligation should be avoided immediately after childbirth or abortion. This is because research has shown that most women who later seek to have the operation reversed, have had the tubal ligation done at this time. Many doctors refuse to do the operation if the woman has less than four children. This is, of course, arrogant of doctors. If a couple decide they want no more children, and are aware that the operation produces permanent sterility – so that if they change their minds later it cannot be readily reversed – then they should have the right to choose.

Two methods are available to perform tubal ligation. The first, which is the most popular, is to use a laparoscope. A laparoscope resembles a narrow telescope. It is introduced into the peritoneal cavity through a 1cm cut at the lower edge of the umbilicus. Once it is inside the abdominal cavity, the doctor can see the uterus and oviducts clearly. By manipulating them he can place a metal clip on each oviduct, thus crushing a section of the oviduct. This prevents the sperm reaching the ovum. If a woman has a clip placed in each oviduct, and later wishes to have her fertility restored, an operation can be performed to cut out the crushed section of the oviduct and to reunite the healthy sections. The success rate (in terms of a live birth later) is better if a microsurgical technique is used, but is not good. For this reason a woman should not decide to have a laparoscopic 'sterilization' performed unless she is completely sure she does not wish to have a further pregnancy. The second method is to make a small incision just below the pubic hairline. The cut need only be 2 to 4cm in length. Each tube is 'fished' for and brought up into the cut. A wedge of the tube is then removed.

Following laparoscopy the woman needs only to stay in hospital for the day (in fact in some places laparoscopic tubal ligation is done without admitting the woman to hospital). After the second method (called a 'mini-lap') the woman needs to stay in hospital for 3 or 4 days. Both methods have a small failure rate, about 2 women in every 1000 who have had a tubal sterilization may become pregnant.

Tubal ligation is a most successful and appreciated method of birth control provided the woman is aware that it is permanent. It is true that an operation to reverse the procedure can be attempted, but at present only a few pregnancies occur after it. In the future, with new methods of microsurgery, this may change, but at present a woman must have made up her mind that she does not ever want a further pregnancy. In certain cases the doctor may suggest that it would be preferable to remove her uterus, which is called hysterectomy, rather than performing a tubal ligation. Before the woman makes a decision whether to choose a hysterectomy she should expect her doctor to discuss the matter with her fully. Provided the woman has had the opportunity to discuss the operation with her doctor and has been counselled properly, few problems occur whether tubal ligation or hysterectomy has been chosen. After tubal ligation more than 99 per cent of women are very pleased they had the operation. There are no side-effects and the couple need take no other contraceptive precautions, confident that pregnancy will not occur.

A few myths persist about tubal ligation. These are that after tubal ligation (or 'sterilization' as it is sometimes wrongly called), the woman loses her sexual urge, her periods stop, she gets fat, and after a few years the oviducts open up and pregnancy becomes possible once more. These 'folk-tales' are all untrue. After tubal ligation a woman has the same sexual desires and urges as before the operation.

Usually a woman's periods are unchanged in amount or in frequency, but if she was taking the Pill before tubal ligation she may find that her periods are heavier. This is because the hormones used in the Pill usually cause a reduction in menstruation so that when the Pill is no longer taken the periods seem heavier. There is also some evidence that a woman's periods are a bit heavier if she has chosen to have tubal ligation done through a laparoscope. A woman does not get fat after tubal ligation – unless she overeats; and the operation does provide permanent protection against pregnancy.

The efficiency of contraceptives

Most sexually active people use contraceptive measures to enable them to enjoy the mutual pleasure of sexual intercourse without the fear of a pregnancy occurring at an inappropriate time.

In her reproductive years a woman may spend periods of time using one form of contraceptive, periods when she uses no contraceptives, periods when she is pregnant and periods when she returns to contraceptive use. She will want to know which of the contraceptive measures available is the most efficient in preventing a pregnancy so that she can make a choice (Table 7/2). It may be that she will choose one of the most reliable methods, such as the hormonal contraceptives or the IUD despite the side-effects. It may be that she will choose a slightly less efficient method (such as the vaginal diaphragm or condom) which has few or no side-effects. This choice may be made as a woman grows older, when her ferility is reduced, secure in the knowledge that should an unwanted pregnancy occur she can obtain an abortion with safety. But it would be irresponsible for a woman to choose not to use any form of contraception and rely on abortion to end her unwanted pregnancies. A single abortion poses little danger to a woman, but repeated abortions increase the danger of damage to her body. This is why I have written that when a woman desires to limit the frequency of pregnancy she should use contraceptives, relying on abortion as a 'back-stop' if the contraceptive fails to prevent pregnancy or when an unwanted pregnancy unexpectedly occurs.

Table 7/2
Failure (i.e. pregnancy) rates over a period of 12 months

	per cent
No contraception	70
Vaginal douche	45
Vaginal foam, jellies, etc.	30
Periodic abstinence	25
Withdrawal	25
Condom	5
Vaginal diaphragm + spermicidal jelly	4
Intrauterine contraceptive device	3
Oral contraceptives:	
Continuous progestogen	4
Sequential	2
Combined	0.3

Induced abortion

Induced abortion has been practised by women since people collected in groups for their mutual protection. When food was plentiful children were welcome; when food became short, either because of famine or population pressures, an additional child could mean disaster. As no contracepive methods were available (apart from sexual abstinence) abortion was used to end an unwanted pregnancy. Few of these abortions were performed under ideal conditions, but most women survived, although many were injured or made sterile by infection following the abortion.

The toll which clandestine abortion took of the health of women has led enlightened legislators, in the past few decades, to change the laws which made abortion illegal, replacing them by laws which permit abortion to be performed with dignity and safety. The change is due to several factors. First, it was apparent that even in nations where abortion was illegal, large numbers of women continued to seek and to obtain abortions. Second, a wealthy woman could always obtain an abortion without humiliation and with considerable safety but her poorer sister was often humiliated and her health placed in jeopardy when she sought the services of a back-street abortionist. The dangers of back-street abortions are demonstrated by the finding that the majority of deaths following abortion occurred if the woman had tried to abort herself or had used the services of an unskilled person; and by the statistic that in certain Latin American countries, between 25 and 50 per cent of beds in maternity hospitals are occupied by women suffering from the effects of illegally induced abortion. Third, the existing laws did not prevent induced abortions from occurring, the more liberal laws, it was hoped, would reduce the dangers of abortion. This has proved to be so.

The change to legal abortion has spread rapidly since 1970, and today 60 per cent of the world's women live in nations where a legal abortion can be obtained, usually with relatively little difficulty or loss of dignity. Experience of legal abortion in the USA and Britain has been carefully documented and analysed. These investigations show that since legal abortion has been introduced, the number of deaths due to abortion has dropped dramatically, so that a woman who has an abortion of a pregnancy which is no more than 10 weeks advanced, performed in an appropriate place by a skilled medical attendant, has only one chance in 100 000 of dying as a result. This is 10–20 times less than the deaths associated with childbirth. The studies also confirm that the longer the duration of the pregnancy the higher is the possibility of complications.

In nations where abortion laws have been made less restrictive, opponents of reform have declared that if abortion was permitted more freely than previously, women would abandon other methods of birth control and would rely on abortion. They foresaw a continually rising frequency of abortion. They were wrong. In Britain the number of abortions rose the first 5 years after the more liberal laws came into operation, but the rate has since fallen. Moreover, fewer than 5 per cent of women who have had an abortion, have returned for a second abortion. The remainder have either become pregnant and have delivered a live baby, or have used contraception to prevent another unwanted pregnancy.

The women, and men, who campaigned for abortion law reform correctly believed that the majority of sexually active women would be protected by contraceptives; that abortion would be used as a 'backstop' for those women who became pregnant through ignorance, illluck or great misfortune; and that most of those women who had had an abortion would subsequently avoid an unwanted pregnancy by using contraceptives. This belief has proved true, and it epitomizes a rational attitude to abortion. This is that women and men should be informed about contraception, that contraceptives should be easily obtained, and couples would use one of the contraceptive measures currently available to prevent an unwanted pregnancy occurring. But should an unwanted pregnancy happen, the woman should be able to have an abortion performed without delay, without the need to beg or risk being humiliated, and in a place where the abortion can be performed by a skilled medical attendant. It also implies that all the people with whom she comes into contact should be sympathetic and understanding helpers, and should give the woman counsel so that any guilt she might feel would be minimized, and inform her about contraception so that she might prevent another unwanted pregnancy.

Organizations, such as Preterm in the USA and in Australia, and similar organizations in Britain, as well as many hospital clinics, meet these criteria. More will do so if women continue to make their voice heard.

It is true that organizations opposing abortion have also become increasingly vocal. They point out that the fetus has a right to life, and if aborted its mortality is 100 per cent. Unfortunately, they also tend to publish selective, inaccurate statistics which make induced abortions appear far more dangerous than they really are, and some of their propaganda induces strong feelings of guilt among women who have had an abortion. This is an affront to the integrity of a woman who has sought an abortion only after careful thought, as most women do.

Before abortion law reform in Britain, fearful women who wanted an abortion resorted to the most useless and sometimes the most desperate methods. Many were misled by friends and friendly pharmacists, when they tried to obtain drugs to induce the abortion of an unwanted pregnancy. An investigation by Dr Martin Cole in Britain in 1964 showed that 'female remedies' could be purchased in 12 out of 15 pharmacies chosen at random, and in 17 out of 22 shops selling condoms or diaphragms. Most of the drugs claimed to bring on menstruation suppressed 'due to colds, shock, fright, strain, etc.'; but they were sold as abortifacients, and were not cheap. The drugs studied contained iron, quinine, purgatives or herbals such as aloes and pennyroyal which tradition held brought on menstruation. They are, of course, all quite useless if a woman is pregnant. None will procure an abortion.

The lack of efficacy of these drugs led women, who could not afford proper care, to try to induce an abortion using the easily available enema (or vaginal douche) apparatus. With considerable contortions, women have introduced the nozzle of the douche into their cervix and have tried to fill their womb with mixtures of soapy water or caustics. In all too many cases this led to a medical disaster, and often to the death of the mother. In other instances desperate women have introduced a domestic instrument – crochet hooks, button hooks, knitting needles, or pieces of wood – into their womb in the hope that it would bring about an abortion. Often it did – but often the women also became infected.

When a woman went to a back-street abortionist, her chance of obtaining an abortion, while avoiding death from haemorrhage, or sterility from infection, varied with the training and skill of the abortionist. The best trained were fairly efficient and used gynaecological instruments skilfully. Others used an enema syringe, or introduced an object into the womb to start bleeding so that the woman could then go to the hospital claiming that she was aborting spontaneously. This situation has now changed, and although some women still hopefully and ineffectually try 'home remedies', and some still go to back-street abortionists, most have access to the services of skilled medical helpers. In their hands abortion is very safe, provided it is undertaken in the first quarter of the pregnancy.

Most of the methods of terminating an early pregnancy available are surgical and require invasion of the woman's body. Recently a medical method has been developed which is effective in producing an abortion provided the woman is treated less than 49 days after the start of her last menstrual period. This is the use of a drug called mifepristone (RU-486). The drug is taken by mouth and 48 hours later a tablet of a prostaglandin drug is taken. In most women the abortion starts soon after this and in over 95 per cent is completed quickly. Most women lose no more blood than they do in a normal period, but about 5 per cent of women have a heavier blood loss and need to have a suction curette (see later). One woman in a hundred fails to abort and has to have a surgical procedure to terminate the pregnancy. At present mifepristone is not available in Australia, the UK or the USA.

The advantage of mifepristone and the prostaglandin drug is that the woman does not need to go to hospital, in most cases, and is spared the cost and embarrassment of a surgical procedure.

The safest surgical abortion is one which is performed on a healthy woman, whose pregnancy is less than 10 weeks advanced, by a skilled medical attendant, in a well-equipped clinic or hospital. The earlier the abortion, the safer it is. This has led some doctors to suggest the method of 'menstrual regulation'. In this a woman who is at risk of being pregnant, waits to see if her menstrual period comes on time and, if it does not, seeks help within 7 days. At this time it is impossible to diagnose pregnancy clinically, and laboratory tests (except for a special test) are not helpful. The doctor empties the uterus with a small tube attached to a syringe. The woman may or may not be pregnant so that no moral question is raised and the doctor is only regulating her menstruation.

Menstrual regulation is very safe, but the pregnancy continues in 1 woman in every 100 on whom the procedure is used. Menstrual regulation can be performed painlessly without any anaesthetic. A possible 'disadvantage' of the simplicity of the procedure is that it may prevent some women from using contraceptive methods, although I believe it doubtful. Large numbers of women have been treated by 'menstrual regulation', and the reported results show that only 1 woman in every 250 000 treated has died – a rate three times less than the deaths which follows an injection of penicillin! The safety of menstrual regulation emphasizes the importance of seeking help as early as possible if you think you may be pregnant and do not want to continue with the pregnancy. Even so, it is better, safer and less distressing to prevent pregnancy by using a contraceptive than by resorting to abortion, whether menstrual regulation or some other method is used.

The method of suction is also used by doctors who end an unwanted pregnancy in its first 10 weeks. An injection of local anaesthetic is made into the cervix, which blocks all pain; or else the woman may choose to have a general anaesthetic. A narrow glass, metal or plastic tube, the size depending on the number of weeks the woman is pregnant, is pushed gently through the cervix, so that it lies in the cavity of the uterus. The tube is connected, through a second tube to a vacuum bottle. The vacuum created in the uterus sucks the tiny embryo in its sac from its attachment to the lining of the womb with no damage to the uterus itself. Usually there is no more bleeding after the operation than there is with a normal menstrual period and often there is far less. The woman can go home within an hour or so of the procedure and usually has no further problems, although she is counselled what to do should problems occur.

After the 12th week of pregnancy, suction curetting, as it is called, is not recommended, and if the pregnancy is over 14 weeks complications may be frequent and serious.

Because of these dangers, most gynaecologists recommend that if the pregnancy has lasted for more than 12 weeks after the last menstrual period, surgery should be avoided. Instead, substances called prostaglandins should be used. These substances are injected into the uterus and after a period of time (which lasts on average 16 hours) bring on strong contractions of the uterus, rather like a 'miniature labour' which, after some hours, lead to an abortion. During the interval between the injections and the abortion, the woman may feel nauseated, or develop a fever, as prostaglandins have these side-effects. The process of the abortion is not very pleasant and can be painful though pain relieving drugs are given. It is associated with more complications than occur when the abortion takes places in the first 10 weeks of pregnancy. Both the discomfort and the greater danger of late abortion confirm what I have written earlier in this chapter. This is that abortion is most safely performed in the first 10 weeks of pregnancy.

As the duration of pregancy increases abortion becomes increasingly dangerous to the woman. The mortality rises (Fig. 7/10) and the complications increase. If the abortion is performed before the 10th or 12th week, only 2 per cent of women have complications, usually heavy bleeding requiring a curettage, or fever. When the abortion is

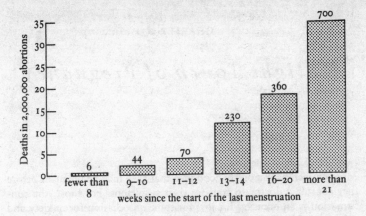

FIG. 7/10   Deaths from abortion. Two million abortions reported in the USA.

performed between the 12th and 15th week, heavy bleeding compli-
cates 5 per cent, and fever 4 per cent of the abortions. As well, there
is some concern that abortions performed in the second quarter of
pregnancy, between the 10th and 19th week, may damage the cervix
of the uterus causing 'cervical incompetence'. This complication is rare.

For these reasons when a woman has made the decision, and discussed it with a counsellor, that she wishes to have an abortion, the
operation should be done with the least delay, with consideration for
her feelings, and in an appropriate place.

Counselling before having an induced abortion is also important to
prevent any adverse psychological effects of the procedure. In general
there are few or no lasting psychological effects following an induced
abortion. In fewer than 10 per cent of women anxiety, guilt or depression
occurs which lasts for more than a month. Only those women who were
ambivalent about having the abortion or were pressured by parents or
partner are more likely to experience regret a year later.

Induced abortion performed before the 12th week of pregnancy by
a skilled doctor in an appropriate place is a safe procedure, both
physically and emotionally.

CHAPTER 8

A Slight Touch of Pregnancy

Most women have a pretty good idea that they may be pregnant before they consult a doctor to confirm their suspicions. For most, the confirmation is an occasion for joy; for some an occasion for anxiety and sorrow. A few women, desperately wishing to become pregnant, can mimic many of the signs of pregnancy, and believe themselves to be pregnant when in fact they are not. Even after the doctor has told the patient that she is not pregnant, she refuses to believe him. These patients have a 'phantom pregnancy', and require sympathetic psychiatric attention.

The symptoms of early pregnancy

Amenorrhoea

The first symptom of pregnancy is usually that the menstrual period fails to occur on the expected date. If a woman has regular periods and has had the chance of becoming pregnant, the absence of menstruation (amenorrhoea) suggests that she is pregnant. But a woman who has regular periods should wait at least 10 days before consulting a doctor, as before this time he will not be able to tell if she is pregnant. If her periods are not regular, amenorrhoea is less helpful in making a diagnosis of pregnancy.

Pregnancy is the most usual cause of amenhorrhoea in women aged 16 to 40, but it is not the only cause. Menstruation may be delayed or suppressed by weight loss and emotional stress, some illnesses and if certain drugs are taken. Apart from pregnancy, weight loss and emotional stress are the usual causes of amenorrhoea in a woman who previously has menstruated regularly. Emotional stress may be due to 'fear' that the woman is pregnant, a fight with a loved one, or a new and difficult job. Weight loss and emotional stress suppress the release of the brain hormones which control menstruation (see p. 343).

Breast changes

Many women experience breast fullness and discomfort just prior to their menstrual period. If pregnancy occurs, these symptoms persist and are increased. The breasts become fuller, firmer and more tender. Occasionally they throb and the nipples tingle. The degree of these symptoms is quite variable, but as pregnancy advances the fullness of the breasts increases, and the nipples become larger and darker. The area round the nipple, which is called the areola, also becomes larger, darker and rather swollen. In this area there are tiny openings to milk ducts and minute glands. In pregnancy the minute milk glands and ducts enlarge to form small protuberances or follicles – which are named Montgomery's follicles after an Irish obstetrician who first described them. These are rarely noticeable until the pregnancy is 8 weeks advanced.

The changes in the breasts are caused by the female sex hormones oestrogen and progesterone produced by the placenta. These hormones cause growth of the ducts and milk sacs of the breast, and lead to fat being deposited around them. The tingling and throbbing occasionally felt is due to the increased flow of blood through the blood vessels which supply the breasts.

Nausea and vomiting

In about half of pregnant women some degree of nausea or vomiting occurs. Usually this is quite mild, and occurs in the morning. Occasionally, however, it is more severe, and vomiting may occur at any time of the day. When this occurs, it usually starts about 2 weeks after the first missed period, and lasts for about 6 to 8 weeks. The cause of the nausea is not known, but it seems probably that it is due to the increases in the amount of sex hormones produced in pregnancy. It usually goes by the 12th week of pregnancy as the body adjusts to the higher hormone levels.

Bladder 'irritability'

In early pregnancy the kidneys work over-efficiently, and the bladder fills with urine more quickly. This leads to frequency of urination, which is an early symptom of pregnancy.

What the doctor looks for

The patient visiting her doctor in early pregnancy will be asked about the symptoms just mentioned, and will then be examined. As will be described in the chapter on antenatal care, the examination includes a careful assessment of the patient's general health, in which the heart is listened to, the breasts are examined, the abdomen is palpated, and an 'internal', or pelvic, examination is performed. This examination need not be feared, as it is quite painless. The patient lies on her back with her legs bent and her knees apart. She breathes slowly and relaxes all her muscles. The doctor first examines her vulva and then gently introduces a small instrument, called a speculum, into the vagina so that he may look at the cervix. Many doctors take this opportunity to take a sample of the cells which cover the cervix, so that these may be examined in the laboratory. This is called the 'Pap smear' (cervical smear) test, after Dr Papanicolaou who first described it. Abnormal cells are found in about one sample in every 200 examined. These patients have to be investigated further in case the abnormal cells indicate a very early cancer of the cervix. The doctor then removes the speculum and putting on a plastic glove, inserts two fingers into the vagina. With his other hand he presses gently on the abdomen just below the umbilicus (Fig. 8/1). In this way he can feel the shape of the uterus and tell if it is enlarged, as would be expected in pregnancy, or if there are any other swellings which may require treatment. The pelvic examination is most informative when made between the 6th and 10th week of pregnancy.

Immunological tests

Immunological pregnancy tests are now available which can diagnose pregnancy before clinical signs are detectable. The tests, which rely on advanced technology, can be made on a sample of the woman's blood or her urine. The tests measure the level of the 'pregnancy hormone', human chorionic gonadotrophin. The blood test can detect if a woman is pregnant before she has missed a menstrual period. The test on urine becomes positive within three days after the menstrual period is missed.

A SLIGHT TOUCH OF PREGNANCY

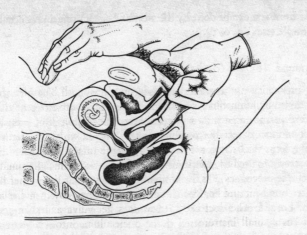

FIG. 8/1   The diagnosis of early pregnancy.

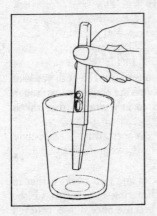

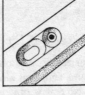

NOT PREGNANT
You are not pregnant
if after 4 minutes only
one dot is showing in
the small upper round
window of the test.

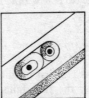

PREGNANT
You are pregnant if
after 4 minutes dots
appear in both
windows of the test.
Even if one of the dots
is very light, it means
that you are pregnant.

To perform the test you will need some urine, which should be collected in a clean glass. You may use either first morning urine or a sample taken at any other time of the day.

Remove the pink cap from the test stick. Dip the **thin end** of the stick slowly into the urine and hold it there for about 5 seconds. Make sure that this smooth part **up to the horizontal line** is completely covered by the urine.

Replace the pink cap **immediately after** dipping.

FIG. 8/2   The immunological diagnosis of pregnancy.

The urine test can be done by the woman herself using a very accurate, but simple test (Fig. 8/2).

Ultrasound

Early pregnancy can also be diagnosed by ultrasound. The ultrasound is produced by a machine. The sound waves 'echo' off different tissues and can be translated into a picture. From the 7th week of pregnancy ultrasound can detect the presence of the 'sac' in which the fetus lies and the fetus itself. It can also give a picture of the fetal heart beat. It is sometimes used to identify if the pregnancy is in the Fallopian tube (an ectopic pregnancy). If the woman is unsure of her menstrual dates an ultrasound picture enables the doctor to determine when the baby will be born. From about the 15th week of pregnancy, ultrasound can detect twins, and later is used if the doctor is uncertain whether the baby is a breech. Ultrasound is also used to detemine the position of the placenta, and by taking readings at intervals, it is possible to determine the speed of growth of the baby.

The symptoms and signs of later pregnancy

As the uterus grows, its size becomes obvious. After the 16th week of pregnancy, other symptoms and signs also indicate pregnancy, although by this time it should be pretty obvious to any woman that she is pregnant.

'Quickening'

At about 18 to 20 weeks in first pregnancies and two weeks earlier in subsequent pregnancies, the first faint fluttering movements of the baby are felt. This is called 'quickening' because once it was believed that the baby only became alive at this time. It is reflected by the Biblical reference to the 'quick and the dead'.

Movements of the fetus become strong and more frequent as pregnancy advances, and the mother may notice that her baby has periods of activity and periods of rest. In the rest periods, it probably sleeps. Provided the periods of activity and rest coincide with the same periods in the mother, all is well; but some babies seem to take a perverse delight in having their active periods at night, to the annoyance of the mother! If the movements are very active, lumps appear and disappear on the uterus and are noticed by the mother. They are caused by the baby's limbs stretching the muscles of the uterus. Many babies are less active, and sometimes a day or more passes without movements being felt. This does not mean that the baby is dead, but if the woman feels no movements for a longer period, she should consult her doctor, who will listen for fetal heart sounds. A machine, called a Fetal Heart Detector, has been developed which relies on the 'doppler principle' of sound waves. This machine can detect the baby's heart beats as early as the 12th week of pregnancy, and is nearly 100 per cent accurate after the 16th week.

Frequency of urination

Frequency of urination, which was a symptom of early pregnancy, ceases after the 12th week, to reappear in the last weeks of pregnancy. In late pregnancy the symptom is due to the pressure of the baby's head on the bladder, and can be quite disturbing, especially at night.

What the doctor finds in late pregnancy

The growth of the uterus

To some extent the doctor can tell how much the pregnancy has advanced by noting the height of the top of the uterus in the patient's abdomen (Fig. 8/3). The method is not very accurate, and various factors such as tenseness of the abdomen or obesity can lead to false readings. At the same time, the doctor gently runs his fingers over the uterus to determine the position of the baby. He should always tell the woman where her baby is lying, outlining the position for her. He usually listens for the baby's heart sounds, but if the woman is feeling the 'movements' of the baby, this is not really necessary.

The growing uterus stretches the woman's abdominal skin, and by the 20th week it will be obvious that she is pregnant. From this time on, small pinkish streaks, about 4cm (1½in) long, may appear over the lower abdomen, especially in the flanks. These 'streaks of pregnancy' are due to small breaks in the lower layer of the skin which is less well able to stretch. They also sometimes appear on the thighs. After the birth of the baby, the colour fades to silvery-

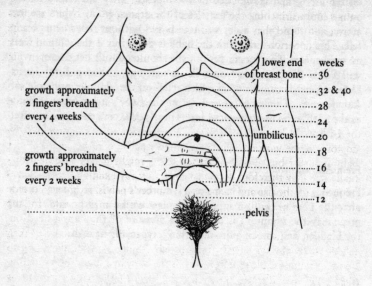

FIG. 8/3 The growth of the uterus in pregnancy.

white, but remains permanently. There is no known way to prevent them, although some women believe that massage of the skin with olive oil helps.

In dark-haired women, another change may be found. This is a brownish pigmented line stretching in the midline from the umbilicus to the pubic bone. It is of no consequence, and fades after delivery, almost disappearing in time.

'Medical imaging'

The development of ultrasound machines in the past 10 years has been a major advance, and has meant that x-rays are rarely required in pregnancy. This is important as babies of mothers who have had x-rays taken during pregnancy have a slightly greater chance of developing leukaemia.

Ultrasound has replaced x-rays in most cases to diagnose twins, to determine if the baby is a breech or is lying transversely, and to determine the maturity of the baby (that is, its gestational age). Many doctors now recommend that every woman should have an ultrasound picture taken either between the 10th and 13th week or the 16th and 22nd week of pregnancy. The argument is that an ultrasound examination (1) establishes accurately how much the pregnancy has advanced, (2) detects the presence of twins, (3) may detect a congenital abnormality in the baby at a time when termination of pregnancy (abortion) is possible and (4) provides the family with the first picture for the baby book!

X-rays still have a small place in obstetric care. Occasionally, the doctor may be worried that the woman's pelvis is rather small or her baby is rather big. Either of these factors might make childbirth difficult. He may therefore decide to have an x-ray examination to determine exactly the size and shape of the mother's pelvis, in order to decide whether normal childbirth or a caesarean section may be safer for the mother and her baby.

Pregnant women sometimes ask if x-rays or ultrasound can be taken to determine the sex of the unborn baby. Since x-rays only show up bones, it is impossible to tell the sex of the baby by x-rays. Occasionally, ultrasound *may* identify the sex of the baby (if the baby's scrotum is visualized), but this is not always possible.

Sex preselection

Can you choose the sex of your child by having intercourse at a certain time; by eating specal diets, or by douching with a special fluid? All these suggestions have been made. Couples have spent time and money visiting doctors who claim that they can help the couple have the boy or girl they want. In spite of much newspaper and magazine publicity, no method has been devised which lets you choose the sex of your child. It happens by chance.

CHAPTER 9

A Wondrous Growth

The fetus

Fertilization occurs in the outer part of the oviduct, when a single spermatozoon penetrates the 'shell' (or zona pellucida) of the egg and enters its substance. The sperm's tail is stuck in the 'shell' and drops off, leaving the sperm head free in the egg. The part of the sperm head, called the nucleus, which contains in twisted strands the information needed to make a new individual, joins with the nucleus of the egg, and they fuse. The first step towards a new individual, who will take half of its characteristics from its father and half from its mother, has been taken. Inside the zona pellucida, the fertilized egg with its fused nucleus divides into 2 identical cells, then into 4 cells, then into 8 cells, then into 16 cells, and again until it looks like a mulberry made up of 64 cells. These divisions take place during the 3 days that it takes the fertilized egg to move gently along the oviduct to reach the cavity of the uterus. Inside its cavity, the fertilized egg develops further, fluid appearing among the mulberry cells, and eventually splitting them into two parts: an outer shell of cells, and a collection of cells at one side. The outer cells will form the placenta; the inner mass will form the embryo. Quite soon after this, on the same or the next day, the zona pellucida dissolves and the fertilized egg, now called a blastocyst, plants itself into the juicy, soft lining of the womb (Fig. 9/1). Nine days after fertilization the blastocyst has burrowed deeply into the lining of the womb and has grown to the size of a pin-head. Four days later, at the time the menstrual period is expected, it has enlarged to be just visible to the naked eye. From now on the growth of the embryo and the placenta proceed apace. From the very earliest time, a fluid-filled space develops around the embryo. This space is lined with a thin, glistening membrane, and this in turn is surrounded by a thicker membrane. The

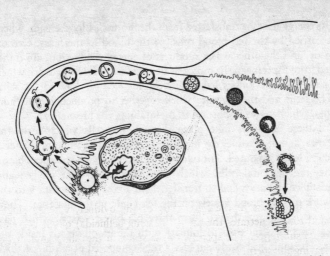

FIG. 9/1 The begining of pregnancy. The diagram shows fertilization of the egg in the oviduct, and its development as it journeys through the oviduct to reach the uterus and implant.

membranes with the contained water from the amniotic sac, or the bag of waters. By the 36th week of pregnancy, 1000ml (1¼ pints) of water surround the fetus. The fetus (until the 8th week of pregnancy, it is called the embryo) is able to move about freely within the amniotic sac, but it is prevented from being injured should the expectant mother fall, as the water absorbs all the shock.

Within two days of implantation, the outer cells of the blastocyst are sprouting in finger-like projections called trophoblast, all round the sphere of the egg. Quite quickly most of them die, and only the disc of cells lying deep in the lining of the uterus continue to grow. This disc forms the placenta, through which the fetus obtains all its nourishment. The placenta is connected to the fetus by the umbilical cord. At first the umbilical cord reaches from the placenta and joins the embryo near its tail, as can be seen in Fig. 9/2, but quite soon the tail curls round and the umbilical cord joins the fetus in the centre of its abdomen, at the place which after birth is the navel, or umbilicus. This is shown in Fig. 9/4. In many ways the placenta and the fetus work together, which is understandable as they form from the same fertilized egg. The placenta acts as the lung, the liver and the kidney of the fetus. Oxygen for its energy needs is transferred from the mother's bloodstream, where it is carried by the red blood cells, to the blood in the fetus. Carbon dioxide, and the other waste products of energy production, are transferred from the fetus to the mother's blood. This reduces the work which the fetal liver and kidney have to perform.

The fetus and the placenta work together to produce various hormones, which are so important in maintaining the pregnancy.

All these activities take place through the cells which form the placenta, and at all times the mother's blood and the blood of the fetus are completely separated. The two bloods never mix. The mother's blood bathes the placental cells, which permits them to take oxygen and nourishment from it, and to transfer them across the placenta into the network of tiny blood vessels on the fetal side of the placenta. These tiny vessels join together to form three big blood vessels, which pass along the umbilical cord to join up with the blood vessels inside the fetus. The umbilical cord is in fact a tube composed of a kind of thick jelly, through which the three vessels (two arteries and a vein) pass to link the fetus with the placenta.

You may be asking a particularly relevant question. If the fetus is formed from chromosomes from the mother and the father, its genetic make-up is different from that of the mother. Why then is the fetus not 'rejected' by the mother in the way that a person rejects a donated kidney or heart unless given strong anti-rejection drugs? It is now believed that a pregnant woman secretes substances, called *blocking antibodies*, which coat the cells which make up the placenta. These prevent the mother's immune system from recognizing that it is 'foreign tissue'.

It is easier to understand the further growth of the fetus and placenta by describing it at intervals: first at 6 weeks, then at 8 weeks, and then every 4 weeks to 40 weeks. In this description, the period is calculated from the first day of the last menstrual period, so the actual age of the embryo is about 2 weeks less. The new individual is called the embryo until week 8, and a fetus thereafter. During the embryonic period, all the structures which make it a normal human are formed; and subsequent development, during the fetal period, consists of growth and development of structures already formed.

To see the embryo and fetus, you have to imagine yourself inside the dark, warm, soft womb, where it grows throughout the pregnancy enclosed in the amniotic sac.

Changes in the expectant mother

While the development of the embryo and fetus is progressing in the dark confines of the uterus, all the functions of the expectant mother's body are adjusting to the needs of pregnancy. The basis of all these changes is the effect of the sex hormones oestrogen and progesterone, which are manufactured by the cells of the placenta from its earliest days. The changes start very early in pregnancy, and most of them anticipate the demands that the fetus will make on its mother for oxygen, for food and to get rid of its wastes. In the early embryonic weeks, when the embryo's organs are forming at an incredible rate, the mother easily supplies the required oxygen and foods; in the later fetal weeks, when its growth is increasing even more, the fetus needs larger supplies of oxygen and nutrients for a longer period. The mother's body adjusts to these demands by quieting-down her own functions, so that nutrients (especially sugars) stay longer in her blood, and are more easily extracted by the placenta for the use of the fetus. Further energy is spared by the placidity which is common in a pregnant woman; her muscle tone is reduced, she does less, and because the energy is not burned-up, it is stored as fat deposited in her breasts, on her thighs and on her hips. But the slowing of her body functions has some disadvantages. Her gut is less active, so that her stomach empties more slowly and constipation is common; her kidneys receive a higher concentration of nutrients in her bloodstream, and more are filtered out to be lost in the urine. This is part of the price she pays, but it is not difficult for her to compensate for this loss by a balanced diet.

She does not need to eat 'for two', as some people believe. A healthy woman needs only to increase her food intake to provide about an extra 420 kilojoules (100 k-calories) a day. This is provided by eating an extra two slices of bread, or an extra slice of bread and drinking 100ml of milk a day.

The need for the placenta to receive a large quantity of blood, from which to extract the nutrients required by the baby, is met by a 40 per cent increase in the volume of the mother's blood, and by its more rapid circulation through her blood vessels. She manages to achieve this by increasing the amount of blood that the heart pumps out with each beat, and by increasing the rate at which the heart beats. This is why some women are conscious of the action of their heart in pregnancy, and complain of palpitations. More blood is pumped around the body more rapidly. The red blood takes up more oxygen in the lungs, and

143

as nutrients are held longer in the bloodstream, these and oxygen can be more readily given to the baby across the placenta.

As has been noted, this exchange takes place through the special cells which form the placenta, and the mother's blood and that of her baby are kept separate at all times. The blood of the fetus passes through its body, then out along the vessels of the umbilical cord and through the network of fine vessels (called capillaries) in the placenta, which you will remember is composed of cells of the outer part of the fertilized egg (see p. 140). The tiny vessels are covered by the cells which make up the placenta. Although the placenta resembles a soup-plate when seen after birth, under the microscope it is composed of hundreds of tiny finger-like projections (called villi), each containing the network of tiny capillaries (Fig. 9/15) through which the baby's blood flows. The surface area of these villi is enormous. It has been calculated to be 11 square metres, or 12 square yards. The villi hang into a lake of blood. The lake is filled with blood which comes from the mother's circulation, reaching it by passing through the blood vessels which supply her uterus. The lake lies deep within the uterus, and is in fact lined with tissues made by the placenta, rather as a swimming pool is separated from the garden by a concrete basin. Each time the mother's heart beats, her blood is pumped in spurts into the placental-bed lake, carrying with it the nutrients and oxygen. As it flows between and around the weed-like fronds of the placenta, the oxygen and nutrients are taken from it by the placenta cells, and the waste products from the fetus are discharged into the mother's bloodstream through the placental cells. In fact, as you can see, the placenta acts as a very efficient lung, kidney and bowel for the fetus.

Cleaned of its waste products and enriched with nutrients and oxygen, the blood in the capillaries of the villi is returned to the fetus along the umbilical vein, and enters its body again at the umbilicus. Meanwhile the mother's blood, with its extra load of waste products, is pumped out of the placental-bed lake and re-enters the mother's circulation to be cleaned by her kidneys, to take up more oxygen from her lungs and nutrients from her gut and liver.

In this way the fetus takes the first pick of what is available to the mother, and even in a famine when the mother is starving, the fetus will get a reasonable amount of food and will not be much underweight at birth.

Other substances, such as drugs and alcohol cross the placenta. Antibiotics, in a concentration half that in the mother's blood appear in the fetal circulation within 60 minuts. Some drugs which cross the placenta may affect fetal growth and development.

In general, an expectant mother should avoid taking drugs during pregnancy unless her doctor says that they are necessary. Alcohol also crosses the placenta and when the expectant mother drinks excessively, it may cause damage to her baby. However, small amounts of alcohol – for example, less than two glasses of wine two or three times a week – are harmless. Perhaps more important are the antibodies which cross the placenta. If a person is infected by a germ, he forms substances in his body which attack and destroy the same germ if it infects him again. These substances are called 'antibodies'. Antibodies made by the mother cross the placenta all the time in the second half of pregnancy, so that when the baby is born it has a fair number of antibodies. These protect him against infections which lurk in the environment, until he starts to manufacture his own antibodies, which he does remarkably quickly.

The growth and development of the baby is an astonishing and prodigious event. From a single cell, containing in code all the information needed to make a new individual, growth occurs over a mere 266 days. At the end of this time, a new human being has formed, which is 8 million times heavier than the original fertilized cell. The cells have developed and differentiated to form special tissues and organs, all of which are co-ordinated and working, so that the child can breathe, digest food, move its muscles, hear sounds, taste flavours, react to stimuli, and develop further. A most wondrous growth!

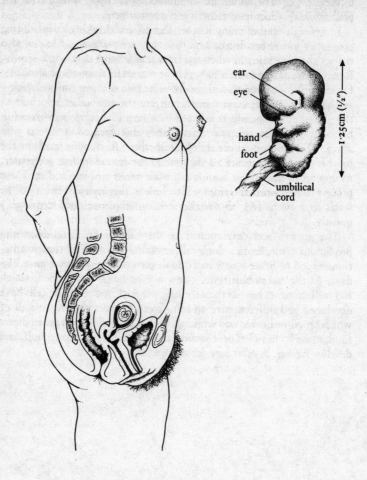

FIG. 9/2 Pregnancy at 6 weeks. The embryo is not recognizably human. It is only 28 days old, as conception occurs 14 days after the first day of the last menstrual period.

6 *weeks*
(Fig. 9/2)

The womb has enlarged, but it is still difficult for the doctor to tell if the patient is pregnant. It has enlarged rather more than is necessary for the size of the embryo; in fact it has *anticipated* its needs. The embryo is 1.25cm (½in) long. Its eye socket has formed, it has a reptile-like head and a tail. Its arm and leg buds are visible, but small and spadelike in shape. The placenta is larger and weighs more than the embryo.

The mother may have nausea and may vomit. Often but not always, this occurs in the morning, which is why it is called morning sickness. She may notice that her breasts are largers and heavier than they were in the past. She may want to urinate more frequently. These are normal symptoms of early pregnancy. Figure 9/12, p. 166, shows the ultrasound picture of a fetus at 7 weeks.

In the picture you can see the sac of fluid in which the fetus lies, and the fetus itself which is 12mm long. When the picture was taken the baby's heart could be seen beating.

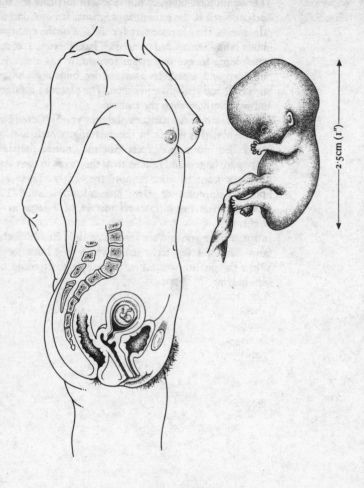

2·5 cm (1″)

FIG. 9/3 Pregnancy at 8 weeks. The fetus is becoming more human in appearance, and is now 42 days old.

8 weeks
(end of the
2nd lunar
month)
(Fig. 9/3)

The embryo is now much more like a human. It is 2.5cm (or 1in) long. The head is large compared with the body, and the external ears are forming. The limb buds have become arms and legs with tiny fingers and splayed toes. The eyes have become covered with eyelids which close across them, and remain shut until the 24th week. By now all the main organs of the body have formed, the heart beats sturdily, blood circulates through its vessels, its stomach is active and the kidneys are beginning to function. The only changes in the organs from now on will be an increase in their size and the sophistication of their function.

The mother may have had a pregnancy test which is positive, or, after her doctor has examined her, may be told she is pregnant. She is likely to have nausea, and her breasts are bigger than before. If this is the mother's first visit to her doctor, the doctor will ask her about previous medical and surgical illnesses, and whether she has a family history of high blood pressure or diabetes. It is usual for the doctor to take a 'Pap smear' from her cervix when he examines her pelvis. The doctor will also check her heart, listen to her lungs and check if she has varicose veins. He should check her breasts and discuss breast-feeding with her. Tests on her blood, and her urine, will be made at this time.

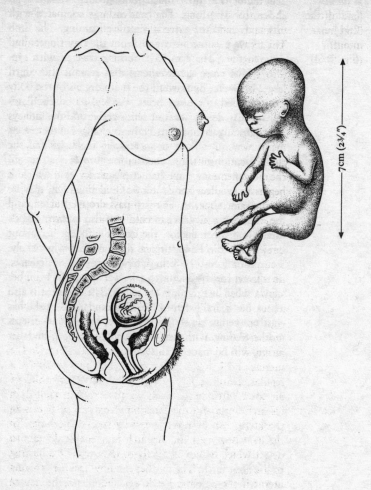

7cm (2¾")

FIG. 9/4   Pregnancy at 12 weeks.

12 weeks
(end of the
3rd lunar
month)
(Fig. 9/4)

The uterus can just be felt peeping out of the pelvis, above the symphysis. The patient is sure that she is pregnant, and the nausea is almost gone.

The fetus, as it is now called, from the Latin, meaning a 'young one', is 9cm (3½in) long, and weighs 14g (½oz). The body has grown, but the head is still over-large. Nails are appearing on its fingers and toes. The external genitals are appearing, but it is still difficult to tell its sex. By the end of this week, the mechanical movements of legs and arms have changed into movements which are far more graceful and purposeful, as the nerve and muscle co-ordination improve, although the movements are tiny. The fetus can now swallow, and begins to swallow the amniotic fluid in which it lives. At the same time, it begins to pass drops of urine into the amniotic sac. The placenta has also grown, and is now about six times the weight of the fetus.

Babies 'breathe' long before they are born, probably from as early as 12 weeks after conception. Of course, no oxygen as such goes into their lungs, but blood spurts through the lung blood vessels rhythmically, at about 80 'breaths' a minute. Babies can also get 'hiccups' in the last weeks of pregnancy, as many expectant mothers know. It is likely that this 'breathing' is the way in which babies prepare their lungs for life outside the uterus, and it has been found that babies who have a regular breathing pattern adjust to 'proper' breathing of air after birth more easily. This is being studied in research units and the 'breathing' pattern of babies in the uterus can be investigated by special machines. In the next few years this research may enable doctors to detect which babies are likely to have trouble adjusting to life after birth. The mother can now feel her growing uterus if she palpates her lower abdomen. The nausea has ceased in most cases, but persists in a few women. At this time her doctor may want to arrange for an ultrasound picture of her uterus, containing the fetus (see Fig. 9/13, p. 167).

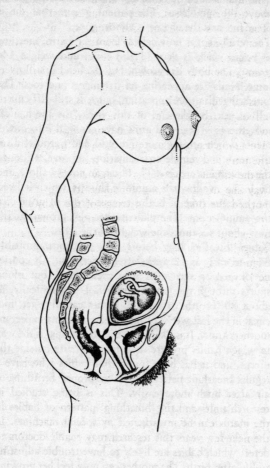

FIG. 9/5 Pregnancy at 16 weeks.

16 weeks
(end of the
4th lunar
month)
(Fig. **9/5**)

The uterus is easily palpable, and reaches almost half-way to the umbilicus. It is beginning to make a bulge!
The fetus is now 18cm (7in) long, and weighs 100g (4oz). The head is still large for its thin body, which is bright red because the blood vessels glow through its transparent skin. Its heart is beating strongly, and its muscles are becoming active. Its sex can be distinguished. The growth of the placenta has slowed down, although its efficiency has increased, and now the weight of the placenta and the fetus are about equal.

The uterus has grown so that it reaches half-way up to the umbilicus, and has begun to make a visible bulge in the mother's abdomen. She may conceal this by the way she dresses or may announce it! She may have noticed the first faint flutterings of the baby's movements in her uterus or these may be noticed later. By this stage most women feel the baby has an identity. In most cases the nausea has ceased and most mothers feel well. Figure **9/14**, p. 168, is the ultrasound picture of a fetus at 18 weeks.

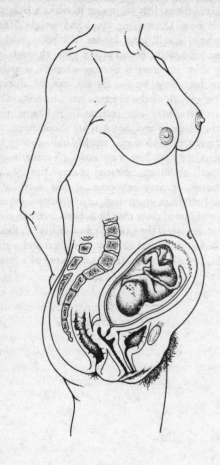

FIG. 9/6 Pregnancy at 20 weeks.

20 weeks
(end of the
5th lunar
month)
(Fig. 9/6)

The uterus has now grown and reaches to the level of the mother's umbilicus. She will feel the movements of her baby as he or she changes position, stretches his arms or kicks his legs in the uterus. She will have noticed that the baby has periods of movement and periods when it is asleep.

The fetus is now clearly human in appearance, and has 'quickened'. It is about 25cm (10in) long, and weighs about 300g (11oz). Its skin is less transparent and is covered with a fine, downy hair (called lanugo), which covers its whole body. Some hair is appearing on its head; it has developed eyebrows, but its eyelids are still completely fused. It is very active in its weightless condition within the amniotic sac. Its internal organs are becoming more mature, but as yet its lungs are insufficiently developed to cope with life outside the uterus. It is a bit like an astronaut in space! It swims weightless in its heat-controlled capsule. Its food and oxygen are conveyed to it and its waste products excreted through its lifeline – the umbilical cord. The placenta and the mother act as its life-survival pack. From this stage of pregnancy onwards, the growth of the placenta slows down, while that of the fetus increases, so that by 40 weeks the placenta only weighs one-fifth the weight of the baby. However, its efficiency as an exchanger for oxygen, nutrients and waste products continues to increase up to the 40th week of pregnancy.

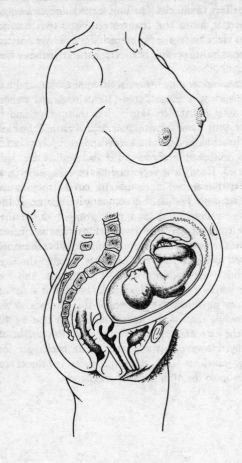

Fig. 9/7 Pregnancy at 24 weeks.

24 weeks
(end of the
6th lunar
month)
(Fig. 9/7)

The mother is obviously pregnant. Although most women feel well, many become tired more easily and sleep longer at night. A few women begin to feel backache as their back muscles stretch. This is because the mother is putting her shoulders back to balance her bulging abdomen.

Some doctors arrange for an ultrasound examination at about this time. Other doctors 'screen' their patient for 'gestational diabetes'.

Her fetus measures 32cm (13in), and weighs 650g (1lb 7oz). Its skin is now less red, and is covered with lanugo, and wrinkled because it lacks fat. From this month on, fat will be deposited in the skin. Its eyelids have separated, but a membrane covers the pupils, which are dull. The head is comparatively large. If the fetus is born at this stage, it will attempt to breathe, but its lungs are not properly developed so that it will have great difficulty in breathing. Its survival will depend on expert care.

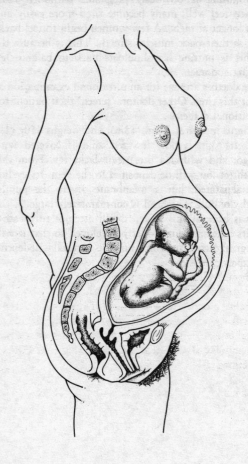

FIG. 9/8 Pregnancy at 28 weeks.

28 weeks
(end of the
7th lunar
month)
(Fig. 9/8)

The uterus now reaches 4 finger-breadths above the umbilicus.

The fetus moves around vigorously within the uterus, and its heart can be heard distinctly by the doctor. Its length is 38cm (15in), and its weight 1000g (2lb 2oz). Its body is thin; its skin still reddish and covered with a protective coating of a creamy, waxy substance, called vernix caseosa, which is manufactured by small glands in the skin. It can open its eyes, and the membrane covering the pupils has gone. If born at this stage, it can now breathe (but with difficulty), cry weakly, but move its legs energetically. In the past most of these babies died, but today more are being saved by treating them in special neonatal intensive care units. In the best units, one baby of this age in every four now survives.

The mother usually feels well but may notice that she sometimes gets indigestion or heartburn. Some women become constipated. She will visit the doctor or the clinic every 2 weeks from now on. At the visit her blood pressure will be taken, her urine examined and she will be able to ask questions which concern her.

The baby moves frequently in her uterus and the mother is very conscious of its 'kicks'. As well she may notice that her uterus contracts, painlessly, at intervals. These painless contractions are called Braxton Hicks contractions.

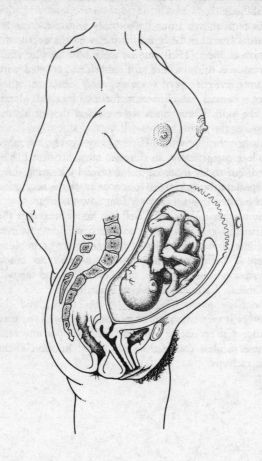

Fig. 9/9   Pregnancy at 32 weeks.

32 weeks
(end of the
8th lunar
month)
(Fig. 9/9)

The fetus is now 43cm (17in) long, and weighs about 1800g (4lb). The skin is still reddened, rather wrinkled, but some fat is being deposited. The bones of its head are soft and flexible. Its lungs have developed and can now support life. It can probably hear loud noises and responds by increasing the movement of its legs and arms. If born at this stage, it has an 85 per cent chance of surviving, provided it receives expert care.

The mother usually feels well, although she may have rather less energy. This is not due to anaemia, as her doctor will have checked her blood to make sure that she is not anaemic. The loss of energy is probably due to an increased amount of progesterone in her blood. Progesterone has many functions in pregnancy, but the most important one is to 'damp' down painful uterine contractions, so that premature labour does not start. The 'painless' contractions many women feel are normal and do not lead to premature labour.

Some women develop swelling of their ankles towards evening.

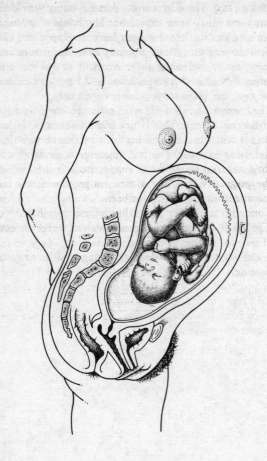

FIG. 9/10   Pregnancy at 36 weeks.

36 weeks
(end of the
9th lunar
month)
(Fig. 9/10)

The uterus now reaches up to the rib cage and the mother may have discomfort, particularly if she eats a large meal in the evening. She may wake up complaining of heartburn. She probably finds it more difficult to turn around when lying down, and it is harder to sit up. If she has varicose veins, these may become larger. She throws her shoulders well back to keep her balance, and she may have some backache.

Most women feel well; some have episodes of aches; a few have marked discomfort. Some women find that they become tired easily and some find that they are less well able to concentrate. Pregnant women benefit if their husband or partner is supportive and involved in the pregnancy. From this time on most mothers are impatient for the baby to be born.

The fetus measures 46cm (18½in), and weighs 2500g (5½lb). It has put on a great deal of weight, 700g (1½lb) in the preceding four weeks. This is because fat has been deposited beneath its skin and around its shoulders. It has filled out; its body has become rotund, and its face has lost its wrinkled appearance. Its fingernails reach to the end of its fingers.

If the baby is born at this time, it has over a 95 per cent chance of surviving.

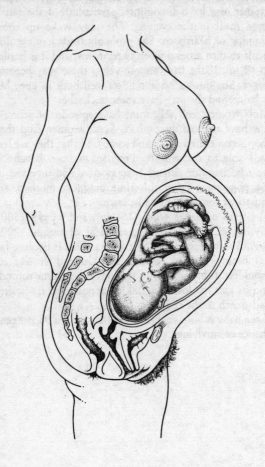

FIG. 9/11 Pregnancy at 40 weeks.

40 weeks
(end of the
10th lunar
month)
(Fig. 9/11)

The pregnancy is now at its full term. The expectant mother awaits the birth of her child with some degree of impatience.

The child is 50cm (20in) long, and weighs about 3300g (7lb 4oz), boys being about 100g (3oz) heavier than girls. There are very wide variations in the birth weight of the baby, and a normal, healthy, full-term child may weigh as little as 2500g (5½lb) or as much as 4500g (10lb). Occasionally the baby weighs even more. Its skin is smooth, and the lanugo which covered it has disappeared, except over the shoulders. The skin is still covered with the greasy vernix caseosa. Its head is covered with a variable amount of hair. The bones of the head are much firmer and are closer together, but the diamond-shaped soft area above the forehead and the Y-shaped area at the back of the head can still be felt. The head is now proportionate to the body, measuring about one-quarter of the body's length. The eyes are open, but usually a dull, slate colour – the permanent colour appears later. The ears may stand out from the head, and the nose is well formed. The genitals are well formed, and if the infant is male, the testicles are in the scrotum.

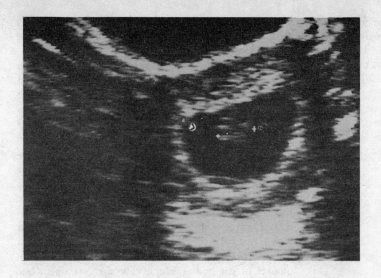

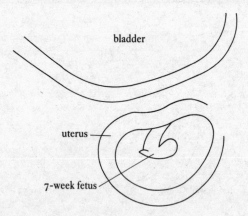

FIG. 9/12 Ultrasound picture of a fetus at 7 weeks. Line drawing shows the identifying points.

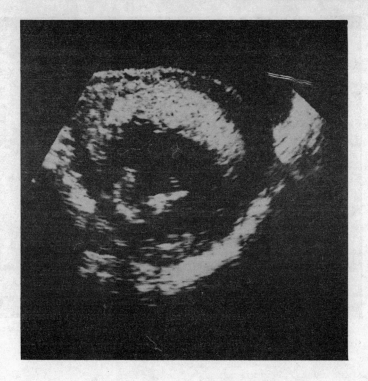

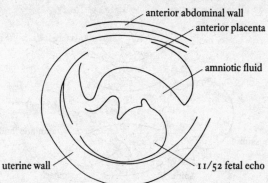

anterior abdominal wall
anterior placenta

amniotic fluid

uterine wall

11/52 fetal echo

Fig. 9/13 Ultrasound picture of a fetus at 11 weeks. Line drawing shows the identifying points.

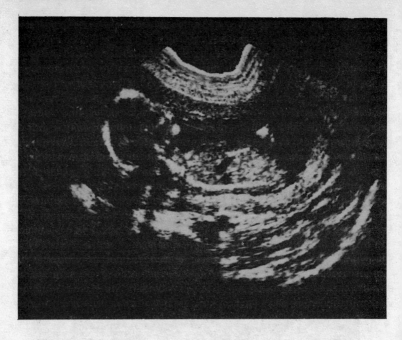

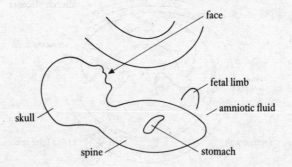

FIG. 9/14 Ultrasound picture of a fetus at 18 weeks. Line drawing shows the identifying points.

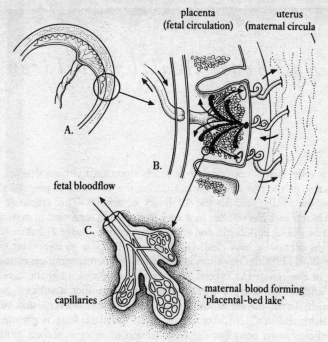

placenta
(fetal circulation)

uterus
(maternal circula

A.

B.

fetal bloodflow

C.

maternal blood forming
'placental-bed lake'

capillaries

FIG. 9/15   A diagram showing (A) the placenta lying attached to the wall of the uterus; (B) a section of the placenta in detail; (C) how blood from the 'placental lake' bathes the villus.

169

CHAPTER 10

And Bears Healthy Children

It is only in this century that as much attention has been devoted by doctors to the care of the patient during the 40 weeks of pregnancy as was previously paid to the 14 hours of labour. This emphasis on antenatal care has resulted in a very considerable reduction in maternal deaths during childbirth, and a very considerable salvage of babies who might otherwise have died. Good antenatal care is so important that the World Health Organization has had two expert committees consider it. In one report the experts said that the object of antenatal care 'is to ensure that every expectant and nursing mother maintains good health, learns the art of child care, has a normal delivery, and bears healthy children'. In other words, good antenatal care is preventive medicine at its best. But the co-operation of every expectant mother and of her medical adviser is needed to achieve this high standard.

During the antenatal period, the fetus relies upon its mother for all functions, and the healthier the mother, the stronger and healthier will the infant be. Indeed, its health in the first years of life, and maybe even longer, is influenced considerably by the condition of the mother during the prenatal months.

For antenatal care to be effective, the pregnant woman must go to her doctor as early as possible in pregnancy, and be seen at regular and increasingly frequent intervals during pregnancy. A good doctor will not only examine her, but will provide time so that he may explain the changes occurring in her body, may answer her questions, and banish any anxieties she may have. The woman must always feel that she can ask her doctor about anything that is bothering her. She is not wasting his time, and it is part of the doctor's duty to try and help her, for her emotional condition is as important as her physical condition. Some of the problems about which she may worry are mentioned in this book; but conversation with her doctor is as important as reading, for points which are not properly understood can receive an explanation in conversation.

Women who receive social and psychological support during pregnancy are less likely than other women to have negative feelings about their pregnancy and about the forthcoming birth. They are more likely to feel that they are 'in control' during the pregnancy, to have a worry-free childbirth, to communicate more effectively with the doctor and the nursing staff, and to be more satisfied with the care they receive.

The first visit

The first visit to the doctor should be made at about the time of the second missed period. Whether the patient chooses a specialist, or a general practitioner (a personal physician, as he is more properly called) or a doctor in an antenatal clinic, is immaterial. What is important is that she has confidence in her doctor, and that he, for his part, is prepared to seek the opinion of a specialist should this be required. If the patient chooses her personal physician, he will already know a great deal about her general health, and many of the investigations mentioned in this chapter will not be required.

Some women dread the first visit, feeling embarrassed that they will be asked 'personal' questions and examined vaginally. While the questions and examinations are necessary, the patient need not be embarrassed, and the doctor will do everything to make the embarrassment as slight as possible. The patient can be reassured that the examination is quite painless.

The questions

The doctor first inquires about the date of the last menstrual period and the duration of the average menstrual cycle. This is measured, as has been mentioned, from the first day of the menstrual period (which is called day 1) to the first day of the next menstrual period. He will also need to know the duration of the menstrual period and whether the character of the bleeding has changed. From this information he can give the patient a prediction of the approximate date of her confinement. The patient can make the calculation herself in this way: to the date of the first day of the last menstrual period add 10 days (counting each month as having 30 days), subtract 3 months from the month in which the period occurred, and add one year. For example, a patient

171

whose menstrual cycle is normal has started her last menstrual period on 12 September 1993. When will the baby be expected?

Last menstrual period	12/9/93
Calculation	+10−3+1
Estimated date of delivery	22/6/94

The baby is due on 22 June 1994.

Another example: the patient's last menstrual period was 24 April 1993. When is the baby due? Here the calculation is a bit more complicated, as the addition of 10 days brings the date into another month.

Last menstrual period	24/4/93
Add 10 days	+10
	= 4/5/93
Subtract 3 months, add 1 year	−3+1
Estimated date of delivery	4/2/94

The baby is due on 4 February 1994.

The estimate date of delivery is accurate to within 14 days in over 80 per cent of women (4 women in every 5), and is a great help to the patient in planning for her confinement.

Having told the woman when her baby is expected to be born, the doctor asks how the pregnancy is progressing, and about any complaints the expectant mother may have. He then enquires about her past health, and lists the illnesses and operations which may have occurred. The purpose of these enquiries is to bring to light any conditions which may affect the course of the pregnancy, and for which treatment can be given. If there have been previous pregnancies (including abortions), the doctor should be told about these, and indeed he will enquire searchingly about them in detail. The purpose once again is to try to anticipate complications, and to find out how well (or badly) the woman was able to cope with her previous pregnancies.

The examination

The remainder of the visit is taken up with the examination. For this it is usual for the expectant mother to strip completely, and to put on a gown provided by her doctor. This is important, as the doctor tries to find out the general health of the woman. Usually he first notes her height and records her weight (see p. 203). Then he examines her breasts, and determines if the nipples are normal. If she proposes to breast-feed her baby, he may prescribe certain manipulations which are done by the patient herself during pregnancy. These manipulations seem to encourage milk production and make the establishment of breast-feeding easier. He then listens to the woman's heart with a stethoscope, gently palpates her abdomen, and observes her legs to see if there are any varicose veins. In early pregnancy, the abdominal palpation is merely to check the tone of the abdominal muscles and to see whether there is any enlargement of the liver or spleen. After the 12th week of pregnancy, the doctor also palpates the enlarging uterus and measures the distance from the top of the pubic bone to the top of the uterus to determine if the baby is growing normally, and after the 28th week to check the position of the baby in the womb. After these examinations, and prior to the pelvic examination, the doctor takes the woman's blood pressure. It is left until this stage as emotions can often cause a rise in the blood pressure, and the doctor is trying to obtain a baseline blood pressure against which to measure changes. The estimation of the blood pressure is a most important investigation and is made at every visit, since a rise in blood pressure in pregnancy warns the doctor that pregnancy-induced hypertension (pre-eclampsia) may be starting. Its exact cause is not known, but it is known that the arteries which supply the uterus and the kidneys go into a spasm. If the spasm becomes severe, the blood supply to the placenta is reduced, and the baby may fail to grow properly, or may even die in the womb. The severity of the spasm can be reduced if pre-eclampsia is detected early. Appropriate treatment at this time will control the disease before it becomes a danger to the well-being of the baby.

Finally, the doctor performs a pelvic examination. It was noted in Chapter 8 that this examination is neither painful nor embarrassing if the patient co-operates. The doctor first introduces a speculum into the vagina to inspect the cervix and to take the cervical smear. He then gently performs a pelvic examination with two fingers introduced into the vagina.

Laboratory investigations

No first antenatal visit can be considered complete until the doctor has made certain laboratory tests. Just before the pelvic examination, the doctor will have asked his patient to empty her bladder of urine. Many doctors ask for the urine to be passed in a special way. The pregnant woman is given a small moist cotton-wool swab with which she cleans the entrance to her vagina, wiping from the front backwards. She then starts to urinate, and when the flow of urine is running, she collects the 'midstream' specimen in a sterile container which has been given to her. This method is only necessary at the first visit. At all other visits, the patient either brings the urine specimen with her, or passes it into a container in the normal way. The purpose of the midstream specimen is to enable the doctor to find out if the patient has a hidden infection of the urinary tract. This hidden infection often becomes obvious in pregnancy, causing kidney infection, and many doctors believe in giving prophylactic treatment to cure it. The specimen of urine is also examined for the presence of protein and sugar. The presence of the former is another sign of impending pre-eclampsia. If sugar is found in the urine, investigations are made to find out if the patient has diabetes.

Recently many doctors have stopped testing the urine for sugar, because sugar is often found in the urine of normal pregnant women. Instead, doctors are recommending checking for a form of diabetes which occurs in pregnancy and then disappears. This is called 'gestational diabetes'. The test for this is to measure the glucose level in a woman's blood at her first antenatal visit and again at the 28th week of pregnancy (when blood is usually taken for a second time to check for anaemia). Some doctors prefer to give the woman 50–75g of glucose in orange juice, to take a sample of blood one hour later and to measure the level of glucose in the sample. This test is performed when the woman is between 20 and 24 weeks pregnant.

Several important tests are made on a sample of blood taken from a vein in the arm. Pregnant women tend to fear this procedure, but the discomfort is only momentary and the information obtained is very valuable. The blood is examined by a special test to determine if the patient has syphilis. It is important to detect the disease early in pregnancy when its cure is relatively easy. If left untreated, syphilis may damage the baby severely. In late pregnancy, the germs which cause syphilis pass through the placenta and multiply in the fetal tissues, either killing the fetus or damaging some of its organs. Those children who are the victims of congenital syphilis can be treated after birth, but treatment is not always successful. But if the disease is detected in early pregnancy and treated adequately, congenital syphilis will be prevented.

The specimen of blood is also examined to find out the mother's blood group, particularly whether she is Rhesus negative. Rhesus disease is considered in Chapter 17.

Many doctors also arrange for the blood to be examined for rubella antibodies. If they are present, it indicates that the woman has had rubella (German measles) and need not be concerned that her baby will be affected should she come into contact with a case of rubella. Ideally, the rubella test should be made before a woman decides to become pregnant, so that a vaccine can be given if the test proves negative, to protect her against rubella.

If the woman comes from a part of the world where hepatitis B is common or if she is a drug addict, blood is tested to find out if she has been infected and is still infectious for hepatitis B. The reason for this is that she may infect her baby and the people attending her in childbirth if her blood enters their body through a break in the skin. Today most doctors and nurses who look after pregnant women are given injections of hepatatis B vaccine to prevent this happening. The baby of a mother who has hepatitis B antigen in her blood is also given the vaccine soon after birth so that he is protected from developing liver cancer when he becomes an adult. She may also ask to be tested for AIDS.

Finally, the specimen of blood is examined to estimate the haemoglobin concentration. The haemoglobin concentration measures the amount of iron in the red blood cells, and so is an index of anaemia. It is important for the doctor to know if anaemia is present, as the expectant mother requires extra iron because the fetus also has to obtain a considerable amount of iron from the mother during pregnancy. If the haemoglobin concentration is low, the doctor will be able to treat it before it has any serious effects. Since the baby takes most of its iron requirements in late pregnancy, the haemoglobin estimation is repeated twice more during pregnancy, at the 28th week, when the baby is beginning to increase its demand for iron, and again at the 36th week. Thus if the mother has become anaemic, she can be treated adequately before her confinement.

The summing-up

The examination and tests are over, the expectant mother has dressed again, and sits talking to her doctor so that he can discuss the diet she should eat, the exercise she should take, and can clear up any doubts she may have. She should not hesitate to ask her doctor about any matter which is bothering her. Some women obtain misinformation about pregnancy from acquaintances, whose experiences invariably seem to have been gruesome. Much of the information is erroneous, some of the advice harmful, so that the expectant mother is anxious, bewildered and confused. The person to clear up her confusion is the doctor. She should ignore the gossip of well-meaning busybodies, and should feel able to ask her doctor for accurate information at all times. He, for his part, should always be ready, and have time, to discuss the pregnancy with the expectant mother.

If a woman has previously given birth to a baby with Down's syndrome or is over the age of 35, then the chance of having an affected baby increases considerably. Two tests are available, to diagnose the condition. The first of the tests is *chorionic villus sampling*, the second is *amniocentesis and cell culture:*

Chorionic villus sampling (CVS): Between the 9th and 11th week of pregnancy a small tube is inserted through the cervix under ultrasound guidance. A sample of the tissue covering the sac in which the fetus lies (the trophoblast or chorionic villi) is sucked out through the tube. The sample is examined in a laboratory. Twenty-four hours later, it can be determined if the baby has Down's syndrome.

Amniocentesis: This test cannot be done until after the 15th week of pregnancy. A thin needle is introduced into the uterus and a sample of the amniotic fluid which surrounds the baby is removed. This is called amniocentesis. The sample is examined in a laboratory, but it takes about three weeks to find out if the baby is affected or not.

Following either procedure, about one fetus in every 100, will spontaneously abort.

The advantage of chorionic villus sampling over amniocentesis is that if an abnormal baby is found, the woman may choose to have the pregnancy terminated by abortion, at a time when the procedure is less traumatic and safer.

Recently there has been an attempt to detect another congenital condition in early pregnancy. The condition is one in which the baby has a neural tube defect. This may involve its brain, which is only partly formed (the condition is called anencephaly) or its spinal cord (spina bifida). In some countries blood is taken from each pregnant woman and examined for a substance called alphafetoprotein. If the level of alphafetoprotein is raised, the blood test is repeated and an ultrasound picture is taken. If these tests also suggest that the baby has a neural tube defect, a sample of the amniotic fluid is examined for alphafetoprotein. If the level is raised, the baby is affected. The problem is discussed with the woman and her husband or partner. Following the discussion they may decide that they would prefer that an abortion was induced.

Subsequent visits

If she is otherwise normal, the expectant mother will make an antenatal visit to her doctor every 4 weeks until she is 28 weeks pregnant (7 lunar months), every 2 weeks from then until she is 36 weeks pregnant (9 lunar months), and every week from then until she has been confined.

Some doubt is now being voiced if this number of antenatal visits is necessary. It is probable that they can be reduced without affecting the well-being of mother and baby. This would leave more time for each visit so that other concerns of the pregnant woman could be talked about. If any complication arises, or if the patient has previously had some illness, such as diabetes, 'blood pressure' or a heart condition, the doctor will want to see her more frequently.

Many doctors (but by no means all) arrange for the woman to have a routine ultrasound examination made. There is no real agreement about the best time for the examination, but most obstetricians think if it is made at about the 18th week of pregnancy the most information can be obtained. At this time the ultrasound examination will determine the exact size of the baby and confirm when she or he is due to be born; it will detect twins and it will identify some congenital abnormalities.

At each of the visits during pregnancy, the doctor is concerned about two people – the expectant mother who is carrying the baby, and the fetus as it floats nearly weightless in its heat-controlled, waste-disposal and food-intake controlled capsule (the amniotic sac) within the uterus. At each visit the doctor will seek to find out how the patient is progressing, and how she is enjoying her pregnancy. He will answer any queries, and if he detects that all is not progressing normally, will give advice. At each visit the expectant mother's weight is noted, and a weight gain of more than 4.5kg (9lb) in the first 20 weeks, or more than 0.5kg (1lb) a week in each of the last 20 weeks is usually frowned upon.

An increasing number of obstetricians question the value of weighing an expectant mother at each visit. Previously this was done because it was believed that an excessive weight gain between visits indicated that she might be developing pregnancy induced hypertension (PIH) and a small weight gain indicated that her baby was growing slowly and might be born 'growth retarded'. Both these beliefs have been found to be untrue. However, many women are concerned about their weight gain in pregnancy and are reassured if they are weighed at each antenatal visit.

The ankles and legs are examined for swelling and varicose veins, the blood pressure is recorded, and the urine tested.

The doctor then turns his attention to the baby. He estimates the height of the uterus, as was described previously, and he palpates it gently to find out the exact position of the baby. He will probably find that up to the 28th week (7th lunar month), the baby will be in a different position each time. It may be head down (called a cephalic presentation), or with its head in the upper part of the uterus and the buttocks in the lower part (a breech presentation), or it may be cross-ways (a transverse or shoulder presentation) (Fig. **10/1**). This is because at this early stage of pregnancy there is a relatively large volume of 'water' (really amniotic fluid, which does not have quite the same composition as water) in the amniotic sac, and the baby can therefore move about easily. After the 30th week of pregnancy, the great

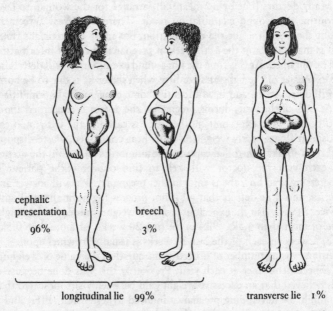

cephalic
presentation
96%

breech
3%

longitudinal lie 99%

transverse lie 1%

FIG. 10/1 How the baby lies in the uterus. The percentages given for the different presentations are those found just before labour begins.

majority of babies settle with the head over the mother's pelvis, and their buttocks in the wider upper part of the uterus. By the 40th week, also called 'term', 96 per cent of babies lie in this position as cephalic presentations, and between 3 and 4 per cent lie as breech presentations. In some cases the back of the baby is on the right side of the uterus, and in others on the left. It makes little difference to the progress of labour, and the baby can change positions between two examinations. The gentle palpation of the uterus distinguishes these points, and enables the doctor to determine whether the baby is lying as a cephalic or a breech presentation (Fig. 10/2). This is of some importance at about the 34th week, as the doctor may wish to try to 'turn' the breech baby into a cephalic presentation with head down. At every visit the doctor should tell the expectant mother where the baby is, and should help her to feel it if she wishes. If he listens to the baby's heart, and she wishes to hear her baby's heart beat, he should try to arrange for her to do this using his stethoscope or with a machine called a 'fetal heart detector'. The baby's heart beats much faster than the mother's, averaging 120 beats a minute, but varying a bit.

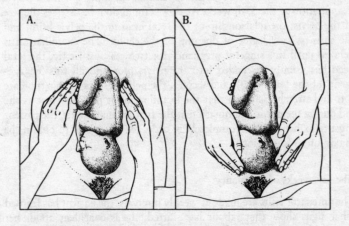

FIG. 10/2   How the doctor finds the position of the baby. (A) Feeling the back; (B) detecting the baby's head.

179

Lightening

By the end of the 36th week, most women carrying their first baby (primigravidea) feel 'lightening'. This is because the baby's head 'drops' into the pelvic cavity; consequently the upper part of the uterus drops, relieving the pressure under the ribs and making breathing easier. Lightening often occurs suddenly, the expectant mother waking up one morning relieved of the pressure and discomfort she has experienced previously. Unfortunately, the descent of the head into the pelvic cavity is often associated with pressure on the pelvis, and an increased vaginal discharge, so that she exchanges one set of mild complaints for another. At this time, too, the painless uterine contractions which have been felt for some weeks become more frequent. They are called Braxton Hicks contractions.

In women who have had previous children, 'lightening' takes place later, either in the week or 10 days before labour starts or in the early stages of labour.

Pelvic examination

The descent of the fetal head into the pelvic cavity is a good indication that the pelvic size and shape are normal. The doctor uses this information to be sure that this is so. It is usual for him to make a pelvic examination at the 37th week. At this examination, he assesses the size of the pelvis, the relationship of the fetal head to the pelvic brim, and the softness and degree of opening of the cervix. The examination is delayed until this stage of pregnancy for two reasons: firstly, the fetal head has usually descended into the pelvis (doctors call this 'engagement' of the fetal head); and second, the pelvic tissues at this time are soft and stretch easily, so that the examination is painless. Just as she did during the pelvic examination at the first antenatal visit, the patient must relax her muscles completely in order for the doctor to obtain the maximum information.

The last weeks of pregnancy

The antenatal visits are made at weekly intervals; the patient has learned what signs show that labour has started; she is confident about her doctor, she is fit and well; she has a knowledge of what happens in labour; she has prepared the baby's clothes, she has visited the hospital;

and the doctor has answered all her questions. In short, she is a healthy, knowledgeable mother, who has learned the art of child care, who knows the sequence of events she may expect in labour, and she is about to have a normal delivery and bear a healthy child.

CHAPTER 11

An ABC of Hygiene in Pregnancy

The conditions discussed in this chapter are all 'minor', that is they are minor in that they do not cause serious disease. To the expectant mother they may be major problems. Since so many body systems may be involved, it seems appropriate to list the conditions alphabetically for more ready reference.

Pregnancy and adjustment to parenthood are periods of emotional stress for all women, although the amount of stress varies very considerably. Some women find pregnancy a joyous period of their life, others become emotionally distressed. Still others are concerned about the mood changes they experience. Stresses which would be coped with easily when the woman is not pregnant may become distressing during pregnancy and an expectant mother may overreact emotionally to a real or imagined insult. Other women, who are usually mentally active, find that during pregnancy they become mentally lethargic and thinking is an effort.

In the early weeks of pregnancy most women identify with the tiny fetus; they talk about 'my' pregnancy rather than 'the' pregnancy or 'it'. This is because the fetus is perceived as part of the woman's body, and has no separate identity. Between the 15th and 20th week of pregnancy, a change occurs. The fetus begins to move, and to develop an identity of its own. The woman's enlarging abdomen tells her, and her friends, that she is really pregnant and she now begins to be interested in the fetus as 'her baby'. In late pregnancy, from about the 35th week, a further change occurs. Now most women become impatient with the pregnancy, bored with their swollen abdomen, anxious to give birth and to see, touch and care for the newborn baby.

As pregnancy advances, with its attendant minor discomforts, many women are concerned that their increased fatness, lethargy, distended abdomen and pendulous breasts may adversely affect their husband's love. The way a man can reassure her partner is to kiss and cuddle her and to be interested (as he should be) in the continuing pregnancy and the growth, in the mother's uterus, of their baby. After all, the start of pregnancy was a joint pleasure; its continuation should be shared too!

Alcohol

Women who drink more than three standard drinks (30g of alcohol) a day during pregnancy may give birth to babies which are small-for-dates, or have the 'fetal alcohol syndrome' in which the baby is small, mentally retarded and has characteristic features. The current evidence is that the fetal alcohol syndrome may occur if a pregnant woman drinks in excess of six hard drinks a day.

Because of this, pregnant women should avoid alcohol, or drink no more than two glasses of wine (or its equivalent) two or three times a week.

Anaemia

In most developed countries few women become anaemic in pregnancy, although tests may suggest that the woman is anaemic. This is due, in part, to an increase in the total volume of blood which occurs in pregnancy, so that the woman's blood seems 'anaemic'. But as true anaemia could cause problems, doctors routinely measure the level of haemoglobin in the blood and make several other tests on the same sample of blood. Usually the doctor makes the blood tests at the first antenatal visit and again at about the 28th week of pregnancy. Many doctors insist that all pregnant women take iron tablets but there is some doubt if this is really necessary if the woman eats a good diet. A few women, particularly if the woman is carrying twins need an anaemia-preventing vitamin called folic acid, but most women do not.

A compromise is for a pregnant woman to take the iron tablets as often as she remembers, unless the tests show that there is a true anaemic state, when investigation and treatment is needed.

Backache

In late pregnancy particularly, the pelvic joints and ligaments relax. At the same time the growing weight of the uterus changes the centre of balance, so that the expectant mother has to stand with her shoulders further back than normal. This position has been called 'the pride of pregnancy'. However, it and the relaxed ligaments produce backache to some extent in most pregnant women, but more so in multigravidae (pregnant women, who have previously had one or more pregnancies). The backache increases during the day and is felt most towards evening, and at night when it may prevent sleep. The pain is usually felt low in the back or over the sacro-iliac joint. Treatment is largely to prevent the condition from becoming severe. If the expectant mother's posture is bad, she should seek advice. High heels tends to aggravate the strain on the back, and should be avoided whenever possible. If the backache is marked, analgesics may be needed, but the doctor should be consulted first.

Bathing

Showers are recommended in preference to long baths, or tub baths, as the Americans call them, in the last four weeks of pregnancy, when the bath water may conceivably enter the vagina. Before this time long baths are perfectly safe and pleasantly relaxing! Swimming in general is permissible, and may be continued as near term as the expectant mother wishes.

Body image

Many women have an enjoyable and joyous pregnancy, accepting the change in their body shape as evidence of their capacity to nurture the baby growing in the uterus. Other women find pregnancy an uncomfortable time, and are unhappy that their body has become fat and bulbous. This loss of pleasure in their body can lead to anxiety and to a feeling that they are no longer attractive to their husband or partner. The loss of a pleasing body image can be reduced if the woman's husband or partner shows that his feelings towards her are unchanged, by his behaviour to her, by cuddling her and sharing their pregnancy.

Breasts

Care of the breasts in pregnancy helps the establishment of breast-feeding. The nipples should be stroked and drawn out gently for about two minutes a day from early pregnancy. If the expectant mother wishes, she may rub in some bland lanolin ointment, particularly if the nipples

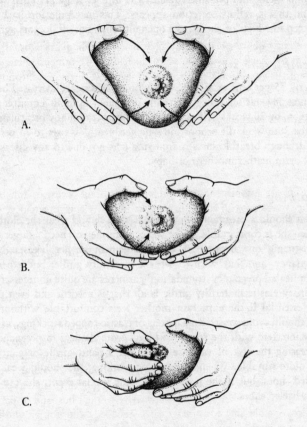

FIG. 11/1   The care of the breasts in pregnancy.
A. How the hands are placed at the start of expression, to enclose the breast at its margin
B. The hands move inwards towards the areola, firm pressure is exerted on the whole breast. The movement is repeated about 5 to 10 times.
C. The breast is fixed by one hand and the milk ducts are compressed with the other hand, the thumb above the fingers below. The pressure empties the milk ducts. At the end of the expression, the nipple is drawn out with the fingers.

are dry. From about the 32nd week (8th lunar month), the breasts may be 'expressed' by placing both hands with the palms widely spread around them, and pressing towards the nipples (Fig. 11/1). It will be found that a yellow secretion appears. This manipulation is thought to keep the ducts of the breasts open although not all doctors agree.

Breathlessness

Nearly 75 per cent of all pregnant women experience increased breathlessness on exertion. It begins in early pregnancy in about a quarter of the women, by 20 weeks half of the women are occasionally breathless, and by the 30th week the proportion who get breathless rises to 75 per cent.

Although breathlessness is annoying it is not due to any disease and will harm neither mother nor baby.

Clothing

What should a pregnant woman wear? She should wear the clothes in which she is comfortable. If she wears a bra she will need a larger sized, well-fitting one because of the enlargement of her breasts due to pregnancy, and may wish to wear a maternity girdle; but expensive, complicated pregnancy 'foundation' garments are quite unnecessary. An ordinary elastic maternity girdle is all that is needed, and even this is not essential if the expectant mother feels comfortable without one. She should avoid constricting garters or elastic-topped stockings, as these may interfere with the return of blood from the legs in pregnancy, so increasing the risk of varicose veins, but a panty-girdle or pantyhose are quite suitable. When at home or working, she should wear low-heeled shoes, but if she goes out to some special event, she can wear high-heeled shoes.

Constipation

You have two kinds of muscle in your body – the voluntary striped muscles, and the involuntary smooth muscles. The striped muscles make up the muscles of your arms and legs, and respond to your control. If you want to pick up a saucepan, a message goes from your brain and your arm muscles move your hand forward. If you find the saucepan is too hot, you voluntarily stop the movement! The smooth muscles make up the muscles of your heart, your gut, and your womb. These muscles work without voluntary control, and you cannot voluntarily alter their action. However, they do respond to some drugs and hormones. Progesterone, the special hormone of pregnancy, relaxes smooth muscle. In one way this is useful, as it enables the uterus, which is mainly composed of smooth muscle, to grow without attempting to expel the fetus prematurely. In other ways smooth muscle relaxation can be annoying. The muscle tone of the gut is lowered throughout pregnancy, which leads to constipation. In late pregnancy, the tendency is aggravated by pressure on the lower bowel by the enlarged uterus. If the expectant mother is worried about constipation, she should increase her fluid intake, and re-establish the 'habit' by attempting to open her bowels regularly just after a meal. Many doctors now recommend that women who are constipated eat about two tablespoonsful of coarse bran daily and choose wholemeal bread instead of white bread. These two measures have the effect of making the stool bulkier and reduce the time it takes for food to pass from the mouth to the time the residue is passed out as stools. Both these changes reduce constipation and eliminate the need for drugs. But if a woman does not want to eat bran and the other suggestions I have made fail, her doctor will give her 'Senokot' (standardized senna) or the contact stool-softening laxative, bisacodyl. She should avoid self-medication with strong laxatives, or oily laxatives.

Dental care

Care of the teeth does not differ in pregnancy from that at other times. The old notion that each child cost a tooth is a relic from the time when regular visits to the dentist were not made. In areas where fluoride is not added to the drinking-water, the use of one tablet per day containing 1mg fluorine taken from the 20th week of pregnancy will protect the infant against dental caries. A few women develop swelling of the gums at the base of the teeth (marginal gingivitis, as it is called). This is not abnormal, and disappears after childbirth, but if in any doubt the expectant mother should consult a dentist.

Diet

More rubbish has been written about diet in pregnancy than on almost any other medical subject. In the years before World War II, the influence of diet on the growth and survival of the baby was thought to be considerable. Recent studies have cast doubt on this, and present opinion is that within the normal range of diets available, their influence on the birth weight and survival of the baby is minimal. As far as the obstetrical efficiency of the expectant mother is concerned, the diet she ate in her own infancy and childhood has much more importance. This is the reason the World Health Organization's Expert Committee on Maternity Care said that one of the objectives of antenatal care was to help the expectant mother 'learn the art of child care'. This includes giving her child a properly balanced diet, rich in protein.

By and large then, the effect of diet on the outcome of pregnancy has been exaggerated in the past. Fanciful, vague, complicated diets have been ordered which had little value and were often confusing. I do not suggest that a pregnant woman should not pay attention to what she eats. She should! In pregnancy she has to provide the nutrients necessary for the growth of her child, as well as for her own needs. This does not mean that she needs to 'eat for two' and, as will be seen later, *excessive weight gained in pregnancy is very hard to take off*. It does mean that she should understand what she is eating and why.

Basically the diet provides *carbohydrates and fat*, which produce the energy needed for life; *protein*, needed for the formation of new tissues; *vitamins and minerals*, which help in the complex chemical processes in the body. All foodstuffs contain one or more of the above nutrients. Unfortunately, the cheaper foodstuffs are the energy-supplying carbohydrates, while the tissue-building protein, the vitamins and some of the minerals come from relatively expensive foods, like meat. Because of this, poorer people, and most of the people in the developing countries, eat too little protein, vitamins and minerals, and barely enough carbohydrate to provide the energy needed for their daily tasks. This energy is measured in a unit called a calorie or a kilojoule (kJ) and the average pregnant woman needs about 2200 calories (9500kJ) a day. In the affluent lands, most women eat too much, particularly carbohydrates such as bread, sweets and sugar and fats in cakes, confectionary, ice-cream, and fatty meats (sausages, hamburgers, pies). Their calorie intake is excessive for their needs, and the excess is stored in the body as fat.

Pregnancy puts an increased demand on the body for protein, and unless the expectant mother alters to a diet which provides more protein, she may not get sufficient, while still eating too much carbohydrate.

The nutritional needs of a pregnant woman have been considered in great detail by high-powered committees in many countries, and the optimal, or best, daily allowance for a woman weighing about 55kg (121lb) has been worked out to be:

Kilojoules	9000 (2200 Cals)
Protein	51g
Calcium	1000mg
Iron	30mg
Vitamin A	750μg
Vitamin D	10μg
Vitamin B:	
Thiamine	1.0mg
Riboflavine	1.5mg
Nicotinic acid	15.0mg
Vitamin C (Ascorbic acid)	50.0mg
Folic acid	0.3mg

To the average expectant mother, the above table is so much jargon, but it can easily be translated into foodstuffs. This is shown in Table 11/1, and is summarized here: (1) *Dairy products:* The expectant mother should drink 600 to 900ml (1 to 1½ pints) of milk a day, either raw or made up in drinks or used in cooking. If she wants, she can substitute cheese for milk, 30g (1oz) being equivalent to 200ml (⅓ pint). (2) *Meat and eggs:* She should eat 60 to 120g (2 to 4oz) of meat, fish or poultry a day, and usually have an egg. (3) *Vegetables:* She should eat green leafy vegetables, cooked for less than 10 minutes in a minimum of water, at least three times a week, and other vegetables as she wishes. (4) *Bread, cereals, sugar, sweets, potatoes:* Bread and cereals are complex carbohydrates which provide energy but do not put on weight. Potatoes contain complex carbohydrates and are a valuable food. They do not put on weight. Sugar and sweets are simple carbohydrates which put on weight and should be eaten sparingly. (5) *Fruits:* She should eat an orange or a grapefruit each day, and any additional fresh fruit she fancies.

How the woman divides up the foodstuffs, having what at which meal, must be her decision. How well, or badly, she cooks the food is the result of her upbringing. How efficiently she chooses and buys the proper foods is the result of her education. If a mother wishes her child to be a good housekeeper, she will have the opportunity over the years to teach her, and this teaching will be reinforced in the schools. To start the lessons, the expectant mother can remember most of what is needed about diet and nutrition in pregnancy if she recalls the

Table 11/1
Nutritional Needs in Pregnancy

Food		Calories	Protein (g)
Dairy products	A daily total of 600–900 ml (1 to 1½ pints) of milk, either raw or used in cooking or in hot drinks. Cheese can be substituted, 30g (1 oz) being equal to 200ml (⅓) of milk.	600	32
	Butter or margarine can be taken as required (say 60g, or 2oz).	480	—
Meat products	The meat product may be *lean* meat, poultry, fish or liver. A serving of 60–120g (2–4oz) a day will provide for the needs. More meat may, of course, be eaten if desired. It is best grilled, roasted or stewed, rather than fried.	250	20
Egg	One a day (or at least most days).	90	6
Bread and other cereals (including sugar as required)	Three to four slices, which is equal to 120g (4oz) is probably sufficient. A half-full teacup of breakfast cereal equals one slice of bread. Wholemeal bread is preferable to white bread. Sugar or jam, say 60g or 2oz.	320	10
		240	—
Vegetables	*Potato:* One to two medium-sized potatoes (150–300g, or 5–10oz). The potato can be cooked in any way, but the most nutritious are those cooked in their skins. If desired, potatoes can be replaced by squash, pumpkin or turnips. In working out a diet, the bread and potato are changeable.	140	5
		50	3
	Vegetables: Salads and other green or yellow leafy vegetables, peas, beans and lentils contain valuable vitamins if they are cooked properly. About 60–120g (2–4oz) should be eaten daily.		
Fruit	The adage 'an apple a day keeps the doctor away' applies in pregnancy. For variety, the apple can be replaced by citrus fruits (orange, grapefruit) or by tomato juice, which are all rich in vitamin C.	50	1
		2220	77

following slogan: 'Buy all you can afford from the butcher, the bread shop, the greengrocer and at the dairy; spend only little at the confectioner, the grocer and the chemist.'

Douching

Vaginal douching is a peculiarly American habit, founded on an exaggerated need for so-called 'personal hygiene'. The vagina is self-cleansing. Douches are usually unnecessary at any time, and particularly in pregnancy, when they have a slight danger. So do not douche!

Drugs in pregnancy

After the 'thalidomide' tragedy, doctors have been even more careful in prescribing drugs to pregnant women. It will be remembered that thalidomide was given in early pregnancy as a sedative or to alleviate nausea. Later it was found that it had prevented the development of the arm and leg buds of the fetus, so that the affected babies were born alive but without arms or legs.

No new drugs are now prescribed for pregnant women unless they have been investigated by the most exhaustive tests, and most doctors only give expectant mothers drugs which they *really* need. The mother herself, particularly in the first 12 weeks of pregnancy, should avoid taking any drug unless she has checked with her doctor, and then only if it is really required.

Today, an expectant mother can rest assured that none of the drugs commonly prescribed during pregnancy has any damaging action on her growing baby. But she should remember that nicotine from smoking tobacco and alcohol are also drugs, and may affect her baby's growth and development.

Employment

Provided that the expectant mother enjoys her work and that it does not subject her to too great a physical strain, the job may be continued throughout pregnancy. In many countries legislation has been enacted which gives paid maternity leave for the last 6 to 8 weeks of pregnancy. After delivery it is usual to be given paid leave from work for 4 to 6 weeks, so that the baby may be cared for, and the mother may adjust to her new duties.

Exercise

Pregnancy is a normal event and should be treated as such. Exercise should be encouraged if this is the usual habit of the patient, but if the expectant mother normally takes no exercise beyond housework, she need not change her habits. The average woman takes a reasonable amount of exercise, and can continue to take it in pregnancy. If she enjoys swimming, she may swim. If she plays tennis or golf, she may continue until the enlarging uterus prevents accurately placed strokes! If she enjoys walking or gardening, then she should continue to walk or garden. In general, she need not alter the pattern of exercise to which she is accustomed, just because she is pregnant. If she has an existing exercise programme she may continue it, modifying it as pregnancy advances.

Exercise in pregnancy has several benefits. Some women find that exercise increases their body awareness. Others use exercise to increase their muscle and joint flexibility. Others use exercise to reduce or prevent some of the discomforts which occur in pregnancy, such as backache. Exercise is beneficial if used sensibly. A woman should not take such strenuous exercise that her body temperature increases unduly, and should seek advice before undertaking strenuous exercise programmes.

For women interested in using a safe pregnancy exercise programme, a videotape *Pregnancy Exercise Workout* is available in Britain from Potentialpointe Productions, P O Box 462, Blackheath, London SE3 7UP and in Australia from Forest Home Films, P O Box 1586, Sydney, 2001.

Fainting

Fainting attacks, palpitations and headaches occasionally occur in pregnancy, and are due to the alterations in the expectant mother's circulatory system produced by the pregnancy. Although annoying, they have no sinister significance, and in Victorian days a faint was the way the modest wife announced to her husband that 'a little stranger was on the way'!

Fatigue

Many women find that they tire more easily or sleep for longer in the second half of pregnancy. The feeling of tiredness increases as the end of pregnancy nears. Different women find different ways of coping with fatigue. Some rest or take a nap in the afternoon, others go to bed earlier. Others take short rests from time to time during the day. It helps to know that most pregnant women feel tired, and if you do, try to work out the method of coping which suits you.

Frequency of urination

Irritability of the bladder is quite common in early pregnancy, and occurs again in the last weeks when the baby's head presses into the pelvis. Nothing much can be done about it, except to pass urine more often. If urination is associated with pain and scalding, the expectant mother should consult her doctor.

Haemorrhoids

Haemorrhoids, or piles, often occur in pregnancy or at childbirth. They are more common in multigravidae, and seem to occur in families. The usual complaints are of bleeding during a bowel motion, the presence of a tender lump noticed during the use of toilet paper, or pain. Constipation and straining to empty the bowels aggravate these complaints. The expectant mother can reduce the discomfort of haemorrhoids by avoiding constipation, and making sure that the stool is never hard. Her doctor will be able to prescribe ointments which relieve the pain and reduce the swelling of prolapsed piles.

Heartburn

Heartburn is an annoying and fairly common complaint, which is more frequent in late pregnancy. It is due to the passage of small amounts of stomach contents into the lower part of the food tube (or oesophagus), which leads from the mouth to the stomach. In pregnancy this occurs because the valve guarding the entrance to the stomach relaxes, and because the enlarging uterus pushes up against the stomach. It is often worse at night, when the burning sensation in the upper abdomen can be quite depressing. Despite its name, it can be seen that heartburn has nothing to do with the heart. The expectant mother can relieve heartburn by eating small meals more frequently, and by taking a glass of milk to bed with her, and sipping this if heartburn occurs. She would also be wise to sleep propped up on one or two extra pillows. If heartburn persists, her doctor will prescribe one of the many antacid tablets or liquids. The more modern ones, based on aluminium or magnesium, are preferable to those containing sodium (salt), such as sodium bicarbonate, as this increases the patient's intake of salt, which may not be advisable.

Immunization

All immunization programmes can be carried out as required in pregnancy. Indeed, because of the apparently increased risk of poliomyelitis to pregnant women, the expectant mother should be immunized against this disease if she has not previously taken her Sabin vaccine. Since the vaccine is given by mouth, it is quite painless and devoid of side-effects. There is a belief, too, that pregnant women are more susceptible to chest complications of influenza, and some doctors recommend that pregnant women should receive anti-influenza injections if an epidemic is expected. I am doubtful of the truth of this, as so many strains of the influenza virus exist, and the injection may only protect the patient, if it does, against one strain. Moreover, the injections are painful. In case of doubt, the patient should consult her own doctor.

Incontinence of urination

About 50 per cent of pregnant women find that when they cough or laugh a small amount of urine is lost before the woman can prevent it. The condition is annoying but no treatment is available and it disappears after childbirth.

Leg cramps

Some expectant mothers develop leg cramps in late pregnany. These occur mostly at night, and the cause is not known. Treatment is not very satisfactory, and there is some evidence that excessive milk intake may be the cause. This is why the total milk intake recommended was 900ml (1½ pints). However, the evidence that excessive milk is the cause of leg cramps is not very secure, as leg cramps occur in Asian women who do not habitually drink milk. If the patient has leg cramps, a drink of milk from the allowance may help. Recently a doctor has suggested that the cramps will be less if the foot of the bed is raised 25cm (10in).

Maternal prenatal influences

A considerable literature has grown up about how maternal influences can affect the baby. This obstetric superstition has been propagated from antiquity, and sought to explain the birth of deformed or blemished infants. This tribal myth has been used by playwrights and novelists to tell dramatic stories, and is still widely believed. It has, of course, no substance. There is no evidence that maternal impressions can affect the baby in any way. The reasons are many: first, there is no nervous connection between the mother and her baby; second, the blood of the mother is quite separate from that of the baby; and third, the infant is completely formed by the 8th week of pregnancy, so that for the impression to have any effect it must occur before this time. In most cases, the 'shocking experience' which the mother 'knows' is the cause of her baby's birth defect occurred much later. The truth is that maternal impressions have no effect on the growth or development of the baby. The baby will not become a famous television actor if the expectant mother spends hours watching television. The infant will not be exceptionally gifted musically if the mother persisently listens to, or plays, music during pregnancy; nor will he be a famous sportsman if her husband insists that she watches all the ball games she can over the 40 weeks of pregnancy; nor will the sight of a one-eyed black cat crossing the road mean that her baby will be born one-eyed and black!

It is true that a few babies are born with congenital defects, but the number with a defect is less than three in every hundred. None is due to prenatal influences. This means that 97 of every 100 babies born are perfectly formed, and of the three which have defects, most can be treated. But it is not true that the defects are due to prenatal influences. A few cases are due to an inhertited defect in one of the genes which make up the new individual. Occasionally, the defect is due to infection by the rubella virus occurring during pregnancy. This is the virus which causes German measles, and the problem is discussed further on page 302.

Nausea

About 50 per cent of pregnant women experience some degree of nausea, and a few vomit. This complaint occurs in the first 12 weeks of pregnancy, usually disappearing at the end of this time, but sometimes recurring in late pregnancy. The cause is almost certainly a sensitivity to the hormones of pregnancy, but the condition may be exaggerated if the expectant mother is over-anxious or emotionally stressed. Most often the nausea occurs in the morning, hence the name 'morning sickness', but it may occur at any time of the day. Nausea in the morning is more common than at other times of the day, because the stomach contains the overnight accumulation of gastric juices.

Most women are able to overcome the nausea by simple means. The composition of the diet should be adjusted to exclude greasy, fatty foods, and fried foods should be avoided. Small carbohydrate-rich meals are taken at more frequent intervals, the first being brought to the wife by her husband as soon as possible after waking. This may consist of toast or biscuits, and tea. After this, small meals are eaten every 3 hours until bedtime. Some women find it better to avoid drinking at meals and to take the fluids, either as sweetened fruit drinks, weak tea or milk and soda-water, at other times.

An example of a suitable diet for the day is:

On waking A slice of toast or two cream cracker biscuits, with a drink of weak tea.
8.00 a.m. Light breakfast of cereal, or toast with honey or jam, and perhaps weak tea. If the expectant mother feels she can eat more, she adjusts the diet to her own needs.
10.00 a.m. Toast with a glass of milk, tea or a fruit drink.
12.30 p.m. Lunch. Soup with toast or cream crackers; rice or noodles with lightly boiled vegetables.
3.30 p.m. Tea. Toast, jam, fruit juice, and perhaps plain cake.
6.30 p.m. Dinner. Lean meat or chicken, green vegetables, potatoes, salad and rice pudding.
9.30 p.m. A drink of tea, cocoa, warm milk, or milk and soda.
To bed A drink and cream crackers to take if the expectant mother wakes up during the night.

This is only an example, and a great number of variations can be chosen by the individual herself. If the nausea is troublesome, the expectant mother should consult her doctor. Although many and varied drugs have been prescribed in the past, doctors today are very wary of new drugs in early pregnancy. In some cases of nausea and vomiting, however, drugs help the expectant mother feel better and cope more easily. If nausea predominates, an antihistamine drug (such as cyclizine or meclozine) is helpful. In more severe cases, particularly when vomiting is a problem, a drug called metoclopramide, taken three times a day, usually helps.

A few women have such severe, intractable vomiting that they need to be admitted to hospital. This condition is called *hyperemesis gravidarium*.

Nose bleeds

Slight bleeding from the nose is not unusual in pregnancy. It is due to the increased blood supply which occurs, and in most cases needs no treatment. It does not mean that the expectant mother has a high blood pressure.

Pica

For some reason, which the psychiatrists try to explain, bizarre cravings for strange foods may occur in pregnancy. Unfortunately, each group of psychiatrists has a different explanation, so the *fact* of bizarre cravings remains, but the *reason* remains unknown. If the craving is for substances other than foodstuffs, the craving is called 'pica'. The word comes from the Latin term for 'magpie', a bird which collects strange articles. Severe craving is not very common, and true pica is rather rare. Most women who do have cravings want carbohydrates, either sweets or laundry starch, or large amounts of fruit. A few have cravings for more exotic things, such as pickles, caviare or avocados. The very few who have true pica may urgently crave to eat coal, clay or pencils. If the expectant mother develops strange cravings for foods in pregnancy, she must realize that she is not going mad, but that the cravings exist and need to be controlled.

Placidity

To the annoyance of the intellectually-alert expectant mother, she may note an increasing placidity and drowsiness as pregnancy advances. She no longer has the clarity of mind and precision of thought she had before pregnancy. Even small intellectual matters become a trial; to do anything is an effort and she fears she is becoming bovine. The cause is the increased circulation of the pregnancy hormone progesterone, and she can be reassured that the placidity will pass once the baby is born.

Seat Belts

Pregnant women should use a three point seat belt when travelling in a car. The seat belt should be placed above or below her pregnant uterus so that if a car crash occurs the restraint does not directly put pressure on the uterus and the fetus.

Sex in pregnancy

If the expectant mother's pregnancy is normal and she has no tendency to premature labour or repeated abortions, sexual intercourse may continue at a frequency which is normal for that couple. Some women find that they desire more frequent coitus in pregnancy; others find they are less stimulated. The reason for the reduced sexual interest experienced by many pregnant women, particularly in the last weeks of pregnancy, is not clear. Some women are fearful that sexual intercourse may damage the baby or bring on labour prematurely. Others fear that an orgasm, however produced, may do the same thing. Other women are embarrassed by their enlarged breasts and swelling abdomen, and feel that they are unattractive and not 'sexy'. Still other women want body contact with their partner but prefer not to have coitus.

Most of the problems will be reduced if the couple can talk to each other about the sexual needs and desires. The couple can enjoy sexual intercourse throughout pregnancy, but the man should be considerate and gentle during penile thrusting. In the second half of pregnancy the woman may find that penile entry into her vagina from the rear is more comfortable and satisfying. Alternatively, sexual desire may be satisfied by non-coital methods. The man may help his partner reach orgasm by manipulating her clitoral area with his fingers or by caressing it with his tongue (cunnilingus). These varieties of sexual technique are both enjoyable and safe, except that a man should never blow into a pregnant woman's vagina during cunnilingus. This is because air may enter a blood vessel causing a fatal air embolism.

Sexual activity, including coitus, can continue throughout pregnancy, right up to the time of confinement and can resume after childbirth as soon as the woman wishes and finds it enjoyable. There is no truth in the myth that sexual activity, including orgasm, in normal pregnant women can produce premature labour or abortion, nor will it lead to infection of the fetus if continued up to the expected time of delivery.

Shortness of breath

In late pregnancy a number of expectant mothers find that even moderate exertion causes shortness of breath. Provided their doctor has checked that their heart and lungs are normal, the shortness of breath, although inconvenient, is without danger.

Smoking

The influence of cigarette smoking on pregnancy has been studied in the last few years. The evidence at present is that cigarette smoking, particularly if more than 10 cigarettes are smoked per day, has an adverse effect on pregnancy. There seems to be an increased risk that abortion will occur, and the birth weight of the baby is likely to be less than that of a baby born to a woman who does not smoke. As well, babies of women who smoke during pregnancy have nearly three times the risk of being born with a cleft lip. Expectant mothers should stop smoking when they are pregnant, so that the increased risk to their baby and to themselves are avoided. In Australia a campaign to induce pregnant women to stop smoking and avoid alcohol and drugs has begun. It is called 'The Pregnant Pause'.

Stretch marks

Fine wavy, pinkish lines appear on the abdomen, the breasts, the upper arms or the thighs of susceptible women during pregnancy. These are so-called 'stretch marks', although they are not due to stretching. They also occur during adolescence, in obesity and in some chronic illnesses. They are probably due to an increased secretion of adrenal gland hormones which, in susceptible women, shatter the elastic fibres in the skin. There is no treatment nor does massaging the skin with oil prevent their occurrence. For some reason they hardly ever occur in African or Asian women.

Sweating

In late pregnancy, many expectant mothers find that they sweat more easily and in hot, humid weather 'feel the heat intolerably'. Sometimes night sweats occur, the expectant mother waking up in a 'lather of sweat'. The excessive sweating is due to dilated blood vessels in the skin, which in turn dilate because of pregnancy. No specific treatment is available, and all that the expectant mother can do is to avoid excessive exertion, to take frequent rest periods, and have frequent cool

199

showers. Because of the increased fluid lost by sweating, the expectant mother should increase her fluid intake.

Swelling of the ankles and legs (oedema)

Retention of fluid in the tissues of the body is normal in pregnancy. The average expectant mother retains between 3 and 6 litres (6½ to 13 pints) of fluid, half of it in the last 10 weeks of pregnancy. Swelling of the ankles, the lowest part of the body, is therefore common. If it occurs in the evening, it is not serious, and all that the expectant mother needs to do is keep her feet up. Women who are overweight for their height by the 20th week of pregnancy, and overweight women who gain more than 0.5kg (1.1lb) per week after the 30th week, have almost a 50 per cent chance of developing evening oedema. In general this is unimportant, but if these women, and all others, develop swelling of the legs earlier in the day, it is a warning sign that pregnancy-induced hypertension may be developing, and the mother-to-be should hasten to see her doctor.

Travel

Apart from the restriction by airlines on carrying women more than 32 weeks pregnant who have no certificate of fitness from their doctor, an expectant mother can travel wherever she likes during pregnancy. She may safely travel by aeroplane, by ship or by car – or at least as safely as other motorists will let her! The only problem may be that she may go into labour at her destination, and will have to find a new obstetrician.

Urinary tract infection

About 5 per cent of women have a hidden infection of the urinary tract, which causes them no trouble until they become pregnant. In pregnancy, owing to the muscle-relaxing effects of progesterone, the collecting area in the kidney and the tube which connects the kidney to the bladder becomes larger. Urine tends to stagnate in these areas, and in the bladder. Women who have hidden urinary tract infection (called 'bacteriuria'), unless treated, have twice the chance of developing anaemia, a raised blood pressure, and of delivering a 'premature baby'. It is usual for doctors to examine the urine in early pregnancy for the presence of bacteriuria and, if this is found, to give treatment. This treatment will also prevent the onset of kidney infection, or pyelo-nephritis. The collecting area of the kidney is called the renal pelvis, or *pyelos* (a Greek word meaning a trough). If the urine becomes infected, the kidney pyelos and the kidney tissue itself may become inflamed – which is why this type of kidney infection is called pyelonephritis.

The symptoms of pyelonephritis are pain in the loins, fever and shivering, sweating, and painful urination. Should these symptoms occur in pregnancy, the expectant mother should call her doctor without delay, as treatment using antibiotics is very successful.

Vaginal discharge

During pregnancy the normal secretions which keep the vagina moist are increased, and additional secretions derived from the glands of the cervix add to the quantity. About 30 per cent of expectant mothers are conscious of the increased vaginal discharge. If the quantity necessitates the wearing of a pad, the mother-to-be should consult her doctor, so that investigations may be undertaken to determine if the discharge is merely an exaggeration of the normal; if it is due to infection by the fungus, *Candida albicans*, which causes thrush; or if it is due to infection by a small parasite, the size of the point of a pin, called *Trichomonas vaginalis*. Usually infection with either of these causes an irritating vaginal discharge, but occasionally it does not. The doctor can only determine the actual cause of the vaginal discharge by examining a smear taken from the vagina with a cotton-wool swab. He looks at this under a microscope, and is then able to prescribe the appropriate treatment.

Varicose veins

Pregnancy provokes the appearance of varicose veins in the legs of women who are predisposed to them. The veins may appear at any time during pregnancy, but on the whole tend to enlarge and become more obvious in the later months. They may appear either as enlarged, worm-like tubes beneath the skin, or as spider varicosities around the ankles and behind the knees. The legs feel heavy, look ugly and may be painful or swollen. Most of the veins disappear once the baby is born, which is why doctors do not recommend surgical treatment in pregnancy. Some remain, however, to enlarge in subsequent pregnancies. Treatment is to keep the feet up as much as possible. As well as this, well-fitting supportive stockings, which are today indistinguishable from normal nylon stockings, should be put on each morning before the expectant mother puts her feet out of bed.

Vitamin and mineral supplements

It is the habit of doctors, encouraged by the beautiful advertisements which appear in medical journals, to insist that all pregnant women receive tablets of vitamin and mineral 'supplements'. This habit is approved by convention, and the majority of women (at least in the USA) would feel that their doctor was being rather incompetent if he failed to prescribe a 'pregnancy pill'. The pregnant dietary supplementary pills often contain a multitude of minerals (for some of which it is admitted that no use has been found) and a variety of vitamins. These pills are swallowed with fair regularity by pregnant women, and I suspect in most cases the contained minerals and vitamins emerge from the other end unaltered, to join the vast concentration of the contents of swallowed pills and potions in the sewage.

The question which has to be answered in the affluent countries, and particularly among the more affluent citizens in these countries, is: 'Are the pregnancy dietary supplements necessary? Would not the money expended be better spent on some other natural foods?' The answer must be a qualified 'Yes'! The great majority of women do not need pregnancy supplements provided they eat a reasonable diet. At the most they need to take each day a single pill containing iron. The 'submerged' 10 per cent of poor women in the affluent societies and the 90 per cent in the developing countries do need supplements, particularly of iron, but even more they need additional protein. These people are the very ones who all too often receive little antenatal care, usually get inadequate food, and most often receive no dietary supplementary pills in pregnancy. Their need is great; that of their affluent sisters is minimal.

The expectant mother should eat a balanced diet; she should obtain proper antenatal care; she should have the haemoglobin concentration of her blood tested, as described previously; and she should be given a prescription for a tablet containing an iron salt (and it does not matter which iron salt). She should take one of these tablets each day from about the 14th week of pregnancy, but if she happens to miss a couple of days, it does not matter much. In fact there is now evidence that women who eat a healthy diet probably do not need iron tablets during pregnancy as they obtain all they need from their food.

There has been some discussion recently about whether pregnant women should be given a particular vitamin called folic acid. It is called 'folic' acid because the vitamin was first found in the leaves of green vegetables, and *folium* is a leaf in Latin. This vitamin is need for the growth of cells, and since little is stored in the body, a steady intake is required. In pregnancy the demand increases considerably, particularly in the last 10 weeks, and the level of folic acid in the mother's blood tends to fall. If the diet contains green or yellow leafy vegetables, lightly cooked using only a small amount of water, there is generally no need for additional folic acid tablets. But because the baby demands and takes so much folic acid from the mother, it may be wise to give supplements to the mother who is carrying twins. The dose she needs is very small, and the vitamin is only needed after the 30th week of pregnancy. The vitamin should only be taken after discussing the matter with the doctor.

What then is the situation regarding vitamin and mineral pills in pregnancy? Beyond taking a single iron tablet each day, and in special cases taking a folic acid tablet, a pregnant woman in an affluent society, who is not poor, does not require to take the vitamin and mineral pills so attractively displayed and bottled by enterprising pharmaceutical companies.

Weight gain

It is quite obvious that women put on weight during pregnancy. The question to be answered is how much is permissible. Until very recently weight gain was restricted very considerably, as obstetricians believed that there was a close relationship between weight gain and the onset of pre-eclampsia. While there is a relationship, it is now known that it is by no means as close as was previously thought and the rigid restrictions on weight gain in pregnancy which used to be advised have been abandoned.

To appreciate how much weight gain is normal, it is helpful to analyse the various things which increase the expectant mother's weight in pregnancy. Obviously, the fetus, the placenta and the liquid in which the fetus lives all contribute. Equally obvious is the increased weight of the uterus and the breasts. Not quite so obvious is the fact that the increased volume of blood, which circulates in an expectant mother's arteries and veins, adds to the weight gain.

Two other factors are involved. The first is the increased deposition of fat in the mother's tissues. In part this is caused by the conversion of excess carbohydrate eaten in the diet, but in part is a normal event caused by the hormones of pregnancy. The amount of fat deposited varies very considerably, but averages 2.5kg (or 5½lb). It is believed that evolution of man led to this deposition of fat in pregnancy, so that the mother had extra energy stored which might later be needed for the care and feeding of her baby. Finally, and again because of the hormones of pregnancy, water is retained in the body. Again the amount varies, but about 4 litres, or 6¾ pints, is retained, half of it in the last 10 weeks of pregnancy.

It is possible to make a table showing how the various factors lead to weight gain in pregnancy (see below). As can be seen, a total of 12.0kg, or 27lb, is a normal weight gain in pregnancy. Because of this, the doctors who restricted severely the patient's weight gain were being unnecessarily harsh.

The weight gain is not spread equally throughout pregnancy. After the 20th week, the fetus gains weight more rapidly, fat is deposited in greater amounts, and fluid is retained more readily. In fact, the expectation is that in the first 20 weeks a weight gain of 3.0kg, or 7lb, will occur, and in the last 20 weeks a weight gain of 9kg, or 20lb, can be considered normal. Of course, there are individual variations. The expectant mother who is underweight for her height may be encouraged to put on more weight, and the overweight mother will be firmly told not to put on so much weight.

Apart from these groups of women it is questionable if a pregnant woman needs to be weighed at each antenatal visit, as was mentioned on p. 177.

A final point: if an expectant mother gains more than 16kg, or 35lb, in pregnancy, she will find it almost impossible to lose the extra weight. Her clothes will not fit, her sylphlike figure will be a memory.

Fetus, placenta and amniotic liquid	4.0kg	(10lb 8oz)
Uterus and breasts	1.2kg	(2lb 10oz)
Blood volume increase	1.2kg	(2lb 4oz)
Fat deposited	up to 3.4kg	(7lb 10oz)
Water retained	up to 2.2kg	(4lb 10oz)
Total	12.0kg	(27lb)

CHAPTER 12

The Three Stages of Labour

The process of childbirth is usually called 'labour'. The term is appropriate, for labour is a time of work. Considerable energy is expended in the contractions of the uterus. For this reason the pregnant woman is in ways like an athlete. If she has had proper training during pregnancy, so that she knows what to expect and what to do in labour; if she is in good physical condition; if her mental attitude to labour is good, the process of childbirth is relatively easy. One of the objectives of good antenatal care is to enable her to reach this peak of fitness at the time labour is due.

Before we consider the process of labour from the viewpoint of the expectant mother, it is helpful to consider what happens in labour. With the aid of diagrams, we can see how the baby is expelled from its heat-controlled capsule, to journey down the dark curved birth-canal, and to be pushed out into a world where it has to use many functions for which it had no need while in the uterus. It has to obtain its oxygen from the atmosphere, not from its mother's blood. It has to get rid of its own waste products. It can no longer depend upon its placenta to act as a liver and a kidney. It has to obtain food instead of depending on the transfer across the placenta of required foodstuffs from the mother's blood to its own blood. In all these functions, the newborn baby succeeds admirably. However, the more normal the process of childbirth, the easier it is for the baby to adjust to independent life.

The last few days of pregnancy

In late pregnancy, just before the onset of labour, the baby has grown to an average weight of 3400g (7½lb), and is 50cm (20in) long. It has occupied more and more space in the amniotic sac, and the amount of amniotic fluid has been reduced from a maximum volume of 1000ml

(1¾ pints) at 36 weeks' gestation, to about 600ml (1 pint) at 40 weeks' gestation, or 'term'. If it a first pregnancy, the baby's head is likely to have settled into the mother's pelvis. The uterus is becoming increasingly sensitive to stimuli, and increasingly active. The cervix is soft, has shortened in length, and is likely to have begun to open a bit, usually about 1 to 2 finger-breadths. If a doctor performs a pelvic examination at this stage, he will feel the 'bag of waters', which is the inexact term used for the amniotic sac, and in it he can feel the baby's head. If he could see the baby, he would find in more than three-quarters of cases that its face was looking towards the mother's right or left hip bone (Fig. 12/1).

The first stage of labour

For reasons which are quite unknown, at a specific point labour starts. The uterine contractions initially are not very strong, and only occur at long intervals. However, with the passage of time, they become stronger and more frequent. This phase of labour does not distress the patient unduly, and is called the quiet phase. It lasts an average of 8 to 9 hours in a first labour, and 4 hours in subsequent labours.

With each contraction, the muscle fibres of the uterus shorten a tiny fraction, so that a pull is exerted on the cervix, which is the weakest

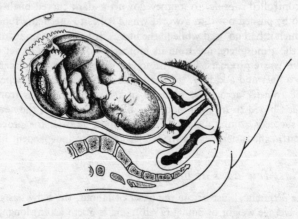

FIG. 12/1   The baby in late pregnancy. Its head is 'fixed' in the mother's pelvis and it 'looks' towards one hip bone. The cervix is soft but not yet drawn up.

part. This is because the muscle is thickest in the upper part of the uterus, and becomes less thick in the lower part. The cervix has only 10 per cent of muscle.

The pull on the cervix first shortens it until it no longer hangs down into the vagina like a cuff, but is drawn up flush. Doctors call this 'cervical effacement'. The pull then opens the cervix, and it slowly opens wider and wider. This the doctors call 'cervical dilatation', and patients may hear nurses or doctors saying that the cervix is so many finger-breadths, or so many centimetres dilated. The quiet phase of labour usually lasts until the cervix is 2 to 3 finger-breadths (or 4 to 5 centimetres) dilated. Three fingers, or 5 centimetres, means that the cervix is half-way to its complete opening, which doctors call 'full dilatation'.

During the quiet phase, the baby's head flexes more so that it tucks in its chin, and the head moves more deeply into the pelvis. This can be seen in the illustration. It will be noted that the 'bag of waters' is still intact (Fig. 12/2). The end of the quiet phase is heralded by a change in the character of the uterine contractions. In the active phase, they become stronger and more frequent, and the expectant mother may request drugs to reduce the pain. The cervix continues to dilate, and the baby is pushed further into the

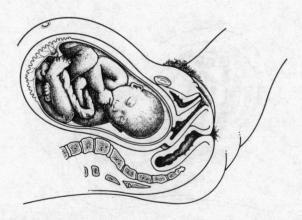

FIG. 12/2   The baby in early labour. Note how it has tucked its chin well in. The cervix has been drawn up, and the bag of waters is still intact.

pelvis, where it may cause pressure on the bladder and back-passage (Fig. 12/3). As the dilatation of the cervix becomes nearly complete, the contractions of the uterus are quite strong, but the degree of discomfort felt by the expectant mother will depend on the adequacy of her preparation for labour, and on her attitude to labour. This period between 8cm dilation and full dilatation is called the *transition stage*. During this stage, as has been mentioned, the contractions are strong and painful; the desire to push is present; backache and pelvic discomfort may be quite severe. However, the mother should resist the urge to push as the cervix is not fully dilated. At this time she should use the techniques she has learned in childbirth classes, or may choose to have an epidural analgesia.

When the cervix is fully dilated, the uterus and vagina together form a curved passage, along which the baby can pass, aided by uterine contractions and the mother's additional use of her abdominal muscles.

The period of time from the onset of labour to the full dilatation of the cervix is called the *first stage of labour*. It lasts, on an average, 10 hours in the first labour, and 7 hours in a subsequent labour, although, of course, the duration of the first stage varies very considerably between different expectant mothers.

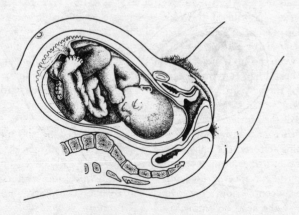

FIG. 12/3   Late in the first stage of labour. The cervix has almost completely opened and the bag of waters bulges in front of the head.

The second stage of labour

The second stage of labour is the time when the mother-to-be has to help. In the first stage she helps most by relaxing during contractions, and by reading, talking, listening to the radio, or watching television. In the second stage she has work to do. She has to aid in the expulsion of the baby from the birth-canal, which is formed from the uterus and the vagina. The second stage usually lasts less than 1½ hours, extending in time from the full dilatation of the cervix to the birth of the baby. If the second stage lasts longer than 1½ hours, the attending doctor usually helps the birth by forceps (see Chapter 19). The beginning of the second stage is announced frequently by bursting of the 'bag of waters', with a resulting gush of fluid from the vagina. The bursting of the 'bag of waters', called by doctors 'rupture of the membranes', may occur much earlier in labour, or occasionally not until the baby is ready to be born. Usually, however, it occurs at the very end of the first stage of labour.

At the same time the expectant mother gets the urge to push. This is caused by the pressure of the baby's head on the tissues in the middle of the pelvis. A message is sent to the brain, which makes the mother want to fix her diaphragm, and contract her abdominal muscles to push her baby out into the world. The baby is therefore pushed downwards, and because of the shape of the muscles which stretch across the pelvis, its head turns so that it comes to look backwards (Figs. 12/4 and 5). Evolution has caused this, for when man expanded his brain and developed a round skull, he made childbirth more difficult. The widest diameter at the entrance to the bony pelvis is the one stretching across it between the hip bones, and the baby adjusts so that the long diameter of its head (that from the forehead backwards) fits into this. In the lower part of the pelvis, the longest diameter is from before backwards, and the baby's head rotates to fit this so that its face now looks backwards towards the mother's back.

With each contraction of the uterus, and aided by the mother's 'pushing' efforts, the baby's head moves nearer the vulval cleft. Soon the top of its head can be seen by the doctor who will deliver the baby. The head advances a bit with each contraction, and retreats a bit between contractions, but overall the advance continues, more and more of the head becoming visible. The mother is working very hard during this time, her pulse rises, she sweats from the effort, and between contractions she rests, dozing and obtaining energy for the

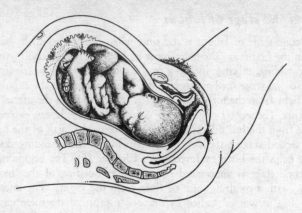

FIG. 12/4   The early part of the second stage of labour. The child's head is beginning to turn so that it faces towards its mother's back. The bag of waters has 'broken'. The mother feels pressure on her bladder and rectum, and she has the desire to push.

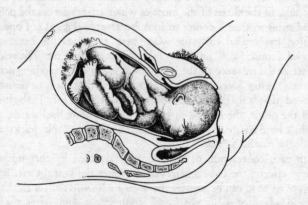

FIG. 12/5   Late second stage. Labour is nearly over. The baby's head appears at the vulva, and the shoulders are turning to fit into the bones of the pelvis. The face is turned completely towards the mother's back. The mother's perineum is being stretched.

next effort. And despite this, it is said that women are the 'weaker sex'! Finally, the head stretches the vaginal entrance and the tissues between it and the back-passage (or anus). This area is called the perineum, and it becomes tightly stretched over the baby's head which bulges through it. This is quaintly called 'crowning of the head'. At this point the doctor may inject a local anaesthetic into the tissues of the vulva, if he has not done so already. This prevents the mother from the pain of stretching of the tissues, which many say feels as if their bottom were about to burst. It is also said that it resembles the feeling of trying to open the bowels after being constipated for a month! The next contraction pushes the baby down further, and the head sweeps over the vulval tissues, the forehead, the eyes, the nose, the mouth and the chin appearing successively (Fig. 12/6).

The birth of the baby's head can be seen in the series of drawings (Fig. 12/7), and it can be noted that once the head is born, it turns back to face the mother's hips. This has been arranged by evolution so that the shoulders of the baby and the rest of its body can slip out of the birth-canal easily. The baby is born! The mother, no longer expectant, looks delightedly at her baby, and as its first cry echoes, she fondles it and then relaxes and may sleep momentarily.

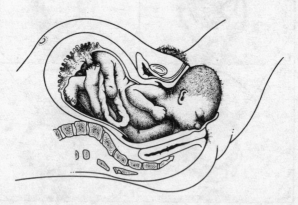

FIG. 12/6   The baby's head is being born, emerging from the vagina and sweeping the perineum backwards.

The third stage of labour

Little more remains but to wait for the expulsion of the placenta, or afterbirth, so-called for obvious reasons. This has separated from its attachment to the wall of the uterus as the baby was born. The doctor either awaits its expulsion or, as is more usual today, aids its rapid removal by giving an injection of a drug called ergometrine, or one

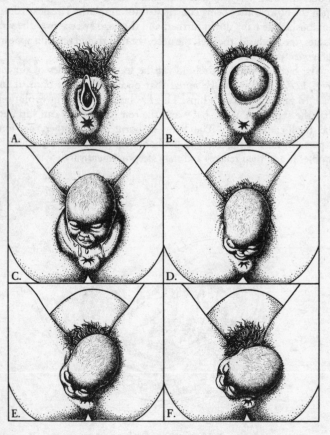

FIG. 12/7   The birth of the baby's head as seen by the doctor. Note how the perineum is stretched by the baby's head before it is born.

called syntometrine which makes the uterus contract firmly. This reduces the blood lost by the mother, which is desirable. The injection is given either as the baby's head is being born or as the baby's shoulders emerge.

CHAPTER 13

Childbirth Without Pain

In the year 1847 in the city of Edinburgh, in the dining-room of a house in Queen Street, three respectable physicians sat sniffing the contents of various bottles. The bottles contained mixtures of chemicals which were said to cause loss of consciousness. They had spent many evenings in this pursuit, sniffing and recording their observations. On a cold, wet evening in November, the group led by James Young Simpson gathered as usual. One of the mixtures that night was a rather pleasant, sweet-smelling fluid. After one large whiff each, the three men became strangely excited and gay; after two, they all became sleepy; and after a third large inhalation, they lay sprawled on the floor, only awakening after a few minutes. In this way the anaesthetic qualities of chloroform were discovered. It was clear to Dr Simpson that chloroform could help to relieve the pain of women in labour – for at that time no pain-relief of any kind was given, and as no patient received antenatal care, labours were often difficult, painful and dangerous. But when Simpson announced, in a paper published in the monthly *Journal of Medical Science*, that chloroform could be used to relieve the pains of childbirth, he was criticized vehemently, attacked in print and from the pulpit by clergy and leaders of the public, as well as by many members of the medical profession. The use of chloroform was against God's will, they cried, for was it not written that because Eve tempted Adam to eat the forbidden fruit, a curse was laid upon her that 'in sorrow would she bring forth her children'? If the pain and sorrow were reduced, it was irreligious. To this Simpson replied that in the Bible the first reported surgical operation had been performed under anaesthesia. The Lord God has caused 'a deep sleep to fall upon Adam; and he slept; and He took one of his ribs, and closed the flesh thereof'. Simpson was told by an American that to give chloroform was to interfere with nature, since the pains of childbirth were a natural function. Simpson agreed but asked, 'Is not walking also a natural function? And who would think of never setting aside or superseding this natural function? If you were travelling from Philadelphia to Baltimore, would you insist on walking the distance by foot simply because walking is man's natural method of locomotion?' An Irish woman visiting Scotland attacked him by saying, 'How unnatural it is for you doctors in Edinburgh to take away the pains of your patients when in labour.' His reply was, 'Madam, how unnatural it is for you to have swum over from Ireland to Scotland against wind and tides on a steamboat.'

Most of the objections were from the clergy; to each Simpson had an answer, and little by little his opponents were silenced, particularly as women appeared to approve of his attempt, in his own words, 'to alleviate human suffering, as well as preserve human life.' The cachet of approval was put upon his method when Queen Victoria was given inhalations of chloroform during the birth of her eighth child. Simpson was vindicated, and when he was later knighted, as Sir James Simpson, the opposition was in disorder. Yet to some extent, although they did not know it, they were partly right. Chloroform, although sweet-smelling, quick-acting and not irritating to breathe, is not a safe anaesthetic, because it may damage the liver. Consequently it is no longer used in obstetric practice.

No one would now deny that women should have the discomfort of childbirth relieved, and countless methods have been introduced in the past. Some were dangerous to the mother, some to the child; but today a reasonable approach has been made, and women need no longer fear the pain of childbirth. There are very real dangers though if the sedation is pushed too far, and the doctors have to find out the point at which adequate sedation and analgesia (that is, pain-relief without unconsciousness) can be given without risk to the mother or baby. It is unfair to promise a mother that all discomfort can be relieved, but it is equally callous for a doctor to allow his patient to suffer unduly, or to permit the nurses, who are so much closer to the patient during most of labour, to appear indifferent to her discomfort.

Today three main methods of relieving the pain associated with childbirth are available. These methods should be discussed with the doctor during pregnancy so that the expectant mother can make her own choice. But it must be emphasized that she can change her mind and make another choice right up to and during her confinement. She must not feel that she is 'stuck' with a particular method. The methods are, first, prepared childbirth; second, analgesic supported childbirth; and third, painless childbirth following an epidural anaesthetic.

Prepared childbirth

The concept of prepared childbirth may include 'psychoprophylaxis', partner supported childbirth, 'natural' childbirth, active involvement in childbirth or a combination of all four.

Childbirth training has broadened in recent years to expand the original technique of psychoprophylaxis. This was first developed in Russia. It is based on the belief that fear and anxiety about pain and danger in childbirth, learned before the woman becomes pregnant and during pregnancy, sink deeply into her memory and produce a 'conditioned reflex'. Because of this reflex, every time a woman thinks of childbirth a mental image of pain and danger is conjured up, so that she enters labour anxious and tense. The tension and fear may increase the pain and delay the birth of the baby. Psychoprophylaxis seeks to eliminate the 'conditioned reflex' and to replace the negative image of childbirth with a more positive one. This is achieved by education during pregnancy in the hope that knowledge and insight will change the woman's perceptions of labour. Psychoprophylaxis also seeks to alter the brain's perception of pain and to convert it into a sensation of discomfort, which can be relieved by muscular activity. It is based on the concept of 'pain dissociation'. Pain becomes less intense if the woman keeps her mind busy by concentrating on something else. The suggested mental activity usually involves concentrating on a learned pattern of breathing, counting breaths, focusing on a particular point in the room or consciously commanding the body to release its tension. However, it is very difficult for most women to maintain control and remain in a calm state during the particularly painful stages of labour. The distraction techniques of psychoprophylaxis are therefore unrealistic and unsatisfactory for many women during childbirth.

As anthropologists, psychologists, physiotherapists and midwives have become increasingly active in the development of prepared childbirth, new strategies for pain management have been developed which offer more than the original psychoprophylaxis concept.

The social environment in which the baby will be born, and its effect on the woman, is now becoming an important consideration. Many women want their partner or some other 'support person' to be with them during childbirth. The presence of an informed loved one during labour gives the woman familiar and personal support to reduce the more clinical environment of a delivery ward.

The discomfort and pain of childbirth is decreased if the attending nursing and medical staff treat the woman as an intelligent individual, who has needs and who can make choices, and who is perceived as a woman having a baby, rather than as a patient requiring medical attention. Some hospitals are trying to make the place of birth as non-clinical as possible by providing a supportive environment with floor mattresses, functional beds, soft fabrics and colours and a shower. These innovations decrease a woman's anxiety and enable her to cope more efficiently with the process of childbirth.

Techniques of auditory and visual imagery provide an additional means of managing pain in labour. Instead of dissociating from her pain (as in psychoprophylaxis) the woman uses the sensations of labour to assist her in creating an image of what is happening inside her body. For example, she may visualize her cervix opening each time she has a contraction. She may visualize the baby's head moving deeper into her pelvis. She may visualize the baby opening her vagina in the second stage of labour.

Another development has been the use of relaxation techniques. In psychoprophylaxis, relaxation was taught as a method of 'control'. The woman used quiet controlled breathing to convince herself that she was not experiencing pain. More recently, relaxation has been used by the woman as a method of 'letting go' and so reducing the pain. She may move and rock to achieve relaxation; she may stamp her feet, or bang her fists to release stress and diffuse the pain. She may discover that for her, the most effective form of pain control is a combination of floor positions, rhythmic groaning and belly rocking.

The proponents of active involvement in childbirth believe that the woman, if possible, should be given a free choice in the position she wishes to adopt and the movements she wishes to make during labour and the birth of the baby. The woman may choose to lie on her side, to squat, or to position herself on her hands and knees. She may prefer to be supported in a nearly upright position, with her partner in front of her or behind her. In this technique there is much less focus on breathing as an 'exercise' or 'pattern', and more focus on breathing as a method which helps the woman 'go with the flow'.

A current approach used by many obstetric physiotherapists is to stress women's differences, rather than adopting a rigid technique. Attempts are made to find out the woman's most preferred behaviours, and to encourage her to use these in childbirth. A woman who is 'tactile', for example, will probably respond well to massage, hot packs applied to her back, and showers and will tend to move about a good deal during labour. Other women prefer 'visualization', eye to eye focusing, or respond to key words such as 'relax', 'go soft', 'let go'. A third group of women are able to relieve the pain of labour more effectively by using auditory strategies. They respond to their support person 'pacing' them during a contraction and to giving themselves positive messages.

When a woman responds to the pain in a way she naturally prefers, her behaviour ceases to be due to a technique or a method. This reduces the anxiety that comes from having to perform a technique with which she is not comfortable, and which she fears she may not perform well.

The philosophy adopted by numbers of childbirth educators is to provide information and to give permission to the woman to be herself. Some women prefer not to attend class or to employ a private childbirth educator. For them, training videotapes are available which enable the woman and her partner to learn at home. One such videotape is *Preparing for Childbirth with Julia Sundin*. It is available from the same sources as the tape mentioned on page 192.

Birthing centres

Hospitals have begun to recognize the need to provide facilities for those couples who wish to have 'family-centred childbirth'.

This expression means that the woman wishes to give birth in as homelike an environment as possible. She wants her partner, and perhaps her other children to share the experience with her, as she believes childbirth to be a crucial event in the life of the family. She wishes to be able to cuddle her baby immediately after birth, so that she may make firm bonds with it. She wants her baby to remain with her after childbirth so that she can learn about it and can breast-feed it when it wants food.

To meet these expectations, a few hospitals have established 'birthing centres'. These are furnished like a bedroom with a double bed, curtains and easy chairs. Any equipment needed for childbirth is kept discreetly hidden.

The woman who chooses a 'birthing centre' has the satisfaction of knowing that she is giving birth in as 'natural' a way as possible, but that if anything goes wrong – such as a change in the rate of the baby's heart, indicating that it may be at risk, or prolapse of the umbilical cord, or haemorrhage – expert medical help and special equipment is available within seconds.

A birthing centre provides all the advantages of home birth without its possible dangers.

In the birthing centre, the expectant mother may be cared for by a trained nurse–midwife or may choose a doctor to help her give birth. In either case the medical attendant involves the family in the experience of labour and childbirth, but has the knowledge, so that if intervention is needed to rescue the baby, action can be taken.

It has been found that women choosing to give birth in a birthing centre require fewer drugs, have fewer operative deliveries and have fewer inductions of labour than women choosing other facilities.

Home births

In the past few years there has been a renewed demand for home birth. Those who have chosen to give birth at home relate the exhilarating experience of giving birth supported by their family, in a familiar environment, in which the woman feels she has control over her body. They compare this with the experience of giving birth in hospital, in a rather regimented impersonal environment, full of regulations and busy staff.

Home birth may have a place in modern obstetric care, but most doctors are concerned that the danger to the baby is increased in home birth. During labour the baby may develop 'distress' indicating that action is needed to deliver him, or after birth he may not be able to breathe properly. In a hospital, the two hazards can be dealt with quickly because of the facilities available, which may not be available at home. As well, a few mothers bleed excessively after birth. In hospital this can be dealt with expeditiously, because anaesthesia and blood are available, but in the home problems may arise.

The dangers to the baby and the risk of postpartum haemorrhage were the main reasons that, over the past 30 years, home birth has been replaced by hospital birth. The experience obtained in 'birth centres' will help doctors evaluate if home birth can be offered to women as a safe choice in childbirth.

Analgesic supported childbirth

While most women in the developing nations receive little or no analgesics during their confinements and because of cultural attitudes have no wish for their husband to be present, the majority of women in the developed nations are given (or, more rarely, choose) the method of analgesic supported childbirth. An analgesic is a drug which reduces or eliminates pain without clouding the consciousness of the person to any significant extent. The principle behind the method is that women in labour should have the pain of labour reduced by being given sedatives or analgesics at appropriate intervals, but the dose of the drugs should be regulated to avoid damaging the fetus.

In the quiet phase of the first stage of labour, the uterine contractions are relatively painless and few women ask for analgesics, although an apprehensive woman may welcome some form of sedation. In the past, barbiturates were widely used but recently some concern has been expressed that the drugs may depress the baby's breathing and the newer sedatives and, more usually, tranquillizers are being given. Many different tranquillizers have been given but, currently, promazine (Sparine), lorazepam and diazepam (Valium) are used most frequently. Promazine is given by injection into a muscle when labour is established, and gives the woman a warm woozy feeling. The other two drugs can be given as an injection or by mouth.

Once the quiet phase of labour merges into the active phase, the uterine contractions become stronger and more painful and most women want an analgesic which will reduce the painful sensations. In pride of place is pethidine (called meperidine in the USA). Pethidine is given by injection into a muscle, usually in the thigh or the upper arm. Within 20 minutes of the injection, the pain is reduced, often considerably, and the woman relaxes and feels drowsy between contractions. The effect of an injection of pethidine lasts from 2 to 5 hours, so that several injections may be needed in the course of labour.

Towards the end of the first stage of labour and in the second stage, the mother may need further help to reduce the discomfort. At this time the woman may choose either to have an epidural or to use a 'gas and oxygen' machine. A commonly used machine is the Entonox machine, which mixes the gases and has a hose with a face mask attached so that the woman can breathe the mixture.

The nitrous oxide gas acts on brain cells to reduce the perception of pain, provided it is given in sufficient concentration. It has been found that a concentration of 50 per cent is the most suitable, but if this concentration is used it must be mixed with 50 per cent of oxygen.

The best relief of pain is when the woman uses the mask properly. She should put the mask tightly over her face and start breathing deeply from the machine as soon as she feels that the contraction is starting. (It is preferable that she holds the mask on her face, not her partner trying to be helpful.) She continues breathing until the pain becomes less, when she takes the mask off her face but holds it ready to be used with the next contraction.

Many women, particularly those delivering a second or subsequent baby, find that the pain relief from pethidine supplemented by inhalational analgesics is all that they need, but some women require more. The only person who can determine the amount of pain felt is the person herself, so that the woman in labour has the right to ask for additional sedation and receive it.

Pain is likely to be more severe in a woman delivering her first baby, as its head presses down and stretches the vaginal entrance. A local anaesthetic injected into the tissues will relieve this pain, so that the 'bursting feeling' is eliminated. The doctor may give the injection into the stretched tissues between the vaginal entrance and the anus. This is called a perineal nerve block. An alternative and better method is for the doctor to give an injection to numb the nerves which supply the vulva as they pass through the pelvis. To do this, the doctor puts a finger in the woman's vagina, and gently pushes to one side until he reaches a triangular shaped bone which is a part of the pelvis. He then pushes a small needle, which is attached to a syringe, along his finger and injects the local anaesthetic around the triangular bony promontory. He repeats this on the other side of the woman's pelvis. This is called a pudendal nerve block. Quite quickly all painful sensations in the vulva and lower vagina are eliminated, so that the baby's birth is relatively painless, although the contractions of the uterus are still felt.

About 50 to 60 per cent of women choose analgesic supported childbirth (or are given the method without any choice); but in many Western nations more women are seeking to have 'painless childbirth' using an epidural analgesic.

Painless childbirth (epidural anaesthesia)

Increasing numbers of woman are now choosing to have an epidural analgesic, so that the childbirth may be relatively or completely

221

painless. An epidural analgesic is made by a trained person, usually an anaesthetist who has a special interest in obstetric anaesthesia. It is usually given when the woman is in the active phase of labour, as if it is given too early it may stop labour progressing. A woman who has had an epidural anaesthetic requires to be observed meticulously as the drug may cause vomiting and, sometimes, a fall in blood pressure. Because the woman has no sensation of pain, she may find it difficult to aid her baby's birth, by using her abdominal muscles and pushing when she has a uterine contraction. This means that the second stage of labour may last longer than in women choosing the other methods, and forceps delivery of the baby is more frequent. Provided that the woman is attended by a skilled doctor this is of no importance but many women are delivered by nurse–midwives who are not trained, or permitted, to use obstetric forceps.

For these reasons the majority of women do not have the opportunity to choose epidural anaesthesia. However, in most hospitals in the developed countries of the world epidural anaesthesia is available. So the expectant mother can make an informed choice she should understand where the injection is made and how it works.

The backbone is made up of separate vertebrae, and protects the spinal cord, which extends as far down as the pelvis through a hole in each vertebra. The spinal cord is made up of millions of nerve fibres, and is linked to all parts of the body. Impulses are constantly passing from all parts of the body to the brain along the spinal cord, and out again from the brain to all parts of the body. A substantial number of the nerves relay to the brain sensations received by the various parts of the body, such as feelings of cold, heat or pain. The nerves relaying these sensations are called sensory nerve fibres, and they pass along different routes from the nerve fibres which bring messages from the brain to the muscles and other structures. Since many of these fibres make the muscles contract, or move, they are called motor fibres. If it were possible to anaesthetize, or numb, the sensory fibres from the uterus without also anaesthetizing the motor fibres to the uterus, labour could be made painless. Luckily, this can be done safely, provided the anaesthetist is an expert.

The spinal cord is surrounded by a glistening envelope (called the dura), for all of its length, and the envelope contains a fluid. Between the envelope and the bony hole in the vertebrae is a space, through which nerves pass from the spinal cord on their way to and from the structures of the body (Fig. 13/1). The anaesthetist inserts a thin needle through the muscles of the mother's back, and with great care gets the tip to lie in the space between the dura and the bone – this is the epidural space. He pushes a fine polythene tube through the needle so that it is in the space, and then withdraws the needle, leaving the polythene tube in the space. He can now give a local anaesthetic into the epidural space, and, if needs be, keep 'topping' it up when the anaesthetic effect begins to wear off. 'Epidurals' have some problems. One of these is that an epidural may cause a fall in blood pressure to a very low level which is neither good for the mother nor her baby. Many anaesthetists try to avoid this by giving the woman an intravenous drip of 500ml of fluid before the anaesthetic is injected. About 10 per cent of women find the epidural does not work effectively and pain is still felt. Another 10 per cent complain that the epidural gives them 'shivers and shakes'.

For most women, who choose to have an epidural after having

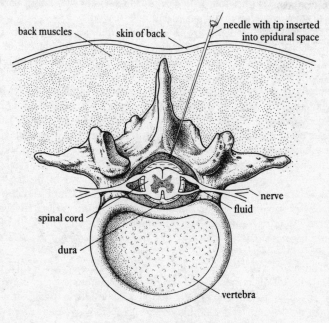

FIG. 13/1   Epidural anaesthesia.

discussed the potential benefits and possible hazards with the anaesthetist, the method relieves most of the pain of childbirth. And with
this type of anaesthesia, the mother has the joy of helping in the birth
of her baby, of seeing it being born, of hearing its first cry and of cuddling
it as soon as it is born.

Choices in pain relief

It is important to remember that a woman has the right to be informed
about the methods available to relieve the pain associated with childbirth, to discuss them with her chosen medical attendant, and to
choose which method she prefers. Whichever method she chooses, it is
the duty of those helping her during childbirth to inform her of the
progress of her labour, to obtain her co-operation and to treat her as
a participant in a wonderful process.

We have advanced a long way from the time when the Biblical curse
on Eve that 'in sorrow would she bring forth her children', dominated
men's minds.

CHAPTER 14

What to Expect in Labour

The mechanical processes which lead to the birth of the baby need to be understood by the expectant mother, so that she may have insight into what happens and what is expected of her. But she also needs to know what happens to her and what she is to do.

Late pregnancy and prelabour

In the last weeks of pregnancy, the baby is settling into its final position preparatory to birth. In the majority of first pregnancies the baby's head has settled into the pelvis and is exerting pressure on the pelvis, the rectum and the bladder. Varicose veins may become more obvious as the blood returning from the legs is dammed back; backache is more common; frequency of urination usual. The expectant mother, too, is becoming impatient. She wants to see and fondle the baby she has nurtured all these weeks. Sleep is less sound, and on hot nights sweating may be a problem. It is quite proper for the expectant mother to ask her doctor for sleeping tablets to help 'tide' her over these last few weeks; but most women adjust to the disturbed nights, and rest during the day to make up for it.

False labour

In these weeks, the uterus is increasingly sensitive, and the painless contractions which have been felt in the preceding weeks become more frequent. Painful contractions may also occur, usually at night and at irregular intervals. This is 'false labour', but it may be mistaken for the onset of true labour, and many an expectant mother has been admitted to hospital, only to be discharged home the next day. The difference between false and true labour is that the contractions in false labour

225

are irregular in duration, occur at irregular intervals, and rather than increasing in intensity, or strength, as times passes, diminish in intensity after a few hours and then disappear altogether. Often they occur at night, and are usually felt in the lower abdomen and back. This is in contrast to true labour, in which there is an increasing frequency and intensity of contractions, which develop an almost predictable regularity as time progresses. But no mother should be ashamed of having gone into hospital in false labour, as sometimes the two types are difficult to differentiate.

What to take into hospital

By this time the expectant mother will have prepared the things which she will require in hospital, and will often have a bag packed in readiness. What she needs depends to some extent on her own desires and local custom. In general, the bag should contain the following:

Nightdress or pyjamas (2 or 3 sets). Many women prefer pyjamas, and wear the top only. In many ways pyjamas are more convenient than nightdresses, particularly if the mother is going to breastfeed. A few hospitals, regrettably, insist that the patient wear a hospital gown. This is generally ugly. The practice is disappearing, and the sooner it goes, the better.

Bras Two nursing bras are usually required.

Bed jacket

Dressing gown. This is essential as 'early ambulation' is now normal, and patients are usually up and about within 6 to 24 hours of childbirth.

Bedroom slippers

Sanitary belt. Sanitary pads are usually supplied by the hospital, but some hospitals ask the patient to supply her own, and to bring them in before labour so that they may be sterilized.

Handkerchiefs or tissues

Toothpaste, toothbrush, toilet soap, washing flannel, nail brush, hairbrush, comb, hand mirror, cosmetics, perfume, talcum powder. Beauty may be in the eye of the beholder, and the new mother has every right to feel and be beautiful. But artefacts help in our society, and why not?

Writing paper, envelopes, stamps and a pen. It is surprising how many letters need to be written once the baby is born.

Books. The lying-in period is a time for rest, interspersed with moments of activity. Books fill in the time, although portable television sets are replacing them.

Baby clothes. A set for dressing the baby on discharge from hospital. Hospitals usually supply nightgowns and napkins (diapers) for the hospital period.

The onset of labour

The onset of true labour is announced by one or more of the following three signs:

(1) The onset of regular, rhythmic uterine contractions, which may be painful.
(2) The passage of a small amount of blood-tinged, sticky mucus from the vagina (the 'show').
(3) The 'gushing' of liquid from the vagina. This is due to rupture of the membranes which form the amniotic sac.

Regular painful contractions

If false labour has been experienced in the last weeks of pregnancy, the expectant mother may be able to detect a change in the character of the contractions, when true labour starts. If no false labour has been experienced, she will be able to determine if this is indeed true labour from the character of the contractions. The contractions of true labour initially last about 30 seconds, and occur at regular intervals of about 15 to 20 minutes. During the contraction, the uterus can be felt to become hard, and some degree of pain is felt, either only in the small of the back, or, as labour progresses, radiating from the flanks into the abdomen. In fact, as a rule the less backache there is, the more efficient is the labour. The pain begins as a small 'twinge', it increases to a peak, and diminishes to fade away entirely. In the opinion of many women, it is like a severe menstrual cramp.

As labour progresses, the duration of the contraction extends from 30 seconds to 90 seconds, the interval between contractions diminishes from 20 minutes to 3 or 5 minutes, and the intensity of the contraction increases.

In general, the woman should go into hospital when the contractions are regular and are recurring at about 10-minute intervals, but of course this is only 'in general', and individuals may feel the need to go into hospital earlier or later.

227

The 'show'

The discharge of bloodstained mucus precedes or accompanies the onset of painful contractions as often as it follows them. What has happened is that the 'plug' of mucus which has filled the cervical canal from early pregnancy is dislodged as the uterine contractions draw up (or 'efface') the cervix and begin to dilate it at the onset of labour. The discharge of the bloodstained mucus is called the 'show', and labour generally starts within 24 hours of its appearance.

Rupture of the membranes

In a few cases, labour is heralded by a sudden gash of liquid from the vagina. This occurs because the membranes of the amniotic sac, which lines the uterus and in which the baby has grown, suddenly rupture. This event may occur before term, or it may occur at term. In either event, the woman should go to the hospital without delay, so that she may be examined, as occasionally problems arise which need to be checked as soon as possible. In general, labour starts within a few hours of spontaneous rupture of the membranes. If labour has not started within 12 to 24 hours and the pregnancy is near term, the doctor will give an infusion of a drug called oxytocin, into an arm vein of the expectant mother, to hasten the onset of labour.

Admission to hospital

From time to time newspaper stories appear of women who failed to reach hospital in time, and the baby was born in the car, in a taxi, or perhaps on the front steps of the hospital. These occurrences are rare, and most expectant mothers get into hospital in good time.

For doctors and nurses a hospital is a familiar workplace; for the expectant mother it can be a strange and frightening place, where unbending people order her to do unpredictable things, and where everyone seems too busy to talk to her and to explain what is being done and why. This authoritarian, inhuman approach is fast going, and hospitals are becoming places in which *people* work to help other people. As childbirth is an essentially normal event, this humanist approach is even more important in a maternity hospital, and happily it is becoming much more common. One way in which an expectant mother can reduce her anxiety is to visit the hospital during pregnancy. Many hospital authorities co-operate in arranging these visits, when she can see the labour ward, or delivery floor, and the type of room, or ward, in which she will stay.

More is needed. Hospital authorities, at all levels, need to remember that a maternity ward must be run for the benefit of an informed woman who wishes to participate in the birth of her baby. Unfortunately some hospitals still 'depersonalize' the expectant mother from the moment of her admission. She is interviewed, apparently irrelevant questions are asked (for example, what is your husband's occupation), her pubic area is shaved, she may be given an enema and she is then put in an ugly, unglamorous hospital 'gown'. Most of this is unnecessary, as you will read.

Hospitals must review their procedures and reorganize their physical arrangements, to meet the expectations of the 'about-to-deliver' couple. The hospital should provide a comfortable, well-decorated lounge, which has coffee and toilet facilities for 'expectant fathers', in which the couple can walk about or sit if they wish, talking to other couples in the early part of labour. Hospitals should ensure that the rooms on the delivery floor are single rooms and are made as 'unclinical' as is compatible with hygiene and safety. The staff should be certain that no woman in labour is left alone at any time. If the woman wishes, the father of her child (or some other close relative) should be able to remain with her throughout the labour, including times when she is being examined.

Once her baby has been born, the child's father should be able to visit her whenever she wishes, and to remain with her as long as she wishes.

In addition, 'rooming-in' should be permitted without question if the mother desires it (p. 248). During the time she is in hospital, information and counselling on parenting, how to cope with the infant in the first weeks at home, child-development and family planning should be provided for her and the child's father. If hospitals do not provide such services at present, women's groups should exert pressure to make sure that they do as soon as is practicable.

What happens at present is that on admission, in early labour, the woman is examined by a doctor on the hospital staff or a nurse, who then informs the patient's own doctor, depending on the custom and staff pattern of the particular hospital. The first thing which is done is to determine if labour is really under way, and how far advanced it is. This information is obtained from the woman's description of what has happened in the preceding few hours, aided if necessary by an abdominal examination to find the position of the baby in the uterus. If labour is not far advanced, it is usual for the woman to change into a hospital gown and to get into bed, so that she may be 'prepared' for delivery. In the past this preparation was fairly complex; the woman had a hot bath, was given an enema, and the pubic and vulval hair was shaved. Today, the hot bath is replaced by a warm shower, if the patient feels she needs one. The enema is omitted, or replaced by the use of a small pill which is inserted into the back-passage, and induces bowel motion with much less discomfort and distress than did the enema. The 'complete' shave is reduced to shaving the area of the perineum, the hair on the pubis merely being clipped short. The old method of a complete shave was uncomfortable (nurses are not very skilful with a safety razor), undignified, the patient feeling that she looked like a 'plucked chiken', and not really necessary unless an abdominal operation was anticipated. It should also be questioned if a woman needs to wear a hospital gown. It is usually ugly, leaves the woman's back and bottom bare and depersonalizes her into a 'patient'. I can see no reason why a woman should not wear her own nightwear which is pleasant to look at and which makes the woman feel comfortable.

When the preliminaries are over, the resident doctor usually reviews the woman's antenatal record if this is available, and checks that she is not suffering from any infectious disease such as a cold. He then examines a specimen of urine and takes the woman's blood pressure. Next he re-examines the abdomen to make sure that the baby is lying normally, and that its head or its breech is fitting into the expectant mother's pelvis. He may also wish to perform a pelvic examination so that he can make a full evaluation of the progress of labour. This examination is in no way different from the pelvic examination performed in pregnancy, except that increased precautions are taken to avoid infection. While the doctor is cleaning his hands, the woman is placed on a sterile cloth and may put on leggings. The doctor cleans the vulval area with an antiseptic solution, and pours some obstetric antiseptic cream into the vagina. This not only prevents infection, but also renders the examination easier. During these examinations the doctor will be able to answer any questions which the patient may have.

The first stage of labour

The first stage of labour is the time during which the cervix must be drawn up and opened fully so that the birth-canal is established. It is a time when the expectant mother can actively do little to aid the delivery of her baby. It is a period of waiting intelligently, with the knowledge of the preparations for the birth of her child which are occurring within her body.

Since it is a period of waiting, more and more hospitals and obstetricians are coming to realize that during the first stage the patient requires to be in an atmosphere which is as homelike as possible, and only when the end of this stage is approaching does she need to be taken to the more antiseptic hospital-like surroundings of the delivery room. To meet the needs of this new philosophy, hospitals are building, or coverting other accommodation into first stage areas, which contain individual rooms and a commonroom, decorated pleasantly, furnished with comfortable chairs, and perhaps with a television set so that the patient may occupy her time more happily, often together with the baby's father.

As I mentioned earlier, some hospitals have developed this philosophy still further and provide birthing centres where the whole of childbirth can take place in a homelike environment.

Unfortunately, a few hospitals have not yet accepted this new approach to labour, and insist that a woman in the first stage of labour is confined to bed. Research has confirmed what midwives have long known, that labour is shorter and more comfortable if an expectant mother is allowed to walk about, to sit on a chair or to lie down during the first stage – using whichever position is most comfortable for her.

As has been noted, the patient who has insight into the processes of labour, and who has perhaps been to 'preparation of childbirth' classes in pregnancy, is much better equipped to cope with the first stage of labour. At some time it is likely that the contractions will become uncomfortably strong. When this occurs, the expectant mother usually wishes to go to bed, and may request pain-reducing drugs, which are readily available. She will also be confined to bed if the membranes have ruptured or if any other complication has been detected. In the first stage the woman should not lie on her back on a hard bed. She should either recline propped up on pillows supported so that she can lie at an angle of 45 degrees to the horizontal or lie on her side, as in this way she improves the flow of blood through the uterus, and provides more oxygen for her baby.

Can a woman have drinks and eat light food during labour? Doctors have different opinions about this, the fear being that if an operation requiring a general anaesthetic is needed, the woman may vomit and inhale the vomit into her lungs. Today with the increasing use of epidural anaesthesia for operative deliveries, the rule that a woman in labour should neither drink nor eat has been modified.

Many obstetricians permit a woman who is at low risk of requiring an operative delivery to drink tea, water or sweet drinks, or to eat toast or lightly boiled eggs during labour. Other obstetricians believe that all feeding, including drinks, taken by mouth should be avoided, and set up an intravenous infusion of fluid.

The second stage

This is the stage of expulsion of the baby from the warm womb into the outside world. This is the period when the active aid of the mother is required to help her baby be born. It is a time of some discomfort, which is reduced by epidural analgesia or by the injection of local anaesthetic into the tissues at the entrance of the vagina.

The help of the mother is needed. With each uterine contraction she takes in a big breath, filling her lungs with air. She then holds her breath, which makes her diaphragm rigid, and by contracting her lower chest and abdominal muscles, she pushes down, adding a further expulsive effort. Often she finds that she can get a better 'push' if she lifts her head and clasps her legs, drawing them up on to her abdomen (Fig. 14/1). During a contraction she works hard, between contractions she relaxes completely. At this time, many women wish to dull the discomfort caused by the contraction. If she does she may choose between breathing 'gas and oxygen' from an Entotox machine, or have an epidural anaesthetic.

At last the baby's head appears, stretching the tissues of the

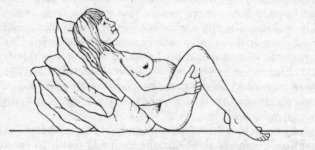

FIG. 14/1   The ideal position for childbirth.

perineum. Rather than allowing the perineum to tear jaggedly, as may happen, the doctor often makes a deliberate small cut with scissors. This is called an 'episiotomy'. It is easier to stitch, is much less painful if stitched properly (in fact using one technique it is virtually painless), and usually heals better, than does a tear.

Unfortunately there are many ways of making and of stitching an episiotomy, and many women find that it causes considerable discomfort, or pain, in the first few days after childbirth. There is also much discussion by women whether or not their episiotomy was done unnecessarily. Studies in Australia and Britain show that between 55 and 85 per cent of women have an episiotomy performed during childbirth. Many women are not told about the operation, or the need for it. In some cases the operation is performed before the tissues of the perineum are stretched by the baby's head. This is too early. Most women have discomfort or severe pain. Twelve weeks after the birth 5 per cent of women still have moderate pain in the perineum, 15 per cent still have discomfort and 15 per cent find that sexual intercourse is painful. Most of these complications can be avoided if the doctor uses a careful technique and does not use an episiotomy as a way of hurrying up the birth.

In view of these findings a woman may find it helpful, during pregnancy, to discuss the whole question of episiotomy with the doctor, so that she can determine his views and learn of the technique he uses.

A final push 'crowns' the baby's head and the doctor now helps in delivering the baby. The expectant mother only pushes when she is asked to do so, instead panting quietly as the baby is slowly and gently born. The birth of the baby from 'crowning of the head' takes about 2 or 3 minutes, and many doctors give an injection at this time to expel the placenta more rapidly. But not all agree that this is necessary.

If the mother wishes, she can see her baby being born. She is propped up with pillows or her partner's help and can watch her baby's head emerging through her vulva into the world. Quickly the baby slips out of her body to lie between her legs. The baby takes its first breath and cries.

The doctor checks that the baby is normal – and over 97 per cent are. The umbilical cord, which has been its lifeline for 40 weeks, ceases to pulsate and is cut.

Most doctors now give the baby to the mother to be cuddled naked against her body so that she and the baby's father can celebrate its arrival and begin the bonding process.

233

Labour should be as pleasant and enjoyable a process as possible and both doctor and nurses should try to make the mother as comfortable as possible by creating a quiet, happy environment. This idea has been extended by the French obstetrician, Dr Leboyer, who believes that the passage of the baby into the world and its adaptation to life outside the uterus should be gentle, or problems will arise later. Some of his views are exaggerated, but the principles he holds are good. The environment of the delivery room should be as 'homely' as is compatible with the need for cleanliness and good observation of the mother during labour. The light in the delivery room should not be more than that needed for the medical attendants to be able to see what they are doing and to ensure the safety of the baby's birth. The attendants should be supportive, communicative and helpful. They should let you see and cuddle your baby; after all you have waited 40 weeks for this exciting moment! De Leboyer believes that a baby should not cry at birth and should be put in warm water until it adjusts to the different environment. There is much dispute about this view, as the cry a baby makes at birth is necessary for it to fill its lungs with oxygen for the first time, and I believe it better for the baby to be cuddled by its mother – so that it has the warmth and contact of her body, rather than the impersonal warmth of a bath. In fact, a careful investigation at McMaster University into Leboyer births and those conducted in a gently conventional manner failed to show that the Leboyer procedure had any influence on the behaviour or the development, mental or physical, of the baby up to the age of 8 months. Nevertheless, the influence of Dr Leboyer is beneficial if it induces obstetricians to think more of the human aspect of childbirth and less of the mechanical processes of parturition.

The third stage

The third and final stage of labour is the time during which the placenta is expelled. It rarely lasts for more than 20 minutes, and is painless. Usually, today, the doctor assists the expulsion of the placenta by pressure upwards on the abdomen just above the public bone, and by gently pulling on the cut cord at the same time. A small amount of bleeding is usual during the third stage, but it is less than 300ml (½ pint) in most cases, particularly if the injection mentioned earlier has been given. The injection makes the uterus contract firmly, and the blood vessels which have supplied the placenta are squeezed tightly in the lattice of muscle fibres.

Labour is over. The episiotomy is stitched. The proper repair of a torn perineum, or of an episiotomy, is important, as the discomfort can make the new mother's first few days uncomfortable and the idea of a 'damaged' part of her genital area can disturb her body image. It is a good idea to ask for a mirror so that you can look at your perineum when the stitches have been taken out (if that needs to be done), so that you can see how normal it is.

The mother, no longer expectant but fulfilled, is washed and powdered. She relaxes and sometimes sleeps while the nurses check that the uterus is contracted, and about one hour after delivery she returns to her room in the lying-in ward. She is emotionally happy. She has done a unique and wonderful thing.

The father in labour

What of the father? It was his spermatozoon which fertilized the egg; it is he who has contributed half of the genes to the child. What is his place in labour? This depends greatly on custom and culture. In some tribal societies the man undergoes a mock labour, is pampered and cosseted during the time his wife, either alone or attended by a single female, delivers her child. In other societies, the man is excluded from the vicinity of the place where the woman has her baby, and is expected to ignore the whole episode, holding that it never happened.

In modern Western society, there is a trend to involve the father in the process of childbirth. He, as well as the mother, reads about the process of growth of the child in the uterus; he learns about the course of labour; together they are involved in the sequence of events leading up to childbirth. This approach has much to commend it. It culminates in the presence of the father during childbirth. In the first stage of labour he remains with his wife, so that in the unfamiliar surroundings of the hospital, she has someone whom she knows, loves and with whom she can share her experiences. An expectant mother should never be left alone in labour. This idea is often difficult to achieve, and the presence of the father can be invaluable. In the second stage of labour, he sits by the head of the delivery bed, or behind her on the bed supporting and attending to his wife, encouraging her, being involved with her. Together they witness the birth of the baby, and together their emotional bonds are strengthened. In using this method for some years, I have observed its value repeatedly; and the look of joy on the faces of father and mother as together they help in the delivery of their child is wonderful.

The question which must be answered is, 'Who decides that the father shall attend the birth of the baby?' The answer is simple, unequivocal: the mother. If the expectant mother wants the baby's father to be present, and *only* if she wants him, may he attend. Certainly it may be necessary to ask him to leave if some operative procedure is required or some untoward event occurs, but if this has been discussed during pregnancy, no difficulty should arise.

Childbirth – a woman's choice

Until very recently women usually went into labour at a specific, but usually unpredictable, time when the pregnancy had lasted about 40 weeks. Labour started and continued for a variable number of hours, interference only taking place if the baby's life seemed threatened or, in rare cases, if the life of the expectant mother was at risk. This 'hands off' philosophy meant that about 1 woman in 10 had a labour which lasted for more than 24 hours, and some women laboured for days. This attitude has changed. Today it is unusual for a woman to continue in true labour for more than 24 hours without help being given to deliver her of her baby, and many doctors intervene if a woman has been in true labour for more than 12 hours. What I have written does not apply to women in 'false labour', so some women continue to feel that they have been in labour for days, usually because no one has bothered to explain what was happening.

The change to earlier 'interference' has been beneficial in that expectant mothers have been spared hours of pain and it has reduced the threat to the baby which occurs if labour is prolonged. It has also had the effect of permitting a different attitude, by doctors, to labour.

Today, a woman can choose one of three ways for her labour to be conducted. These ways are first, 'prepared' childbirth; second, traditional childbirth and third, elective childbirth. Of course, the choice may have to be altered if something occurs in late pregnancy or during the labour which threatens the life of the baby.

Prepared or natural childbirth

In natural (or prepared) childbirth, the woman and her partner have received instruction in antenatal class and have been prepared for childbirth. The woman goes into labour spontaneously and expects to have her partner with her during labour, to receive few or no drugs and to be delivered without the aid of instruments, although she may require an episiotomy. The method is splendid for those women who prefer it and who are attended by sympathetic, helpful, communicative medical attendants. A woman opting for this way of having a baby should be able to choose to have the baby in a traditional hospital delivery room or in a birthing centre. More hospitals should develop birthing centres so that a pregnant couple may have this as a choice for the birth of their baby. Of course, if the labour lasts for more than 12 hours, the doctor may decide to intervene, but usually only does so after discussion with the expectant mother.

Traditional childbirth

The woman goes into labour spontaneously and is given drugs as needed. In the active part of the first stage and in the second stage, she may choose an inhalational analgesic, or request an epidural anaesthetic. If labour is progressing more slowly than expected, she may be given an intravenous drip into an arm vein. This drip contains a drug called Syntocinon which has the effect of stimulating the uterus to contract more strongly, so that the duration of labour is reduced.

Traditionally, the progress of the labour is followed and notes are made by the nursing staff. The nurses make sure that the expectant mother is not becoming dehydrated and check her pulse rate, her temperature and her blood pressure at intervals. They also examine her abdomen to see how deeply the baby's head is settling into the mother's pelvis, and to check on the frequency and strength of the uterine contractions. (These examinations are also made in women who have chosen natural childbirth.)

Recently a change in management has occurred which I believe to be an improvement. The nurses make the same observations, but instead of writing notes, they mark them on a special chart, called a partogram, which gives a visual display of the progress of labour. By studying a large number of partograms, doctors have been able to determine more accurately how labour normally progresses. They have found, for example, that the cervix normally dilates, or opens, at a fairly steady rate, once labour is established, and they can anticipate how much dilated it is expected to be after any chosen number of hours of labour. They have recommended that if the dilatation of the cervix is lagging two or more hours behind what it was expected to be, labour should be encouraged by setting up an intravenous drip containing Syntocinon. If this method is chosen, as it is increasingly, a woman in labour needs to be examined vaginally every 2 hours as well as abdominally so that the degree to which the cervix is dilated can be estimated accurately. The value of using partograms is that the duration of labour is reduced but the doctor only intervenes to set up the drip if progress is slow. Since delivery is often accelerated it is also called accelerated labour.

Elective childbirth

In this method the woman and her doctor decide beforehand on what day childbirth will take place. Of course, the choice of the day is only finally confirmed when everything is ready. This means, in general, that the pregnancy is near term, that the baby's head has settled snugly into the woman's pelvis and that the cervix is soft, shortened and at least 2 centimetres dilated.

On the elected day, the woman comes into hospital early in the morning. The doctor examines her to confirm his findings and then breaks the bag of waters with a special instrument. This procedure is called an amniotomy. At the same time he sets up an intravenous drip containing Syntocinon which stimulates the uterus to contract. Syntocinon is run at a rate which is increased until the uterine contractions occur regularly and strongly at about 3-minute intervals and each lasts about 90 seconds. The rate at which the drip flows is adjusted by a nurse who has to be in attendance constantly so that the dangers of too fast a drip are avoided. If the drip runs in too fast it may make the uterine contractions too strong and too frequent so that the baby fails to get enough oxygen from the mother's blood, and its life is in danger. Many hospitals now use an automatic infusion pump, which automatically regulates the rate of the drip, increasing or slowing the rate if the contractions are too infrequent or too frequent.

Because of the possible risk to the baby from the intravenous drip its heart rate is monitored by a machine called a fetal heart monitor. The changes in the rate of the baby's heart are electronically converted into a pictorial graph on the machine and give a good indication of whether or not it is getting sufficient oxygen.

Once labour is properly established, an epidural anaesthetic is started, so the woman feels no pain. Labour continues in this way and most women can be expected to give birth within 12 hours. If this does not occur the doctor usually recommends that a caesarean section should be performed, or may permit the woman to sleep and repeat the intravenous drip on the next day.

You can see that the advantage of elective childbirth is that you know the day on which your baby will be born, and can plan accordingly; you know that you will only be in labour for 12 hours at the longest and that your baby will be born by the evening. You can also be pretty sure that your doctor will be present to deliver your baby because he or she can arrange his work load better, and can keep himself free of other activities on the day he electively induces your labour and augments the uterine contractions with the intravenous drip.

The disadvantages are that the method requires a good deal of electronic equipment and constant observation by a nurse which makes labour a mechanical, impersonal process. A further disadvantage is that a woman who chooses this method for the delivery of her baby should be aware that although the duration of labour is reduced and she knows that she will deliver her baby on a certain day, the chances of her having a caesarean section are doubled, to between 7 and 12 per cent of all elective inductions, and that a larger number of babies become jaundiced in the first week of life.

It is also essential that the woman and her doctor are sure that the pregnancy has reached its full duration and that the baby is not premature. As I have written earlier, the best way of making sure is for a woman to be examined in the first 10 weeks of pregnancy. But if she has not been examined, or if an ultrasound examination has not been made in the first half of pregnancy, an amniocentesis has to be performed. This involves putting a needle into the fluid surrounding the baby and taking a sample. The needle is pushed into the amniotic sac through the mother's abdomen, and the fluid is tested for certain chemical substances which indicate that the baby is mature.

What I have tried to suggest is that today there are different approaches to labour, but the final choice is the woman's, provided of course that nothing occurs which makes it necessary for the doctor to intervene to rescue your baby from a hostile environment. You are having a baby: you should be able to choose how you want to have it after discussion with your doctor.

The baby after birth

The mother gives one further push, her husband sits beside her encouraging her. Her doctor, or the nurse attending her, gently and skilfully steers the baby's head through her vulva, so that it is born. Mucus streams from its nose and mouth; its mouth moves in sucking motions; and it may open its eyes. A further contraction occurs, the mother gently pushes and the baby slips out, still guided by the doctor, to lie on the bed between the mother's legs. It is born. It blinks its eyes; it jerks its arms and legs, clasping and extending its fingers. The umbilical cord, which has been its lifeline for so long, still beats. The nurse sucks its mouth clear of mucus with a rubber tube attached to a suction bulb if necessary, and the baby is given to its mother to cuddle. It takes in a breath and cries for all to hear.

The baby, which has grown from a single cell only visible under the microscope, has now developed into a living being made up of millions upon millions of cells. Some are formed into complex organs; some into bone; some into skin; some into the blood which carries the life-giving oxygen around the body. Its colour becomes pinker and pinker, the umbilical cord stops beating. It is cut. The baby is an independent, perverse, beautiful, irritating, intelligent, dependent individual. Which characteristics it will develop depends to a large extent upon its inheritance, but to no small extent upon the upbringing it will receive from its mother and father. The attitudes it will adopt will largely be theirs.

What does it look like, this newborn infant, as it lies crying between its mother's legs, or cuddled within her arms? It will be about 50cm (20in) long and will weigh anything from 2500g (5½lb) to 4500g (10lb) – with an average of 3400g (7lb 7oz). Its birthweight depends on several factors, such as the physique of its parents, its race, whether or not its mother was ill in pregnancy, and the socio-economic level of its parents. But between these weights, the baby will be normal and healthy, and cause no anxiety.

Its head is rounded, the bones firm, although still separated to leave a diamond-shaped soft space above the forehead and a Y-shaped edge at the back of the head. The baby's brain will grow in the first years of life, and the separation of the bones enables the skull to expand easily. Its head is likely to be covered with fine hair, but some babies are almost bald. You cannot tell from this how its hair will grow later, nor whether it will be prematurely bald! Its ears stand out firmly. Its nose is developed. Its eyes open and blink, but are a slate-grey colour. The real colour of its eyes come later. Its mouth moves as it makes sucking noises or cries. Its body is rounded; its skin smooth. The lanugo hair which covered it in the uterus has gone, except on its shoulders. Its arms and legs are normal, and the fingers and toes have nails which project beyond their tips. It moves its arms and legs, and if a loud sound is made near it, jerks them convulsively. Its genitals are normal. If a boy, the penis hangs limply, the foreskin projecting beyond its tip, and the testicles are in the scrotum. If a girl, the labia majora are well developed and in contact, so that the vulva is concealed.

It lies peacefully, breathing gently, moving its limbs from time to time. It is this miracle of life which the mother has fed in her womb for the 40 weeks, and has now expelled during the hours of labour (Fig. 14/2).

As soon as possible after birth, the baby should be given, preferably naked, to the mother so that she can touch and cuddle him, and let him suckle her breast. This simple procedure has been found to be

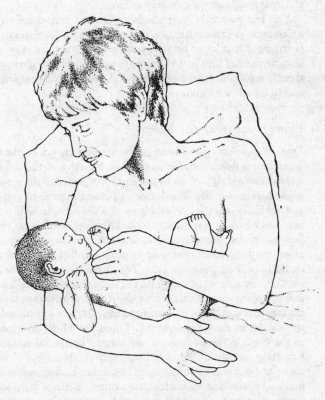

FIG. 14/2   The newborn baby held in its mother's arms.

important in letting the mother and baby interact or 'bond' with each other. The mother, the baby's father and the baby should be given time to learn to enjoy each other and to celebrate the birth. They should be allowed this time before the procedures of checking the baby fully, bathing him and dressing him are done. Mother–baby bonding in this way immediately after birth, and interaction between mother and baby for periods in the first days of life have been shown to influence mothering behaviour favourably for a long period. It has also been found that the baby's behaviour is favourably influenced by bonding. Babies who have had this contact with their mother in the first hours after birth show more affectionate behaviour, such as smiling, laughing and responding, and less crying, at the of 2 months, than babies who are separated from their mother at birth.

You and your baby have a right to interact immediately after birth, unless there is a medical reason that you can't. If, for example, the baby is having difficulty in breathing, or is premature, he may need to be resuscitated and kept in a Humidicrib in a special care nursery. But even then, it is possible for mothers to visit their baby in the nursery, to touch and to 'bond' with him.

Examination of the baby

Over 97 per cent of newborn babies are perfect, but in the remaining 3 per cent a defect may be found. The majority of the defects can be treated successfully, often by surgery, provided that they are detected in the first days of life. The doctor will examine the baby systematically and carefully once its breathing is established. He will examine its head, and look into its mouth to make sure that it has no cleft palate. Because of the pressure on the head of the baby during its passage along the birth-canal, the scalp is often swollen and misshapen, particularly over its posterior part. The swelling is due to congestion of the skin and seeping of fluid into the scalp tissues. It is called a 'caput', and disappears completely within three days. The doctor will then test the movement of the baby's arms and legs, and will pay special attention to its hips, as there is a congenital condition which causes dislocation of the hips. If this is detected and treated by special splinting in the first three months of life, it is completely curable. He will listen to its chest, and examine its abdomen. In particular, he will look at its genitals and make sure that its testicles are normal if it is a boy, and that its vagina is properly formed if it is a girl. Some of the congenital defects cannot be detected by examination – one of these is a strange, and rare, defect called phenylketonuria. If this is not detected early in life, accumulation of a certain substance in the body can lead to mental retardation of the child. Only 1 in 10 000 babies has the defect, but it is now considered that all babies should be tested in the first week of life. The test is quite simple. A sample of the baby's blood is placed on a specially treated piece of paper, which stains if the baby has the defect. Treatment is to give a diet which does not contain phenylalanine, the offending substance.

As many newborn babies have low blood levels of vitamin K_1, which may predispose the baby to bleed internally, most doctors recommend that all newborn babies are given the vitamin, either by injection soon after birth, or by mouth during the baby's first feed.

Bonding

Studies in 1970s, particularly by Dr Marshall Klaus in the USA, have shown that the relationship between parents and their baby is stronger, and the baby thrives better, if they are given the opportunity to 'bond' in the days after birth. If the couple experience labour and childbirth together, and then cuddle and learn about their newborn baby, the problems of failure-to-thrive, of anxiety and even perhaps of baby battering are reduced considerably.

Bonding occurs when the mother and father of the child have close contact with the baby. Ideally, it begins immediately after birth, the naked baby being given so that it may nuzzle its mother's nipple and feel the warmth of her body. The attachment between parents and baby is further encouraged by rooming-in and by the involvement of the parents in the care of their baby while in hospital.

Although early contact between baby and parents is ideal, mothers who for various reasons are unable to make this contact must not feel guilty or deprived, as it is not essential for subsequent good parenting, provided mother, father and baby can be in close contact in the first days after birth.

The first bath

It was traditional that soon after birth the baby was weighed (everyone wants to know its weight!) and then bathed. The white, greasy vernix was washed off with soap and water, and the baby powdered and dressed, to be admired by all. It is now known that this method of bathing the baby removed all the protective grease from its skin, and permitted the germs in the air, or blown from its mother's mouth and nose, to settle on the skin, to grow and cause infections. Today, in general, babies are not bathed. Their skin is cleaned with a cleansing agents which is also antiseptic, called pHisohex, but not all the vernix is removed, a fine, invisible layer remaining. Since hospitals have used this method, the incidence of skin infection in babies has dropped very considerably.

Circumcision

The Jews circumcise their boys on the 8th day of life to fulfil Abrahams's covenant with God; the Muslims circumcise their boys at puberty as a symbol of reaching manhood; Aboriginal tribes in the Australian desert circumcise their boys, partly ceremonially as an initiation to manhood, partly for hygiene as the desert sand can irritate the foreskin. Circumcision of males has a long religious tradition; but in modern times, in the USA and Australia particularly, it has become a routine performance, not for religious reasons, but because it is the custom. It is said that mothers demand it, doctors profit by it, and babies cannot complain about it. The reasons given are that removal of the foreskin makes the penis cleaner, prevents masturbation, makes it less sensitive so that ejaculation is delayed in coitus, prevents cancer of the cervix in women, and prevents cancer of the penis in men. The evidence for all these arguments, except the last, is very shaky. The normal foreskin is adherent to the glans of the penis until the infant is 2 to 3 years of age. There is no need to try to pull back the foreskin until the boy is 4 years old, when gentle retraction may be practised. By the age of 5, the boy can be taught to do this when he is in the shower or a bath. This will keep the penis 'clean'. It will not fix his mind on sex. Nor does the absence of a foreskin prevent masturbation, which anyhow is a normal activity. Circumcision does not improve a man's sexual performance, nor does it decrease it: it has no effect. There is no evidence, at all, that secretions which may be found under the foreskin cause cancer of the cervix in women, although many researchers have tried to prove this. The only men who develop cancer of the foreskin are those who are unhygienic. If as children they had been taught to draw back the foreskin and to clean it, cancer would not have occurred.

None of the so-called medical reasons for circumcision are valid, and there is strong evidence that the foreskin *protects* the glans of the penis, which is a delicate, sensitive structure. Circumcised babies may develop tiny ulcers around the 'eye' of the glans, and in a few cases have developed a tightness of the opening, which causes pain on urination. Although these are minor happenings, they suggest that the foreskin has a protective function, especially in infancy.

The decision whether the baby shall be circumcised is, of course, that of the parents, but they should consider the evidence before they decide, and not decide just because 'everyone has it done, and he will feel different from his friends if he hasn't been circumcised'. That is not a reason at all.

CHAPTER 15

Lying-in and Going Home

The puerperium is the time during which the genital organs, particularly the uterus, slowly return to their non-pregnant state, and when all the other changes which occurred in pregnancy disappear. This period lasts about 8 weeks.

Traditionally the first part of the puerperium was a time of 'lying-in'. It was a time when the woman was kept away from others (particularly men) because she was losing a bloody substance from her vagina and was therefore 'unclean'. It was not realized at that time that the bloody substance, called lochia, was a mixture of blood and the breakdown products of tissues discharged as the uterus slowly became smaller and more like a non-pregnant uterus. The tradition of segregation during the lying-in period has largely gone, but many of the surrounding influences, such as the belief that the woman was unclean, have persisted until quite recently.

Up to thirty years ago, women in the first weeks of the puerperium have been treated as ignorant, idle, ill women who required careful discipline so that they did not damage themselves, and who were expected to fit into hospital routine, however ridiculous, with humbleness and without question. The medical staff 'knew' that if the patient got up before the seventh day after childbirth, prolapse of the uterus would result. So the patient was confined to bed, she found difficulty in passing urine and became constipated. When she did get out of bed, her muscles were so weak that her first steps were faltering. These changes confirmed in the medical attendants' eyes that a puerperal woman was a 'sick woman'. They knew this despite the evidence that in many lands women started work very soon after childbirth without ill effect. Women are often emotional after childbirth which is, after all, a most moving experience, and the mood changes again confirmed the opinion that the patient was ill. For three decades, the baby was separated from the mother and placed in a nursery to be observed by the father like watching fish in an aquarium, and to be brought out for feeding to the mother, who was treated like a battery hen.

Today a new and more sensible approach dominates the care of the puerperal woman. This new philosophy recognizes that the puerperal woman is an intelligent, healthy individual, who has just achieved a most memorable event: she has given birth to a live, healthy baby. She is a person who is subject to emotional moods, for childbirth is a heady thing. She will have to adjust to the demands which the infant will make on her life. This can be difficult, but is less so if she is treated with helpful understanding in the early days of puerperium, and has received adequate instruction in the 'right approach to parentcraft' during pregnancy.

She is a person who is anxious to see, to touch and to care for her child with the helpful co-operation of the nursing staff. Of course, there may be problems, but most of these can be readily overcome.

The new approach to the puerperium makes three main points. First, although more rest is needed in the early days, the patient should be able to get up and walk about as soon as she wishes. Second, it is far better from many points of view for the baby to 'room-in' with the mother. Third, mother and baby can go home not on a fixed day, but when conditions are most suitable for them.

Rest

Immediately after the drama of childbirth and the excitement of celebrating the birth of the baby most women are full of emotional well-being and rather tired. Most women sleep for a while, a few asking for a sedative as they are too excited to sleep. When the mother wakes she will certainly want to see and hold her baby, and from this time it may well join her in her room. She can get out of bed when she likes, but many women prefer to stay in bed for the first 24 hours, and luxuriate in rest! After this time she should get up, and walk about. It improves the tone of her muscles, it increases the blood flow through her tissues, and it enhances the drainage of the lochia. Moreover, women who practise early ambulation feel much fitter. Swabbing rounds and bed-pans (which are revolting but necessary things) are no longer required. The new mother still requires rest, but she can get this by having a siesta of two hours between lunch-time and visiting time. In many hospitals visiting hours are becoming much more generous, as they should be, and children are allowed to visit their mother and newly born brother or sister.

Rooming-in

Rooming-in means that the baby remains in a cot beside its mother's bed for all, or most of the day and night The advantages of rooming-in are that it helps the mother become accustomed to her baby, to adjust to it, to learn its behaviour and to interpret its needs at a time when experienced help is available to reassure her that she is coping appropriately. Rooming-in also has the advantage that the mother-and-baby are treated as a single set or unit and the dangers of cross-infection between babies is reduced to a minimum. Rooming-in helps in the bonding process between mother and baby, and makes it easier for the mother to establish breast-feeding.

While rooming-in should be offered to all mothers and its adoption actively encouraged, some mothers may prefer to leave the baby in the nursery, either because they are too tired, or anxious or, sometimes, after a caesarean section. In some cases, the baby may have to be cared for in a nursery because it is premature or ill. But most mothers choose 'rooming-in' so that they can see, touch and cuddle their baby when they want, rather than seeing him through the nursery window and only touching him at feeding time.

Getting to know your baby

Unfortunately some hospitals seem to be organized more for the benefit of the staff than for the mothers and the babies. Hospital routines become fixed and are followed without thought for the real needs of the mother. Such routines can be destructive to the period of adjustment every woman has to go through as she gets to know her baby.

Rooming-in helps a good deal and even more important is the help given by informed, unhurried, communicative staff. It may surprise you that many women find that at first they do not feel an overwhelming love for their newborn baby. They have been taught that once the baby is born, they will find that they have a sudden burst of mother-love, ony to be disappointed, when the baby has been born, that it is not there. The baby is neither as exceptionally beautiful nor as cuddly as the new mother had expected. The lack of a surge of mother-love can induce guilt, but a woman should know that this is normal. Mother-love does not happen instantaneously. It takes time to get to know your baby, and you will find quite quickly that you have fallen in love with it. The development of mother-love is helped by rooming-in and particularly by cuddling, yet in some hospitals neither is encouraged. Cuddling, which means body contact, is a strong force in helping you create the bonds of love which unite you with your baby. Touch, body contact, is equally important to your baby because it gives it the feeling of warmth and security it needs. The cuddled baby is the contented baby. You cannot cuddle your baby too much. You will not spoil it, whatever the old wives say.

The lochia

The three most obvious indications that the mother is no longer pregnant are that her stomach is at last flat, or at least flatter than it was, that she has a baby to feed and care for, and that she is discharging lochia. The lochia is the bloody discharge from the uterus which is now shrinking back (or involuting) to its normal size. During pregnancy the uterus was the capsule within which the fetus lived and grew. It protected the fetus from the outside environment; it provided for its nourishment through the placenta; and finally, by its muscular contractions it expelled the baby into the world. Now these functions are over, the uterus undergoes involution. Immediately after birth it weighs 1000g (2¹/₅lb) and can be felt as a firm, globular bulge reaching up to the umbilicus. By the 14th day after childbirth, it will have shrunk to 350g (11oz), and can no longer be felt in the abdomen. By the 60th day (8 weeks) after childbirth, it is back to normal size. Involution is brought about by a shrivelling-up of the muscle fibres and the absorption of their substance, partly into the bloodstream and partly into the lochia. The lochia is made up of blood from the site where the placenta was attached, and the crumbling of the lining of the uterus which had developed so greatly in pregnancy. In the first 5 days after childbirth, the lochia mostly consists of blood, and is consequently red in colour. For the next 5 to 10 days, it is reddish-brown as the blood loss lessens and more of the uterine lining is expelled. By the 12th day, it has become pale, either yellowish or white; and the discharge may persist, varying in amount, for up to six weeks. However, in most cases the discharge has ceased by the end of the third week. The duration of the red lochia varies very considerably, and occasionally it continues for 10 or more days, or episodes of red lochia may recur in the following weeks. They often follow urination, particularly when the mother is not breast-feeding her baby. If the red lochia persists for longer than three weeks, if it becomes as profuse as the amount lost on the first day of a menstrual period, or if clots are passed, the doctor should be consulted.

Perineal pain

If a woman has had a tear of the perineum during the birth of the baby or had an episiotomy (page 233) she is likely to experience pain in the perineum. This may be mild or severe and may persist for several weeks, and sometimes for months. Perineal pain is discussed on page 233.

After-pains

After delivery, the uterus does not stop contracting. The contractions continue painlessly for the most part, but in some women, particularly multigravidae, painful contractions persist in the first few days of the puerperium, and may require analgesics. They are especially likely to occur during breast-feeding.

Backache

Backache affects one woman in five in the weeks (or occasionally months) after childbirth. Backache appears to be more common if the woman has had an epidural anaesthetic or a long second stage of labour. Some women also report having an ache in the neck or shoulders. There is no specific treatment and the backache gets better by itself. Whilst it persists the woman should avoid lifting heavy objects if this is possible.

Bowels

In the past constipation was a problem, but today with early ambulation it is less so. Should a patient become constipated and feel uncomfortable, she should ask for treatment. Usually a gentle laxative, such as Senokot, or a rectal suppository, such as bisacodyl, is given.

Haemorrhoids

As mentioned on page 193, haemorrhoids often occur during pregnancy. They may also occur during childbirth. Although the haemorrhoids usually get smaller in the post natal period, in a number of women they persist and cause discomfort. Treatment is to use analgesic ointments and to try to push the haemorrhoids inside the anal canal after the woman has opened her bowels.

Urination

In the first 24 hours after childbirth, the mother sometimes finds it difficult to pass urine because of the stretching during delivery of the vaginal tissues and the tissues around the bladder. Early ambulation helps, and in fact most women have no trouble.

Urinary incontinence

Some women find that they have difficulty in controlling their urine and have episodes of wetting themselves in the weeks or months after childbirth. The condition is improved if the woman starts 'pelvic exercises' soon after childbirth.

Diet

The old music hall song 'A little bit of what you fancy does you good' applies in the puerperium. Most women want a meal, certainly a cup of tea, after delivery; and in the puerperium a good wholesome diet, rich in protein and vitamins and complex carbohydrates, is needed. Most nutritionists recommend that the puerperal woman who breast-feeds should get at least 2500 calories (10 500kJ) a day. The diet of a puerperal mother should be as generous as that she took during pregnancy, with an additional 500ml (1 pint) of milk a day (some of which may be used in cooking).

Third-day blues

On about the third day of the puerperium, the excitement of the new baby has diminished a bit. The mother has found that she has an independent, demanding infant to cope with, milk may be filling her breasts, which may be tender, and the emotional sensitivity noted earlier may produce a reaction. Depression, mood changes or fits of crying occur. Everything is going well, but suddenly the patient bursts into a sobbing fit, and after the episode feels better. The thing to remember is that 'third-day blues' (which may occur on the fourth or fifth day) are not uncommon, and need sympathetic understanding from the husband and the medical attendants. Often the 'third-day blues' merge into the 'crisis of parenthood'.

Exercises

After giving birth whether normally, or following a forceps delivery or a caesarean section, the mother is encouraged to get out of bed and, within reason, to begin normal activities.

In nearly all maternity units and hospitals, postnatal exercise classes conducted by physiotherapists are available. In these classes the focus is on such things as postural dynamics, abdominal muscle restoration, pelvic floor re-education, and relaxation and stress management. A physiotherapist is available to assess the woman's body mechanics and identify specific postnatal problems, such as backache or incontinence, and adapt the exercise programme accordingly. Advice is given on each woman's exercise needs and preferences on returning home, and a printed sheet of essential postnatal exercises to be done in hospital and at home is given to each woman.

Guidelines for exercise programmes in the longer term include six main considerations.

(1) The exercise programme must not compromise the lower back before it has regained its normal strength and function.
(2) The abdominal muscles need to regain their normal strength and tone.
(3) The pelvic floor muscles need have not only to support the pelvic and abdominal contents and maintain bowel and bladder (sphincter) control, but also have to withhold the added stress being placed upon them by exercise.
(4) Postural awareness needs to be part of the exercise programme.
(5) The exercise programme needs to have positive psychological benefits.
(6) The exercise programme should not interfere with the emotional relationship between the woman and her baby.

For those women who have never exercised, and may never exercise, it is of value to be reminded of the wondrous healing nature of the human body. They need to be aware of their posture and learn to incorporate pelvic floor exercises into their daily routine, and take care to lift and carry correctly, leaving the heavy things for their partner. They need to rest when their body tells them to, take time out just for themselves sometimes, and they need to be patient with themselves as they adjust physically and emotionally to this new phase of life.

Visitors

In the matter of visitors, attitudes are changing. At one stage only the husband might visit, and this had a venerable tradition. In the seventeenth century, a great French obstetrician referring to the habit of holding a party on the third day of puerperium when the child was baptized, wrote, 'Though there is scarce any of the company, which do not drink her health, yet by the noise they make in her ears, she loses it.'

Today it is realized that this attitude is unnecessarily restrictive. The husband should be allowed to visit at any time of the day, and it is nonsense to say that this interferes with hospital routine; the hospital is there for the patient, and not the patient for the hospital. Other visitors should be permitted at specific times each day, but should inquire first if they may visit. Each woman feels differently about visitors: some women want very few, preferring to be with their husbands; others want to keep in touch with their friends. But the friends should realize that the demands of a young baby, and the odd schedule of early waking found in hospitals, may make the mother very tired. For this reason, visits should be cut short. The visitor can always see the mother when she goes home, and nowadays this is tending to be sooner after childbirth.

Adjusting to being a parent: the 'crisis of parenthood'

Unfortunately in most maternity units or hospitals, the mother is not encouraged to ask the questions which trouble her, and has little opportunity to make any real contact with a changing, busy nursing staff (who often give conflicting advice) and a busy, often uncommunicative doctor. Because of the routine of many hospitals, which excludes rooming-in and restricts the time her husband or some other close relative can visit her, the mother may have difficulty in learning to know her baby and to understand the altered relationship she will have with her husband on her return home.

After her return home, 5 to 10 days after childbirth, she may become increasingly isolated, particularly if it is her first child and if her relatives live at some distance. Because of costs of land, houses and high rents, most young couples have to live in the newer suburban areas of cities, where public transport is inadequate, and shopping, mainly in supermarkets, can only be done if the woman has a car. The isolation is intensified as she realizes that she has to cope with mothering a new and unpredictable baby, whose needs fill her time by day and often by night. Even those visitors who come to see her, give her conflicting advice, and if she seeks medical help she often has to wait for an hour or more for a five-minute consultation. Her isolation and the feeling of strain in trying to cope are intensified if her husband is uncooperative, and leaves most or all of the household tasks to his already overburdened wife. No one has told her, neither during her upbringing nor during pregnancy, that mothering is not an instinct but has to be learned. No one has bothered to explain that she will have to adjust to her new role: that of being a mother, responsible for a 'small, utterly dependent creature', as one mother wrote to me. She had expected motherhood to be instantaneously joyous, but she found that the joy was often less than the tears and feelings of inadequacy. When extended families were usual, one or more people were immediately there to help to reassure and to comfort the anxious new mother. In our Western urbanized society, the nuclear family, mother, father and children living in suburbia, distant from relatives, imposes increasing strains on new mothers, so that exhaustion is common.

At unpredictable hours the baby asks to be fed, needs to be changed and cries. Crying may be a demand for food, for changing, for mothering and/or cuddling, which gives the baby the tactile stimulation so needed for its development. But it is difficult to distinguish, at least in the first weeks, between a hunger cry, a discomfort cry and a cry for mothering.

Faced with the problems of learning how to mother her infant, often lacking knowledge and understanding of the baby's needs; more important, lacking support, the new mother begins to feel that her baby's demands are excessive, and that she is never going to be able to satisfy them. Many babies cry a great deal more than the mother expected, many sleep far less than expected, particularly at night. Because of this the new mother lacks sleep, and becomes increasingly exhausted. In her exhaustion she wonders if she will ever be able to be a good mother and why it is that she lacks the ability other women appear to have to cope with the small, selfish, continually demanding infant. She feels a failure and begins to be resentful towards the small infant who has disrupted her life so effectively, and may be damaging her relationship with her husband, even if he is particularly understanding.

She resents that she has been brought up to be a housewife *and* a mother, but now has not time to keep the house as clean and tidy as she would wish, and care for her intrusive child at the same time. This compounds her sense of failure. Her resentment towards her child may be replaced by temporary hostility. As one woman wrote 'you try to do everything to please the little leech, but it sobs and seems to reject everything you do, yet it dominates your life'. The new mother may feel helpless and believe that her failure to cope is a reflection on her. This may be followed by brief feelings of violence towards the baby, and depression.

The baby, in turn, seems to notice the hostile environment. It vomits after feeds, it cries even more, it may have diarrhoea. All these suggest to the already harassed mother that she is not caring for it properly despite all her efforts. Her depression can worsen and she has periods of crying, periods of exhaustion, periods of irritability and even of irrationality.

Any sexual feeling she may have is dampened by the depression, and this in turn aggravates her anxiety as she worries about her husband's feelings towards her. If she is breast-feeding she wonders if it is weakening her and whether her milk is 'suiting' the baby. She may change to bottle-feeding only to find that the bottle-fed baby continues to make the same demands. Her anxiety and depression worsen and can last for weeks. She is in the 'crisis of parenthood'.

How do you cope with the 'crisis'? How can the problems of adjusting to parenthood be reduced?

Coping with the 'crisis'

It will help you if you remember that the period of adjustment is short, and that each day you and your baby learn to know each other better. In the first weeks you may find you have to feed your baby every two hours, but you can be sure that by six weeks he will have found his feeding pattern. If your baby cries 'too much' at first, you can be sure that he will cry less as time goes on. And a baby which cries, because he wants to be cuddled and to see and hear what is going on about him, instead of being left alone in a cot, is likely to be a more interested, intelligent child. You can go on doing the things you have to do and still cuddle your baby if you buy a baby-sling. Most peasant women carry their babies all the time and still do hard work in the home or in the field. Why not do what they do, put your baby in a 'mei-tai', either on your back, or, if the baby is very young, across your front? The baby will like it and you will not feel so impatient if you are able to do what you have to do. If your baby cries a lot at night, wanting food or company, bring him into your bed and let him sleep with you, warm against your breathing body. You will not lie on him or smother him. Babies wriggle and move, so that if you started to lie on him, he would wake you within moments. If, at times, you feel guilty because you think that you hate your baby for demanding so much from you, do not worry. You do not really hate your baby and the hostile emotion was only a brief reaction to your tiredness.

In any 'crisis' it helps to have a sympathetic person with whom you can share your problem. If you and your husband have a close relationship, he will care for the baby and will relieve you of some of the chores in the house. He will cuddle the baby, change the nappies and be generally supportive, so that you can rest more. He will know that during the period of adjustment the baby controls your lives, and he will understand and help. Also, if you have a near relative who can help you care for the baby, or who can relieve you so that you can get out of the house for a while, ask her. But if you have not, join one of the community helping organizations which exist. These are the Nursing Mothers Associations, the Childbirth Education Association and Parent Education Centres in Australia, the La Leche League in Britain and the USA, and Play Group Associations. This supportive help can make all the difference. Make sure you find out the addresses and telephone numbers of one of the organizations before you leave hospital and that you join it. The organizations provide 24-hour telephone counselling and home visiting when needed.

Reducing the problems of adjusting to parenthood

The way to do this begins long before the baby is born. When I was researching this part of the book I wrote asking women if they had difficulties in adjusting to parenthood. The women were members of the Childbirth Education Association or the Nursing Mothers Association of Australia. The response was tremendous, and the suggestions which follow were made by them.

- In schools and at home, education for parenthood should be part of the curriculum for both boys and girls. The course should include discussions of the emotional and psychological changes which occur during pregnancy and after, as well as the physical changes which occur, so that women can build up confidence in themselves as mothers, and so that men can learn that as fathers they have an important role in helping their wives during the period of adjustment to parenthood.
- In the prenatal months expectant mothers and expectant fathers should have the opportunity to learn about adjusting to parenthood so that both are involved in the process, and both understand that supportive help is needed, especially by the new mother.
- Mothers must remember that they are not superwomen and so must their husbands! It is almost impossible to care for home, husband and baby as efficiently as a woman would like. You cannot be a full-time housewife and a full-time mother, one function has to be neglected during the period of adjustment to some extent at least, and that must be the role of housewife.
- Mothers must remind themselves that their feelings of inadequacy are shared by large numbers of other mothers and they are neither alone nor abnormal.
- Women must exert pressure to make sure that there are centres in hospitals and in the community where they can meet other mothers, share experiences, obtain confidence, and where they can meet experienced, helpful counsellors. In the future it is to be hoped that in every community there will be a Resource Centre or a Family Health Service which will supplement the work of existing organizations.
- Women should work to see that in each community a baby-sitting service and an emergency home help service is provided for mothers, at a reasonable cost.

If women go on using their influence, we may obtain what Caroline Pearce of Adelaide sees as needed to supplement the other suggestions. She says that the corner shop should be 'restored to its rightful place as a convenience', and as a social contact point. She believes that home

257

deliveries of household goods should be encouraged. She asks that town planners help to reduce physical isolation by locating shops sensibly, by designing them well, and by making them accessible to mothers with babies and small children.

She writes: 'In our society, women need help and support so that they may develop healthy relationships with their children, who may in turn be capable of healthy and meaningful relationships with others.'

Going home

The day of discharge should vary to suit the particular mother and her baby. If the mother is normal, as is likely, she should be able to go home whenever she feels fit, once lactation is established, confident that she can cope with the baby. During her stay in hospital, she will have learned to bath the baby, and will have acquired the confidence that he is not as fragile as she had thought. She will have learned to interpret his cry, and to know which cry means 'I'm wet, change me', which 'I'm hungry, feed me', and which 'I'm full of wind, burp me'! She will have learned how much the baby depends on her, and yet how much it has its own character.

It is wise to remember that babies feel atmosphere. Quite often the change from the noisy hospital to the quiet home is noticed but not understood by the baby. Because of this, in the first two days at home he may be irritable and fractious. The mother may think that her milk 'isn't doing it any good', but this is not the reason, and is no occasion for changing to a formula milk. What the baby wants is to feel secure. This he does when he is held close to his mother and cuddled. The prescription for fractious babies in the first few days at home is frequent cuddling.

The postnatal check-up

It is usual for the doctor to request that the puerperal mother return to see him between 6 and 8 weeks after confinement. This postnatal check-up is of considerable importance, as it enables the doctor to make sure that all is well, and it gives the mother the opportunity to discuss any problems which may still cause her anxiety. Many doctors want to see the baby as well as the mother.

The examination is quite painless, and the extent of the investigation which need to be made depends on whether the pregnancy and labour were normal or complicated. If they were normal, the doctor will merely palpate the mother's abdomen, examine the cervix with a speculum, and perhaps take a further cervical smear. He will also do a pelvic examination so that he can determine if the uterus has involuted properly. If the mother has any complaints, he will deal with these.

In recent years, the postnatal visit has provided the opportunity to discuss with the doctor the subjects of birth control for herself and immunization programmes for her baby. These two matters are today probably the most important aspects of the postnatal visit.

Postpartum (postnatal) depression

Between 8 and 12 per cent of women are unable to adjust to parenthood and become so depressed that they seek medical help. Other depressed women try to carry on. The clinically diagnosed depression usually occurs in the first 3 months after childbirth. Women who have an increased risk of developing depression after childbirth are those:

- who have a family history or a personal history of a depressive episode.
- who lacked experience in parenting when a child or an adolescent (for example having no siblings to care for).
- who had an unstable or abusive family during childhood and adolescence.
- who lacked positive support from husband or partner during and after pregnancy.
- who are cut off from a near relative or friend who could care for the baby from time to time.
- possibly who had negative experiences in their contact with health professionals during the pregnancy (for example lacking communication and information).

In other words women are more likely to develop postpartum depression if they are socially and emotionally isolated or have had recent stressful live events.

Postpartum depression is not related to any hormonal or biochemical change or to any nutritional deficiency. If a woman feels that she is depressed or if her close relatives or friends notice that she is becoming depressed she should seek help. Some of the signs of depression are sadness, inability to sleep, poor appetite, poor concentration, a

259

feeling of being unable to cope, fatigue, irritability and anxiety.

The woman needs help from a sympathetic doctor who is prepared to listen to her and give support and encouragement, not drugs, at least at first. The doctor may arrange for assistance in caring for the baby so that the mother may have 'time out'. In some cases admission to hospital for a few days for support and group therapy may help. In more severe cases, psychiatric consultation may be needed.

Sexual relationships after childbirth

After childbirth, a woman's sexual desire and activity are subject to a number of factors. Some women, who are finding the strain of parenthood and the need to adjust to being a mother onerous, have reduced sexual desire and arousal. Other women who are sexually aroused, are deterred from sexual intercourse because of a painful episiotomy scar or vaginal irritation. Still other women avoid sex because of fear of damage to their body.

These negative attitudes to sexuality are felt by some women. Many women are more sexually aroused once the baby is born and would enjoy sexual encounters, but do not because they have not received permission from their doctor. Many women are not informed or are misinformed by doctors about sex after childbirth.

A couple can enjoy non-coital methods of sexual pleasuring as soon after childbirth as they both wish. These activities help both partners adjust to their new relationship now that they have to share each other with their baby.

Sexual intercourse can be resumed whenever the woman feels comfortable about having sex, and the activity is pleasurable. There is no reason to wait until the postnatal visit.

It is interesting that women who breast-feed are usually more sexually aroused and responsive than women who choose to bottle-feed their baby.

A number of women who have been 'torn' during childbirth or who have had an episiotomy, find that intercourse is painful. Often the husband needs to spend more time arousing his wife sexually by kissing, hugging and by mutual pleasuring so that she is fully relaxed and her vagina is wet before they start having sexual intercourse. Sometimes, however, coitus continues to be painful. If this occurs you should see your doctor and explain exactly how and where it hurts so that help can be given you.

The return of menstruation after childbirth

If the mother is breast-feeding, menstruation does not usually return for about 24 weeks, or 6 months. Some 10 per cent of women menstruate by 10 weeks after childbirth, 20 per cent by 20 weeks, and 60 per cent by 30 weeks. Ovulation is unusual before the 20th week after childbirth, but about 2 per cent of lactating women ovulate before this time. However, pregnancy rarely occurs in the first 20 weeks of the puerperium. Even if the menstrual periods start, breast-feeding can be continued as the quality of the milk is not altered during menstruation.

In modern Western society, about 75 per cent of mothers do not breast-feed for more than 3 months. These women are at much greater risk of pregnancy, as in over 80 per cent of them menstruation and ovulation have begun by the 10th week after the birth of the child.

CHAPTER 16

Breasts and Breast-feeding

There are many pressures on women to conform to patterns of behaviour and physical appearance. Much of this is induced by the sexual stereotyping of a male-dominated society. This can be seen in the ways in which these physical stereotypes vary from one society to another and from one period to another. Sexual attractiveness is largely a matter of social conditioning.

Women should therefore try not to be anxious about the size and shape of their breasts conforming to some sexual stereotype. The primary function of the mammary gland is to provide nourishment for the infant, but in different cultures and at different times its sexual significance has predominated.

The development of the breast

The infantile breast in both sexes consists of a nipple which projects from a pink surrounding area called the *areola*. Around the 10th or 11th year of life the areola bulges, and the nipple projects from the centre. The development of the male breast ceases at this point, but the female breast develops further as the sex hormones (oestrogen and progesterone) are secreted by the ovaries (Fig. 16/1). The milk ducts which grow inwards from the nipple, divide into smaller ducts and divide again to form tiny milk-secreting areas called *alveoli*. At the same time fat is deposited around the ducts, so that the breast becomes increasingly protuberant and conical-shaped. After puberty, the development is more rapid, and by the mid-teens the breasts have assumed their adult form, being rounded and firm. In fact, however, they are rarely as round and as firm as our fantasies would have us believe. When a young woman stands up, her breasts hang down slightly, the upper surface is slightly concave and the lower surface

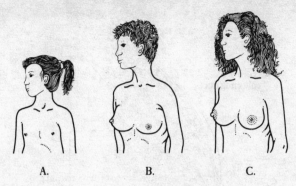

A.   B.   C.

FIG. 16/1 The development of the female breast (a) Prepubertal (b) Late adolescence (c) Maturity.

slightly convex, joining the skin of the chest at an acute angle. Pregnancy leads to a considerable growth of the ducts and the alveoli, and if the mother breast-feeds her baby, the development is even greater. But in the majority of women the breasts return to their non-pregnant size and shape once lactation has ceased.

The adult breast is of variable size, the size having no relationship to the ability to breast-feed. Small breasts can produce as much milk as large breasts. Anatomically the breast is divided into 15 to 25 sections, called lobes, which are separated from each other by fibrous tissue radiating from the nipple, so that the lobes are rather like the sections of an orange. Each lobe has its own duct system, which ends in a dilated area under the areola and extending into the nipple. This forms a tiny milk reservoir when lactation is established. From this a small duct opens on to the surface of the nipple. There are therefore 15 to 25 openings on the nipple. Going backwards, the main duct divides into smaller ducts, and like the branches of a tree, these ducts divide into still smaller ducts each of which ends in, and drains, a collection of 10 to 100 milk-secreting areas (Fig. 16/2). The entire duct system is embedded in a pad of fat, and it is this which gives the breast its shape. The duct system of each lobe therefore resembles a tree, the alveoli being the leaves, the small ducts the branches, and the main duct the trunk.

During each menstrual cycle, changes occur in the breasts, the ducts developing and the alveoli budding in the second half of the cycle. At

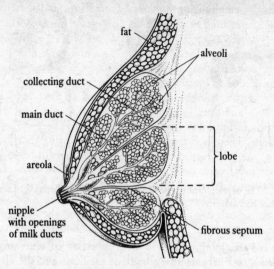

FIG. 16/2   The structure of the breast.

the same time fluid oozes into the fatty tissue of the breasts so that they become firmer and heavier. In some women they may become tender and cause discomfort, which is most marked in the week before menstruation. This is not abnormal, but merely an exaggeration of the normal, and treatment will help. In a few women, the swelling and tenderness persist instead of diminishing during menstruation and disappearing in the first half of the next menstrual cycle. The breasts remain tender and the gland tissue can be felt as irregular lumps. If this occurs, the woman should consult her doctor so that he may investigate fully, and give her treatment to relieve her discomfort.

As the woman becomes older, the breasts tend to get larger and the fibrous tissue bands tend to stretch, so the breasts droop more. After the menopause, the ducts and alveoli become smaller, and the fat starts to go, so that in old age the breasts becomes smaller, wrinkled and floppy.

Is a bra required?

Modern Western women were until recently conditioned to wear a bra. The support has the advantage that it displays the breast more prominently, emphasizing its sexual symbolism, and that it prevents premature stretching of the fibrous supports. However, the need for the bra has been exaggerated, and it is probably only really necessary when the breast has become fully mature and hemispherical, during pregnancy and lactation, and if the breasts are very large. It is doubtful if a bra is needed on medical grounds in the teenage years, or by a mature woman who has normal-sized, firm breasts. If a woman feels more comfortable and attractive in a bra, then she should wear one; if she is more comfortable and attractive without a bra, then she can happily do without. There is little sense in mothers insisting that their young teenaged daughters require a bra: there is no danger of 'drooping', and little to which to give uplift.

In pregnancy, particularly in late pregnancy and during the time a woman breast-feeds her baby, it is advisable to wear a bra, preferably all the time, both day and night. This is because the increased weight of the breasts at these times may cause stretching of the supporting tissues. The size of the bra chosen will need to be increased as the breasts grow in pregnancy, and particularly after childbirth. It may be worthwhile buying 'nursing bras', which have front openings over each nipple and changeable, washable pads to absorb any milk which may leak.

Small breasts

Because of the strong sexual symbolism of the female breast in Western society, many young adults are concerned if their mammary development fails to equal that of their friends, or more important their favourite film or television star. If the breasts have failed to develop at all, a doctor should be consulted; but if the breasts have developed to some extent and menstruation has started, there is little that can be done to increase their size. Many women, beguiled by astute advertising, make use of costly oestrogen creams, rubbed assiduously into the breasts. If menstrual function is normal, enough oestrogen is being made by the girl herself and the extra oestrogen will do little: oestrogen only causes growth of the ducts of the breasts. What the small-breasted girl lacks is the pad of fat. Nothing, except a better diet, will deposit fat in the breasts. Of course, if the girl has a stooping posture, correction of this and exercises to strengthen the pectoral muscle which lies under the breasts will give them the appearance of being larger by 'throwing' them outwards.

A number of women seek the attention of plastic surgeons who introduce disc-shaped moulds of a plastic material (usually silicone) between the breasts and the pectoral muscles. Obviously, this will make the breasts look larger, although it will not improve their function in any way. Since the material is behind the breasts pushing them forward, their feel is unchanged. The operation may do a good deal to make an insecure woman feel more feminine and attractive, and provided the surgeon is skilled it can be most successful. An alternative method, in which a plastic substance is injected should be avoided, as cancer has followed this technique in some cases.

In 1991 silicone breast implants were banned in the USA, Britain and Australia because of concern that they may leak silicone into the body, causing health problems. The ban only applies to well women who have had the implant for cosmetic reasons. Women who have an implant following a mastectomy for breast cancer are not included. Women who have a silicone breast implant do not need to have the implant removed, unless symptoms occur, or the woman is worried about having an implant.

For women who want to have bigger breasts, there is an alternative to silicone implants. This is a silicone bag filled with saline. This breast implant has not been banned but may also leak so that the breast loses its shape.

Until the issue is resolved women should think twice before having a breast implant.

Big breasts

The size of the breasts tends to increase as a woman reaches the age of 35, particularly if she has been pregnant. Most of this enlargement is due to deposition of fat, and although the Western culture approves of large breasts in a young woman, they are not so desirable in later years because instead of being high and firm, they are pendulous and floppy. Exercises are of little help. In many cases, the large breasts cause no problems, except the psychological one of feeling 'different'. When the breasts are very large, some women get high backache, others get shoulder pain, and because of the swings of the breasts during tennis or golf some develop breast pain. The size of the breasts can be reduced by surgery – called reduction mammaplasty. The operation consists of removing an appropriate amount of breast tissue, and usually of moving the position of the nipple. Before deciding to have a reduction

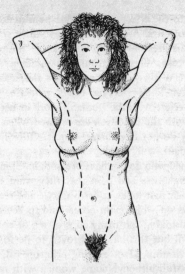

FIG. 16/3   Accessory breasts along the breast line.

mammaplasty, a woman should take careful thought. She may decide that a well-designed and well-fitting bra is all she needs, but if she chooses surgery she needs to select a skilled plastic surgeon to obtain the best result.

Extra breasts

In other mammals more than one breast on each side is normal. In the human, too, a breast (or at least a nipple) can develop anywhere along the breast line, which extends from the armpit to the pubic bone (Fig. 16/3). The most usual site for the extra breast is in the armpit. The extra breast, which has a nipple, appears as a 'tail' of the normal breast. In a few women nipples are found at other places along the breast line. No treatment is required.

Breast tenderness and pain

About one woman in every three notices that her breasts become larger and often tender in the two weeks before menstruation. The breast discomfort is due to the effects of hormones, and tends to be relieved when menstruation starts. A few women have more severe discomfort or breast pain in the premenstrual two weeks, or the pain may persist for three or more weeks. When the woman examines her breasts she finds them 'lumpy', especially in the upper outer part, rather as if she had thick string under her skin. The breasts feel heavy, tender to touch and these symptoms may interfere with the woman's work or her sex life.

Many women with the condition are relieved when they have been reassured that they do not have breast cancer. Only 1 woman in 200 who has breast pain will develop breast cancer, about the same proportion as women who do not have breast pain. Some women suffer so much breast tenderness and pain that they want treatment. It is helpful if the woman first looks at her life style and records, for about 2 months, the days on which pain occurs and its severity. There was a suggestion that drinking too many cups of tea or coffee might be a reason for the pain, but this has not proved to be so. Many women have tried taking vitamin B1 or evening primrose oil, but the results are not very successful, although some women with mild breast pain obtain relief.

At present the most effective treatment is for the woman to take a drug called bromocriptine or one of two similar drugs called danazol and gestrinone respectively. These drugs need to be prescribed by a doctor. Unfortunately the drugs have side effects. Bromocriptine may cause nausea, and the other two drugs produce weight gain, greasy skin or acne in about one-third of users.

The condition is confusing and has been given several names. The one currently favoured is benign breast disease. Older names are fibro-cystic disease and 'chronic mastitis'.

Breast lumps

Rather than a lumpy tender area, a woman may detect a definite lump in her breast. This is of concern because the usual way a breast cancer presents is as a breast lump. However, only one breast lump in five proves to be due to cancer, so that a woman detecting a lump should not panic, but should seek expert help so that a diagnosis is reached quickly.

A breast lump may be detected if a woman aged 35 or more examines her breasts each month (if still menstruating, in the week after her period ceases) and has her breasts checked by a doctor each year. Breast self-examination is not difficult to learn (Fig. 16/4) although its value in detecting an early breast cancer is doubtful. The woman lies down comfortably, and with the tips of the fingers of the opposite hand palpates each breast in turn, systematically starting at the outer upper part and palpating each section of the breast until she has examined it all. The inner half of the breast is examined with the arm raised (Fig. **16/4A**), and the outer half with the arm down at the side (Fig. **16/4B**). If the patient palpates a small lump, she should go to her doctor at once. It may not be cancer, but usually it is necessary to perform a small operation so that the lump can be removed and examined under a microscope.

Breast self-examination or examination by a doctor only detects relatively large breast lumps. Because of this many doctors now suggest that an x-ray technique called mammography is offered to all older

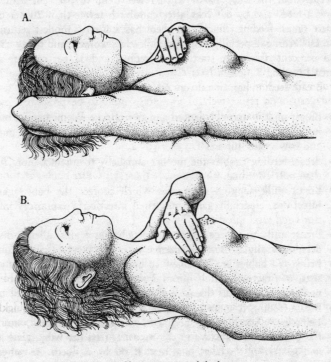

FIG. 16/4   Self-examination of the breasts.

women. A mammogram is made when the woman is between the ages of 45 and 50, and from age 50 it is made each year. If an abnormality is found by mammography further investigations are needed (usually a needle biopsy of the suspicious lump) to exclude breast cancer. Only one woman in every 100 who has a mammogram needs the needle biopsy and only 2 of these women will be found to have breast cancer in the biopsy. The cancer is at such an early stage that cure is very likely. This technique has reduced deaths from breast cancer by about 30 per cent.

Breast-feeding and lactation

About 40 years ago, the number of women who chose to breast-feed began to decline. The lowest proportion of women breast-feeding occurred in the early 1970s when fewer than 40 per cent chose to breast-feed, and by 6 weeks after childbirth fewer than 20 per cent were breast-feeding. Since then there has a been a modest return to breast-feeding, especially among middle-class women, and today about 75 per cent of women start breast-feeding, and 35 per cent are still breast-feeding 3 months later.

Breast-feeding has several very real advantages.

- Breast milk is sterile, balanced and appropriate for the human baby, just as cat's milk is appropriate for a kitten, bitch's milk for a puppy and cow's milk for a calf.
- Breast-feeding enables the mother and baby to interact more fully than bottle-feeding.
- Breast milk supplies substances which protect the baby against infections, especially gastro-intestinal infections, respiratory infections and viral infections.
- Breast milk, to a large degree, protects babies against allergic disorders, especially asthma and eczema.
- Breast-fed babies are less likely to become obese, which, if it persists, is a factor in adult life in coronary heart disease, high blood pressure, gall bladder disease and diabetes.
- Breast-feeding is more convenient for the mother. Unless she has help, if she bottle-feeds, she has to mix the formula feed, sterilize the bottles and teats, warm the mixture, feed her baby, wash out and re-sterilize the bottle and teat. If she breast-feeds she only has to give her breast to her baby to suck.

● Finally, breast-feeding costs less than bottle-feeding, although this factor is unlikely to influence a woman's choice.

Human milk contains slightly less protein and casein than cow's milk. The casein is the substance which makes curd. The curd of cow's milk is dense and difficult to digest, in contrast to the light, fluffy curd of human milk. Human milk contains more milk sugar (lactose) than cow's milk, more vitamins and more balanced minerals. In fact, 'formula milks' made for bottle-feeding have to be modified from cow's milk by the manufacturers in many complicated ways to make them as much like human milk as possible. Furthermore, 'formula milk' requires care in mixing and in storing to keep it sterile and safe for the baby.

With all the advantages, one would think that all mothers would breast-feed unless there was a medical reason for them to avoid this, yet only three-quarters do, and most for less than 3 months.

The reasons for this distaste for breast-feeding have been studied, but no clear explanation has been found. One factor is that the rigid routine of hospitals, in which the baby is kept in the nursery and only brought to the mother at fixed hours, leads to difficulty in milk production because of restricted suckling. Because of this, and because the baby is obviously hungry, extra feeds using formula milk are given. By this stage, after battling with a fractious infant, a stern nurse and a feeling of failure, the mother's emotions further suppress her own milk production and the baby is put 'on the bottle' completely. In hospitals where babies room-in with their mothers and are fed 'on demand', breast-feeding problems are fewer and more mothers breast-feed. But if the mother has had difficulty with a previous baby leading to failure to breast-feed, the memory may deter her from trying to breast-feed the new infant, and she opts for bottle-feeding at once. Another possible reason for the reduced wish to feed may be linked to parental upbringing of the mother when she was a child. Because of the current display of the breast, and its sexual symbolism, many mothers instil the belief into their daughters that the breast is a forbidden zone, to be hidden and never exposed. In a study of English mothers, two psychologists reported that 'modesty and a feeling of distaste' formed a major reason for their preference for formula-feeding, and in the USA another group reported that the mothers they studied were 'repelled' by the idea of giving their breasts to their infants. They were excessively embarrassed at the idea or were too 'modest' to nurse. In other studies of women of higher social groups, reasons for not wanting to feed were that feeding would 'interfere with the mother's social life'; bottle-feeding was so much easier; and breast-feeding would spoil the shape of the mother's breasts. These are selfish reasons, but are nevertheless felt.

If any advice can be given it should be that, for good reasons, breast-feeding is best feeding; but if the mother decides against breast-feeding for whatever reason, the baby will thrive provided the formula milk chosen is a reputable one, and the mother knows how to manage it.

Preparing for breast-feeding

Nearly all women who want to breast-feed can do this successfully. The decision to breast-feed is usually made during pregnancy and it is confirmed after the baby has been born. Breast-feeding has been called a 'confidence trick', and if the new mother is given the confidence that she can breast-feed successfully, she will succeed. Once she has returned home, she will need to have her confidence reinforced by the help she receives from her partner. When you get home it helps to have a friend to call if you have problems, or better still, join one of the nursing mothers' organizations who have informed, helpful counsellors on telephone stand-by at all times.

During pregnancy some women are taught breast manipulations which are believed to make breast-feeding more successful.

The method of preparing your breasts for lactation during pregnancy is quite simple, if you are comfortable about touching and handling your breasts. From about the 30th week of pregnancy put your hands around the outer part of your breasts and gently, but firmly, massage the breast towards your nipple (Fig. 11/1, p. 185). A good time to do this is during a shower or when you are in a bath. After a while most women find that a yellowish substance seeps out of one or more ducts in the nipple. This is colostrum. Some women find the procedure time-consuming and others fail to obtain any colostrum. Don't worry, there is no agreement among doctors that the exercise helps to make lactation easier. Those who believe in the exercise claim that it helps to keep the duct system in order. Breast expression also teaches you how to hand express should you need to do this when the baby has been born.

You should also prepare your nipples for breast-feeding. From about the 30th week when you shower or bathe, wash your nipples with water, dry them carefully and rub a little anhydrous lanolin into them. Then draw out each nipple and roll it gently between your forefinger and thumb a few times. This makes your nipples more flexible and less likely to 'crack' when the baby sucks. Do not believe the myths that you should scrub your nipples or put on methylated spirits to 'harden' them. Nipples should be supple, not hard.

A good way to stimulate your breasts during pregnancy is for your partner to fondle your breasts and to play with your nipples with his fingers, or to suck them, when you make love. It helps prepare your breasts, it makes you closer together and it gives you a warm erotic feeling, which is good!

During the last quarter of pregnancy a few women develop a coloured discharge from one or both nipples. The discharge may be reddish, brown or chocolate. There is no pain and the discharge usually disappears when lactation is established and milk is flowing freely. The cause is unknown. If a woman gets a coloured discharge from her nipples, she should avoid antenatal breast expression and have her breasts examined by her doctor.

How lactation occurs

Once your baby is born, your breasts begin to produce milk because of a hormone, prolactin, secreted by cells in the pituitary gland just below your brain (see p. 23). During pregnancy no milk is made by the alveoli, because prolactin is prevented from acting on the milk-making cells by the high levels of circulating sex hormones – oestrogens and progesterone produced by your placenta. These hormones have prepared your breasts for lactation by their actions on the ducts and alveoli. After the baby is born the level of the sex hormones drops, and messages go to the pituitary cells to start making and releasing prolactin. Prolactin circulates in your bloodstream and is taken up by the milk-making cells of the alveoli of the breasts, so the effect of prolactin is to start and to maintain the manufacture of milk deep in your breasts (Fig. 16/5). At first, only the thick colostrum is secreted, but by 24 to 48 hours after birth, milk appears and the amount secreted is regulated by the baby's demand. The process is helped if you want to breast-feed, and if the baby remains with you so that he can be nursed as soon and as often as he wishes, both during the day and at night.

The secretion of milk continues because prolactin continues to be released when your nipple is nuzzled by the baby or when you cuddle you baby. However, the secreted milk will remain in the milk glands, distending them, unless the milk-ejection reflex occurs. The reflex forces the milk out of the milk glands to run along the ducts towards the milk reservoirs. This 'let-down' of milk is due to contractions of minute muscles which surround the milk glands. The muscles are activated in a complex way, the main component of which is the stimulation of the mother's nipple by a nuzzling baby. A message travels from the stimulated nipple along nerve pathways to the brain, and from there to the pituitary gland. The message tells the pituitary gland to release a muscle contracting substance, called oxytocin, into the bloodstream.

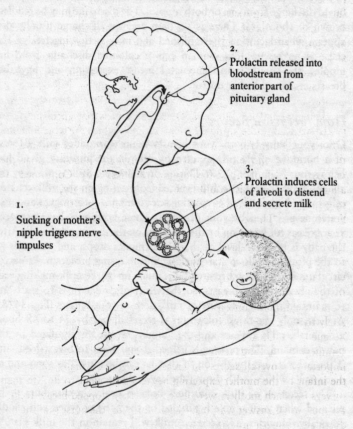

2.
Prolactin released into bloodstream from anterior part of pituitary gland

3.
Prolactin induces cells of alveoli to distend and secrete milk

1.
Sucking of mother's nipple triggers nerve impulses

FIG. 16/5   How milk is secreted

This is carried in the blood to the tiny muscles around the milk glands with the result that the muscles contract and the milk is forced along the milk ducts (Fig. 16/6). Milk-ejection, or 'let-down' has occurred, and is associated with a gentle tingling in the breasts and a desire to nurse. The reflex can also be initiated without actual stimulation of the nipples. A mother hearing her baby cry, for example, may feel the signs of milk-ejection. But the most potent stimulus to milk-ejection is stimulation of the mother's nipple.

If the milk-ejection reflex does not occur regularly and adequately, the secreted milk distends the milk glands and, by pressure, prevents further milk being made, in addition to causing painful breasts. The consequence is that if a mother says she has 'insufficient milk' it generally means that the milk-ejection reflex is not working properly, although her milk production is normal.

As the pathway of the reflex goes through the brain, the release of the oxytocin needed to cause milk-ejection can be affected by the emotions and by other psychological factors. Dr Niles Newton, a psychologist, and her husband, Dr Michael Newton, an obstetrician, talked with 91 mothers, and asked questions to which the women replied in writing. When the answers were analysed, Dr Newton found that those women who subconsciously, or consciously, showed that they disliked the idea of breast-feeding produced less milk. Continued over a number of days, this would lead inevitably to a hungry, crying baby; to greater maternal anxiety and to the decision to put the baby on the bottle because 'I haven't enough milk and it doesn't agree with the baby.' The converse is also true. If a woman really wants to breast-feed she is far more likely to succeed.

The Newtons found that fear about pain, a mother's anxiety about her ability to breast-feed, disparaging remarks about breast-feeding by friends, and an authoritarian, hurried attitude by the nursing staff hindered the milk-ejection reflex and made successful breast-feeding less likely to occur. Dr Applebaum who is medical adviser to the La Leche League in the USA, discussing the problem of good milk-ejection, has commented, 'a kind sympathetic approach by the nursing staff is important to overall success in breast-feeding. Too many nurses hand the infant to the mother expecting her to know what to do.' In many surveys in which mothers were asked why they stopped breast-feeding, the most usual answer was 'insufficient milk' or 'the nurse said the milk doesn't agree with my baby'.

To a large extent the mother's anxiety about successful breast-feeding

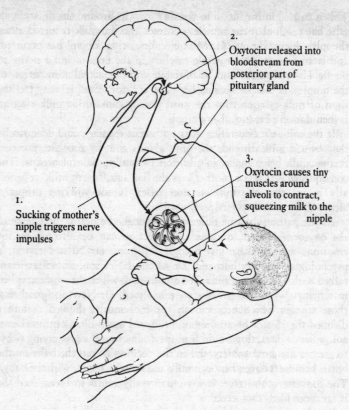

2.
Oxytocin released into
bloodstream from
posterior part of
pituitary gland

3.
Oxytocin causes tiny
muscles around
alveoli to contract,
squeezing milk to the
nipple

I.
Sucking of mother's
nipple triggers nerve
impulses

FIG. 16/6   How milk is 'let down'.

is aggravated by the practice, in many hospitals, of separating the mother
from her baby. In many institutions the baby lives for most of the time
in a nursery and is only brought to its mother at intervals for feeding.
Babies are imitative, so there is generally a good deal of crying in the
nursery. This is interpreted as hunger crying by the nursery attendants.
To quell the noise and treat the supposed hunger, glucose drinks are
given. The wide-holed teat and the sweet drink gives the baby an easy
feed, and it begins to like sweet drinks so that it resists and resents having
to obtain the less sweet breast milk. The partly satiated child, when

taken to its mother, at time intervals chosen by the nursing staff, not the baby, is not interested in suckling. This in turn reduces the milk supply, because the reflex invoked by stimulating the nipple which causes prolactin release is reduced.

Babies fed 'on demand' gain weight more quickly, after the normal initial weight loss, than babies fed 'by the clock'. Only when the mother and baby live together and are treated by unhurried kindly nurses, and when demand feeding is practised, will the emotional bonds between the two become firm. But all too often hospitals seem to be run for the benefit of authoritarian staff rather than for the benefit of the mother and her baby, which in itself is hardly conducive to the establishment of lactation.

The importance of this infant–mother bonding is that the tactile sensations stimulate the baby's sucking reflex and the mother's milk-ejection reflex. The more the milk-ejection reflex is stimulated in the first four days of life, the more successful is lactation likely to be. This in turn suggests that the reflex is started by more than the actual stimulation of the nipples. The close mother–child contact usual in the developing nations, and lost in recent years in our industrialized, mechanized societies, is a further potent stimulus to successful breast-feeding. The practice of 'rooming-in' of mother and baby and to 'demand feeding' is a return to more rational ways and to a greater chance of successful lactation.

But unless hospitals foster and encourage this return to older practices, breast-feeding will continue to decline. Doris and John Haire point out in their authoritative book, *The Nurse's Contribution to Successful Breast-Feeding*, that there is no scientific support for the following practices which were all too common in hospitals in the developed nations:

- Delaying the time of the first feeding for some hours. The fact is an active baby will search for the nipple within minutes of birth, and should do so to practise its sucking reflex. It should then feed 'on demand'.
- Offering the baby glucose water before the first feeding. The scientific fact is that a newborn baby has all the additional fluid it needs in its own body, and needs no extra fluids until breast milk 'comes in' on the 2nd to 4th day It also obtains some fluid (colostrum) from the breast.
- Allowing the mother to sleep through the night before her milk comes

in, instead of letting her keep her baby beside her and put it on her breast when it needs contact and comfort.

- Insisting that the mother only feeds to a 3-hourly or a 4-hourly schedule 'to bring the milk in and keep it good'.
- Preventing 'demand' feeding, which means that the baby is fed when it gives hunger cries. It may need 6 to 10 feeds a day when on demand feeding.
- Offering the baby water sweetened with glucose after it has fed.
- Demand-fed babies rarely need extra water, but if offered it will usually take a small amount.
- Instructing the mother to feed by the clock at intervals of no less than 3 hours when she goes home.

Demand or 'need' feeding

All this suggests that whenever possible a mother should insist that she demand feed her baby. After all, this is what mothers have done since mammals evolved, and it is what the majority of the mothers in the world do today. It was rejected in Western countries about 40 years ago for the routine 3-hourly or 4-hourly feeding, which was more convenient for hospital routine.

Demand feeding implies that the baby is fed when it is hungry, when it needs or demands food. In 'scheduled feeding' the baby is fed at a time decided by the nursing staff, even if this is inconvenient to the mother, and whether the baby is hungry or not. Babies are even woken up to be fed, and, of course, difficulties arise! It is like waking a man at 11 p.m., 4 hours after he has eaten a steak, and telling him he has to eat another steak! Some can, many cannot.

For demand or need feeding to be successful, the baby must 'room-in' with his mother. She is in close contact with him at all times, she cuddles him, she plays with him, she notes his changes in mood, she learns when his cry means hunger. From all these visual, tactile and emotional links, messages are carried to her brain, and the complex system which encourages milk secretion and its flow from the alveoli of the breasts to the collecting ducts is initiated. When the baby is hungry, the mother feeds him, changes him, pets him and then he sleeps. A baby enjoys the breast, he nuzzles the nipples, his hands grasp the breast; and as he drinks his toes curl sensuously, his fingers move rhythmically, and in male babies erection of the penis is common. The mother notices these signs of contentment, she is relaxed, and a further flow of milk occurs.

In the first three days after childbirth, however, milk flow is minimal. The baby has sufficient reserves for this period, and is put to the breast merely to encourage the onset of lactation. He should not be put to the breast for too long, or the nipples may become sore; but he can be put for short periods as often as the mother wishes, since he is living beside her.

By the evening of the third day, or the next morning, lactation should have started, the milk should have 'come in', and proper breast-feeding can begin.

You must make sure that your baby is born in a hospital where the nurses want to help you to breast-feed successfully. You should choose a doctor who encourages you in your desire and who can influence the nurses to encourage you. Choose a hospital where the baby is given to you immediately after birth to cuddle and suckle, assuming of course that its birth has been normal; if it has been difficult you would have to take your doctor's advice. Make sure you can cuddle and suckle your baby for short periods every few hours. If you have prepared your nipples properly you need not worry about the baby's hurting them.

Ask the nursing staff to let you have your baby beside you all night, unless you feel too tired, even before your milk 'comes in', so that you can cuddle him and give him your nipple to suck. This stimulates milk production. Tell the nurses to give your baby only plain water, not glucose water, after a feed if any extra fluid is needed; and then only after talking to you and your doctor. Demand-fed babies do not usually need extra water. Of course, what I have written applies only to a healthy baby. If your baby is very premature or sick you must take your doctor's advice. But talk it over with him. Do not be shy to ask questions. Doctors and nurses are there to help you.

Inverted nipples

The nipples of the fetus in the womb are normally turned in, or inverted. Usually they evert, or pop out, in the last weeks of pregnancy, but occasionally they fail to do so. Inverted nipples may cause embarrassment in these days when many women do not wear a bra, and can interfere with breast-feeding. The reason for the inverted nipples is that instead of being loosely attached to the breast tissues, they are adherent to underlying structures. Exercises are available which will help to make the nipples erect. These may be done if the woman is embarrassed about inverted nipples and especially during pregnancy so that she can breast-feed. You can tell if your nipples are going to remain inverted by gently squeezing your areola between your forefinger and thumb. If your nipple reacts by starting to come out, it is not permanently inverted, but if it shrinks back you may wish to try to get it to become erect. The exercises are fairly easy to do.

Several times a day, the woman places her opposing thumbs, one on each side of her nipple, in the horizontal plane and draws on the areola by moving her thumbs outward. She repeats the exercise several times and then moves her thumbs to the vertical plane, so that one thumb is above the nipple and one below, and does the exercise several times. As the nipple is stimulated and protracts, the adhesions at the base of the nipple are stretched and broken.

Another way to treat inverted nipples is to use specially designed breast shields. They are made of plastic. One side is cone shaped, the other relatively flat with a hole in the centre. You put the shields on your breasts so that the hole covers your nipples; and hold them in place by your bra. The shields put a gentle continuous pressure on your nipple area, gradually drawing the nipples through the holes in the shields. You wear the shields from about the 16th week of pregnancy (it varies, depending on how deeply inverted are your nipples). Start wearing the shields for an hour or two at first and increase gradually until by about the 30th week you can wear them comfortably all day. You should not wear them at night. Sometimes the shields cause the escape of colostrum which makes your nipples moist. If this happens use small pads to absorb the liquid as the discharge can make your nipples sore. You can also coat the nipples with anhydrous lanolin and take off the shields from time to time to expose your nipples to the air.

It has to be said that these traditional methods of dealing with inverted nipples may be useless. A study from Southampton published in 1992 suggests that neither nipple pulling or the use of nipple shields have any benefit. However perhaps another way may help. It has been shown that direct sucking on the nipple area helps to draw the nipple out. If you and your husband wish he can help by stimulating your nipples with his fingers, and gently sucking the nipple area when you are close together. It is a good, happy and erotically stimulating way to prepare your breasts for successful lactation.

The technique of breast-feeding

The most important factor in successful breast-feeding is to be comfortable. It does not much matter whether the mother breast-feeds her baby when sitting up, on her side, or lying down. If she is most comfortable lying down, the baby lies in the bed beside her and she lies on her side facing it. She then adjusts her position so that the baby can nuzzle her nipple and eventually can take the nipple into his mouth. If the baby stuffs it in too far, he may be unable to breathe, and the mother may need to press her breast down from his nose to give him 'air space'.

If she prefers to feed sitting up, she must get comfortable, and often a chair with arms is preferable to one without. She can put a pillow on the arm of the chair, and then has a convenient prop for her arm as she holds her baby. Once again, the baby may need 'air space' when feeding, and she may need to press her breast away from his nose with her fingers.

It is immaterial which position is adopted for breast-feeding, but it is of great importance to make sure that at least some of the areola is inside the baby's mouth. In the diagram on page 282, it can be seen that the duct from each alveolus expands in the areola to form a sinus, or milk reservoir. These storage areas hold the milk, and when the baby squeezes them with his gums, milk spurts out of the nipple and into the baby's mouth. As the baby relaxes his grip to swallow the milk, more milk comes down from the alveoli to fill the sinuses again. In fact, the 'sucking' action made by the baby is only partly responsible for his obtaining milk; the squeezing effect is far more important. Sucking has another purpose, and this is to keep the areola and nipple well within the baby's mouth, and to draw the milk which spurts all over his mouth and into his throat.

If the baby only bites on to the nipple, he will get hardly any milk, will become furious and bite harder. This will give the mother a sore nipple. But if the baby takes the nipple and the areola into his mouth, his gums will grip on the areola, leaving the nipple free, and not damaging it (Fig. 16/7). Should the areola be very large, the mother may have to compress it between her thumb and finger so that the baby can get the nipple well inside his mouth. The mother does not need to hold the baby's head and direct him to the nipple, or to force his mouth open to get the nipple inside; in fact many paediatricians believe that this makes him baffled, bewildered and furious. All she needs to

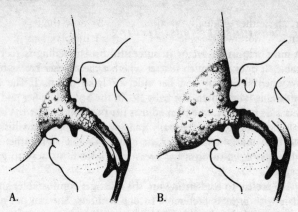

FIG. 16/7 How the nipple should be placed in the baby's mouth A. Correct-nipple sucked well into mouth; gum chewing on areola. B. Incorrect – nipple being chewed.

do is to get the baby comfortably nuzzling her nipple. Once the baby wants it, she must make sure the nipple is well inside his mouth, and that he chews on the areola. Nor should she pull the baby off her breast, because it hurts her and annoys the baby. It is easy to detach the baby from the breast, by simply slipping a finger into the corner of his mouth, between his gums, to break the suction.

The schedule of breast-feeding

This has been mentioned already. In the first three days after childbirth, only a thick yellow secretion (called colostrum) is produced, and as the baby has his own reserve stores of food. It used to be recommended that the baby should be put to the breast for 3 to 5 minutes, between three and six times in the first 24 hours, and then every 4 hours during the next two days to help the milk come in. Recent evidence shows that feeding should not be to a 'routine' but that the baby should be suckled whenever he wants to be fed, at short intervals for as long as you and he want; and each feed should last only a short time. During this time the baby should not be given supplementary feeds either of glucose water or of milk as these are unnecessary and reduce his desire to suckle.

The milk 'comes in' usually on the 3rd or 4th day, but sometimes later, and either gradually or all at once. By now the baby is hungry and much more wide awake than earlier. He may cry, and the mother who 'rooms-in' with her baby rapidly learns to distinguish the cry of hunger, from the cry of discomfort. The baby is put to the breast, and is given alternate breasts first at alternate feeds. He may get sufficient from one breast, or may need to be put on both at a single feed. Usually, too, the other breast leaks milk when the baby feeds. The baby should not stay on one breast for longer than 12 minutes, as he will have got most of the milk in the first five minutes, and if the baby stays on longer the nipple may become sore. If the mother feeds 'on demand', she will generally find it easier than if the baby is fed at fixed times, for the reasons which have already been given.

The frequency which babies 'demand' to be fed is very variable. Some babies want to feed every 2 hours or so while others only 'demand' a feed every 4 hours. When changing breasts it helps to give the baby a short break when he is talked to and cuddled and during this time he may burp. After the feed the baby should be cuddled for a while if he is still awake.

Mothers are concerned that the baby should 'bring up wind or burp' after a feed, and indulge in prolonged back-patting to obtain the burp. This is unnecessary and disturbing to the baby. He will either burp when he is sat up, or cuddled against the mother or he won't. Babies do not usually need to be 'burped'.

The quantity of milk

It is very difficult to decide from the length of time which the baby spends feeding if he is getting enough milk. As the baby usually gets nearly all the milk available in the first five minutes on each breast, he may continue to feed because he is comfortable, or because he is getting a little trickle of milk, or because he is asleep. But if the baby is content, he has had enough. Nor can you tell if the baby is satisfied or still hungry by the fact that he cries after a feed. The cry may be due to 'wind', or because the baby is wet, rather than because he is still hungry. Nor can you tell about the quantity, or the quality, of the milk from the fullness of the breasts or the appearance of the milk. In the first week or two the breasts are usually firm, and appear full, although the quantity of milk secreted is not great. After a while, the sequence of production of milk, the 'let-down' or passage of milk to the milk sinuses, and the balance between demand and production of milk is established, and the breasts appear less full, although in fact milk production has increased.

The best way of telling if there is sufficient milk is to observe the baby. If he is happy, contented and gaining weight (checked every few days, not after every few feeds), there is enough milk. If the baby is fractious and gaining weight, he is getting enough milk but may be guzzling it down too fast and getting 'wind'. Only if the baby is hungry, crying and not gaining weight need there be any worry, and even then inadequate milk supply is only one possible reason.

One of the most important ways of being sure that there is sufficient milk is to avoid being worried. The young mother who is full of anxiety about her milk supply, and who fusses constantly that her baby is not getting enough, may well reduce the amount of milk she secretes. Worry is a good way to reduce the milk supply! Many women rely too much on scales and on formulae for feeding. In the developing countries of the world, millions of mothers who have no scales feed their babies 'on demand'; the babies seem to thrive, and to get all the milk they need. Incidentally, it is almost impossible to overfeed a baby.

The quality of breast milk

The quality of the breast milk of a mother who has a normal diet is high. There is no such thing as 'weak milk'. If the baby is fractious, it is because he has to work to feed, or because he is being suckled in the wrong way – not because the milk is weak. Generally speaking, what the mother eats or does will not alter the quality of her milk. She can continue to eat all the foods she is accustomed to eating, and she can drink alcohol (in moderation, for a drunk mother is hardly a good mother!), tea or coffee. A few substances do cross into the milk and affect the baby. The most annoying drugs are cascara, which no woman needs, and bromides, which can be avoided. A few mothers find that certain foods also affect their baby, although their friends who are breast-feeding find that their babies are not affected by the same foods. It is obviously a peculiarity confined to that mother and her baby, and the simple answer is to avoid that particular food in the future.

Anxiety about the progress of the baby, nervousness and insecurity can reduce the *quantity* of milk secreted, which makes the baby fractious, but this will not alter the *quality*.

Burping or winding

Many women believe that unless a baby burps (brings up wind) during or after a feed he will get colic. To achieve a burp the baby is sat up, or put over the mother's shoulder and his back is rubbed, or patted or slapped until the desired burp occurs.

The need to burp babies routinely has now been questioned. All babies swallow air when they feed but only a few get 'colic'. In the developing countries, where babies are fed frequently, burping is not practised and the babies settle down easily.

The need to burp a baby has been reassessed. Between feeding from the first and the second breast, you should sit your baby on your knee, talk to him and look at him. If he burps during this time, that is fine, but if he doesn't do not worry, offer him the other breast. After completing the feed sit him up and play with him. He may or may not burp, it doesn't really matter.

Contraception during lactation

Although breast-feeding reduces the chances of conceiving, it is not a certain method. Because of this, many lactating women want to know what additional contraceptive measure they should use. The choice of contraceptives was discussed in Chapter 7, and I stressed that a woman should choose what is right for her. But if she is breast-feeding she should avoid the combined oral contraceptives as the milk-supply of some mothers is reduced when taking the Pill, although this is less likely with the new low-dose Pills. Alternatively, she can use the progestogen-only Pill (see pp. 108–9), which is said to increase the milk-supply rather than the reverse. However, it is not the only choice and you may prefer to have an IUD inserted, or to use a vaginal diaphragm. The choice must be yours after appropriate counselling.

Myths about breast-feeding

A reason given by many mothers – particularly French women – for avoiding breast-feeding is that it will spoil their figures, and cause the breasts to sag. These two statements are untrue. A woman who breast-feeds her baby does not need to stuff herself with food – she has already got a store of fat during pregnancy for this very purpose, which she can burn up. Nor do mothers who feed their babies develop sagging breasts. After a pregnancy the breast is a little more mature and soft, rather than being pointed and firm, but it will not sag, particularly if during the last weeks of pregnancy and during the puerperium the mother wears a well-fitting bra, day and night.

Another myth is that breast-feeding 'tires out' a mother. Although the care of a new baby does require energy, and consequently the mother should take an increased quantity of milk (for calcium), protein, vegetables and fruit, breast-feeding is probably less tiring than bottle-feeding. In breast-feeding all the mother has to do is put the baby to the breast; if she 'formula feeds', she has to prepare the formula, keep the milk sterile, warm it, feed the baby, clean the bottle, and get the next feed ready. Some women find that they are uncertain how to care for their baby, and worry about the child's progress. These women are apt to feel 'worn out and tired', and blame this on breast-feeding rather than on the disturbed sleep and additional responsibilities which a new baby creates.

Some women find that when they breast-feed, their sexual arousal and desire are diminished. It is doubtful if this is due to lactation. A young baby takes up a great deal of time and energy so that less is available for other things, one of which may be your libido. But you can be aroused if your husband helps you by being considerate and spends more time in 'pleasuring' you before sexual intercourse begins. Other women find breast-feeding sexually arousing and pleasurable. If it makes you feel randy do not feel guilty; enjoy the feeling! It is quite normal. And with a helpful man you can enjoy both breast-feeding and sex either simultaneously or in sequence.

Do not listen to your 'friends' who tell you that breast-feeding is 'taking too much out of you', or the baby 'doesn't seem to be thriving – it's a bit thin!' or 'why don't you put the baby on the bottle – it's so easy'. Ignore them – you know what is best for your baby. You are the expert!

The final myth is a particularly insidious one. This is that a woman who fails to breast-feed her baby has failed as a mother. This is quite untrue. Breast-feeding offers the most suitable milk for the baby, and it brings the mother and her baby into a close, intimate contact; but for psychologists to say that the bottle-fed baby is deprived and will be less stable and happy in later life is just stupid. The mother can show her concern for her baby by caring for him as she feeds him with the bottle, and she can cuddle him between feeds. If she fails to breast-feed or decides not to breast-feed, she is not 'depriving her child' and need not feel guilty. Bottle-fed babies cannot be identified from breast-fed babies in later life.

Do the drugs you take get into your breast milk?

Lactating mothers often express concerns that drugs they take, or which are prescribed for them by a doctor may be excreted in breast milk and may affect the baby. While most drugs, including antibiotics, do pass into breast milk the amount is small and will neither benefit nor harm the baby.

Only a few drugs may cause damage to the baby. These include *anticoagulants* (given to the mother to treat blood clots) which may cause haemorrhages in the body; *antithyroid drugs* (particularly *thiouracil*) which may depress the infant's thryoid gland; a laxative called *Coloxyl* which may give the baby diarrhoea; *lithium* which may make the baby cold and blue, and *Mysoline* which is sometimes used to treat epilepsy.

If you have been prescribed one of these drugs, stop breast-feeding; if not, you do not need to worry.

Difficulties of breast-feeding

ENGORGEMENT. If the mother determines to follow the plan of 'demand feeding', it may be necessary to put the baby to the breast at regular intervals in the first three days. By the 3rd or 4th day of the puerperium, the milk 'comes in'. This means that milk production is now in full swing, but that the passage of milk into the ducts and out of the nipple is not yet properly organized. In some women the breasts become heavy, tense and warm. In a few women they are painful. The breasts are said to be 'engorged'. Engorgement is only temporary, lasting for less than 24 hours, and the doctors and nursing staff are fully competent to help the mother.

CRACKED NIPPLES. In normal feeding, the infant grasps the areola of the nipple, and not the nipple itself. The nipple lies free in the baby's mouth. How it should be grasped can be visualized if you suck your thumb, so that the end is freely movable in the mouth. If the nipple is free within the infant's mouth, its gums compress the small reservoirs in the lower part of the nipple and milk squirts out of the openings in the nipples. If the nipple is not far enough in the baby's mouth, the milk does not flow easily, the baby becomes frustrated and sucks harder. This may cause cracked, painful nipples. Cracked and painful nipples can also be caused by letting the baby suck for too long. Normally the baby empties a breast in under 7 minutes, and it is pointless to permit him to suckle on that breast for more than 12 minutes. Cracked nipples can be avoided by preparation during pregnancy and by the proper technique of breast-feeding. As well as this, after a feed you should wash your nipples with water (no soap), dry them carefully and put on anhydrous lanolin. If cracked nipples occur, the baby should be taken off the breast for a couple of days, and the breast emptied by manual expression, the expressed milk being sterilized and fed to the baby in a bottle. An antibiotic ointment may be applied to the breast on a doctor's advice.

INSUFFICIENT MILK PRODUCTION. Fear, anxiety, pain, lack of privacy, and unsympathetic attendants can prevent the milk from passing along the ducts within the breasts. In these cases, although milk is secreted, the baby gets very little and cries with hunger. This aggravates the anxiety and a vicious circle is set up. Milk production is best in a mother who is healthy, fairly young, has a good diet and who wants to breast-feed. Milk production is likely to be less if the mother is ill, older and poorly motivated about breast-feeding. Milk production may dimimish if the mother starts taking oral contraceptives, but this varies considerably.

Various foods and drugs have been recommended to improve milk production, but none has been proved to be of any value except one called metoclopramide. Drinking excessive water or milk does not improve milk production, nor does the use of iodine drops, special 'lactation foods', or thyroid tablets. The most efficient way of establishing a good milk flow is a knowledge of how milk is produced; a desire to breast-feed; a healthy, hungry baby; and sympathetic, helpful nurses. Only if this fails to improve lactation should metoclopramide be tried. The drug works by increasing the release of prolactin from the pituitary gland.

MENSTRUATION AND LACTATION. This matter is discussed on page 261.

MASTITIS. Occasionally infection enters the lactating breast, usually introduced through cracked nipples, during the second or third week of the puerperium. The breasts become engorged, hard, reddened, tender and painful. If this happens and you recognize it early enough you should feed your baby more often so that your breast does not become engorged with milk, which encourages the infection to become more severe. As long as you cannot express pus from your nipples you will not infect the baby. This occurs only rarely. In addition, your doctor will give you a type of penicillin which is particularly suitable. It is called flucloxacillin. You take the tablets by mouth.

But remember, an ounce of prevention is worth a pound of cure! Good antenatal preparation for lactation, proper care of your nipples, demand feeding to avoid engorgement and to establish a strong 'let down' will ensure that your breast is empty after a feed. If you take these measures you are unlikely to develop mastitis.

Suppressing lactation

As I mentioned a number of women choose not to breast-feed and a number stop breast-feeding after a few weeks. Unless treatment is given the breasts rapidly become engorged with milk and are painful for two or three days, after which pressure in the milk producing areas, the alveoli, suppress further lactation. To reduce the pain, binders and analgesics have been prescribed, and the mother instructed to limit the amount of fluid she drank. These measures did help, but not a great deal. For the past 30 years, oestrogen tablets have been used, as it was found that oestrogen 'fed-back' to suppress the release of prolactin by the pituitary (p. 273). Recently there has been some concern that oestrogens used in this way increases the chance of a woman's developing a blood clot in a vein and thromboembolism. This led many doctors to refuse to give oestrogen tablets and to go back to breast binding.

Today a drug is available which effectively suppresses lactation and has no dangers. The drug is called bromocriptine. It works by directly stopping the release of prolactin from the hypothalamus.

Although I believe women should breast-feed, I realize that some will not, and a very few cannot. For these women, bromocriptine means that lactation can be stopped without any discomfort. Tablets of bromocriptine are taken daily for 10 to 14 days.

CHAPTER 17

When Things Go Wrong
in Pregnancy

Over 70 per cent of women will experience little trouble during pregnancy apart from feeling nauseated in the first few weeks and pelvic pressure in late pregnancy, but in a proportion of pregnancies things go wrong. This is always of concern to the expectant parents. In this chapter the more common and important of these matters will be discussed.

The first two of these conditions are associated with bleeding (and often pain) in the first half of pregnancy. The third matter is bleeding in the second half of pregnancy. The fourth matter concerns a group of illnesses which most often affect the mother and her baby in the second half of pregnancy. These include high blood pressure, diabetes, heart disease and Rhesus iso-immunization. The fifth group of conditions includes rubella, genital herpes and other infections.

Certain mothers also may have more problems in pregnancy. These include teenage mothers (particularly if younger than 17), mothers whose first baby is due to be born when she is over 35, and women who have had five previous pregnancies. Their problems will be mentioned in this chapter.

Abortion (miscarriage)

Although the proper medical term for a miscarriage in the first half of pregnancy is an abortion, to many women the term means that the pregnancy has been ended by a doctor or some other person. Many women prefer to use the older term 'miscarriage' for a spontaneous abortion.

About one pregnancy in seven ends as a miscarriage, most often between the 6th and 10th week of pregnancy. Miscarriage is less common among women under the age of 25, when 1 in 10 will abort, and becomes more common as a woman grows older. After the age of 35, 1 pregnancy in 5 ends as an abortion.

Most cases of miscarriage are due to the fact that the fetus has not formed properly, and Nature is getting rid of it. In a few cases a miscarriage follows a severe fever, particularly a viral infection, or because of some abnormality of the uterus, particularly a cervix which is 'incompetent', as we shall discuss later. Miscarriages are not caused by fatigue, 'shock', 'excessive' sexual intercourse, a retroverted uterus or an improper diet.

Threatened miscarriage

The first sign of an impending, or *threatened miscarriage* is usually bleeding. The bleeding usually is slight, irregular 'spotting' of blood; this may be followed, after a few hours or days, by a moderate discharge of blood from the vagina, which may resemble a menstrual period. In other cases the bleeding is heavier at the start and may be accompanied by some slight cramping pains, resembling period pains. If a pregnant woman starts bleeding in the first half of pregnancy she should ring her doctor and describe what is happening. The doctor will probably want to see and examine her so that he can decide if the bleeding is due to a threatened abortion or is a sign of some other condition, especially an ectopic pregnancy. The doctor will probably order an ultrasound picture of the uterus, as this often helps to confirm the diagnosis and helps the doctor decide on the most appropriate treatment.

The ultrasound picture may show a normal fetus, of appropriate length for its age, whose heart is beating and who is living in a normal-sized sac. The chance that the pregnancy will continue normally if these findings are made is over 95 per cent. On the other hand, ultrasound may show an 'empty sac', which indicates that the baby has not formed properly; or it may show that the woman has miscarried at least partially.

Women with this ultrasound picture need to have the uterus curetted to remove the remnants of the pregnancy. The ultrasound picture may show an empty uterus, in which case no treatment is indicated provided the doctor has excluded the possibility of an ectopic pregnancy (see p. 294).

In about half of cases of threatened abortion ultrasound will fail to detect a normal live fetus and abortion is likely to occur.

Using ultrasound routinely has helped to make the management of 'threatened miscarriage' much easier. If the fetus is alive and of normal size no treatment is needed, although some doctors still insist that the expectant mother goes to bed for a few days. There is no evidence that this is of any benefit.

Many medications have been recommended to treat a threatened abortion. These include vitamins (especially vitamin E), sedatives and hormones, especially progesterone or one of its chemical substitutes. None of these treatments has been shown to be of any value except as a placebo. In other words their only value is a psychological one, the woman and her doctor believing them to be of benefit. But the best psychological help is for the doctor to explain what is happening and for the expectant mother to be given 'TLC' – tender loving care – by everyone.

Inevitable miscarriage

In this condition, which may follow signs of a threatened miscarriage, or may be the first problem noticed, the woman starts losing a fair amount of blood from her vagina, and has quite severe cramping pains in her lower abdomen. She may expel pieces of tissue. If any of these things occur, the probability is that she is going to miscarry and should contact her doctor or go to a hospital quickly.

The psychological effects of a miscarriage

For most women a miscarriage is a distressing occurrence. During the process many women are distressed by not knowing what the outcome will be; others are distressed by being told to rest in bed without any further explanation. Too little information is given by some doctors both in general practice and in hospital about the reason why the abortion occurred and about the outcome of a future pregnancy. Women need counselling about these matters and need to have an opportunity to express their feelings about the abortion.

A woman who has a miscarriage, and particularly if the miscarriages recur, should know that in most cases the miscarriage occurs because the embryo has not formed properly due to chromosomal defects; that there is nothing that she did or did not do, which led to the abortion, and that after one abortion 8 women in 10 will have a live healthy baby the next time. Even if she has aborted three times in succession (recurrent miscarriage p. 294), she has 7 chances in 10 that her next pregnancy will result in a healthy baby.

Pregnancy after a miscarriage

A major concern of a woman who has miscarried is if her next pregnancy will also abort. After one miscarriage a woman has an 80 per cent likelihood that the next pregnancy will result in a live, healthy, normal baby. If a woman has two miscarriages, the chance of producing a live, healthy baby in the next pregnancy is 75 per cent, and even after three abortions, one after the other, she still has a 70 per cent chance of producing a live, healthy baby with her next pregnancy.

In fact, however disappointed an expectant mother may be, she should not be anxious if a pregnancy ends as an abortion: her next pregnancy has every chance of being normal.

Late miscarriage

Most miscarriages occur in the first 12 weeks of pregnancy, but a few women complain of vaginal bleeding between the 12th and 20th weeks of pregnancy. It is much less common for a woman to abort during this period, but it does occur. These women are sometimes found to have an abnormality of the shape of the uterus which can be detected by an x-ray picture taken (after injecting some oil into the uterus) when the woman has recovered from the abortion.

About 20 per cent of women who have a late abortion, especially if it is not their first late abortion, are found to have a weakness of the cervix (the neck of the womb). Women with this condition, which is called cervical incompetence, usually know only that all is not proceeding normally when the 'waters break' unexpectedly and without apparent reason.

Normally, the cervical canal is quite firm and remains closed, although the uterus is enlarging as the fetus grows. In women with cervical incompetence the cervix begins to open more and more after about the 12th week of pregnancy. As it opens, the bag of waters (the amniotic sac) is pushed through the opening and, unless the condition is detected and treated, it eventually bursts. When this happens an abortion is nearly impossible to stop.

If the doctor is aware that this may happen, usually because it happened before, he can prevent the bag from bursting by putting a stitch around the cervix and pulling it tight, rather like pulling the string around the mouth of a purse. The operation is relatively simple and about three-quarters of women who have cervical incompetence and have the operation can expect to have a live baby. But the condition is rare. In other words, only a very few women have this weakness of the cervix, and the operation is therefore not often needed.

Recurrent miscarriage

This is defined as occurring when a woman has had three or more successive miscarriages (some doctors define recurrent abortion as occurring after two successive abortions). As the woman has a 30 per cent chance of miscarrying again, and a higher than average chance of having a preterm baby, it is wise for her to visit an obstetrician. The obstetrician will investigate to try and find a cause for the recurrent abortions. The investigations may include a hysterosalpingogram (p. 90) to find out if there is an abnormality in the shape of the uterus, and a test for cervical incompetence.

Tests may be made to check that the woman's endocrine glands are working properly. Even with these tests, no cause for the recurrent miscarriages can be found in about 60 per cent of cases. Recently research has shown that in some of these cases the immunological relationship of the couple is too close so that the mother is unable to secrete the 'blocking antibodies' which prevent the fetus from being rejected (see p. 142). This has suggested a treatment. Before becoming pregnant again the woman is given injections of her husband's blood (or another donor's blood). The white cells in the blood stimulate her immune system to make the blocking antibodies should she become pregnant again. Unfortunately, in spite of early hope that the treatment would be effective, recent studies have shown that it is not.

Ectopic pregnancy

Ectopic pregnancy means that the fertilized egg has burrowed into the lining of the Fallopian tube rather than reaching and implanting into the lining of the uterus. As the embryo grows, its placenta eats into the muscular wall of the tube, which eventually bursts. When this happens the woman complains of severe abdominal pain and usually bleeds a little through the vagina. Often she has had some intermittent slight pains earlier. Ectopic pregnancy occurs in about 1 in every 150 pregnancies. An expectant mother who develops pain and slight bleeding should consult her doctor at once as she may have an ectopic pregnancy. The doctor will probably do a highly sensitive beta hCG pregnancy test. He may also order an ultrasound check to see if there is a fetus in the uterus.

Ectopic pregnancy is treated by surgery to remove the damaged portion of the Fallopian tube, or making an incision along the upper surface of the tube, above the ectopic gestation, 'milking out' the tiny fetus and placenta, and so conserving the Fallopian tube. Until recently an incision was made into the abdomen to reach the ectopic but today many ectopic gestations are dealt with through a laparoscope. The operation is less painful and the stay in hospital reduced to a day.

New treatments being tried are to inject a small amount of a sugar solution or a chemical called methotrexate into the ectopic pregnancy and then to let nature dissolve the tissues.

As a woman has two Fallopian tubes she can become pregnant again after an ectopic pregnancy.

High blood pressure (hypertension) in pregnancy

Hypertension means high blood pressure, that is the woman's blood pressure is higher than that normal for most women during pregnancy. Some women, usually older than 30, have hypertension when they become pregnant, but most women who develop a high blood pressure do so in the second half of pregnancy. When this occurs the illness is called 'pregnancy-induced hypertension'. It is also called 'pre-eclampsia' and (wrongly) 'toxaemia of pregnancy'.

Pregnancy-induced hypertension (PIH) may be associated with oedema and, in a few women, with the appearance of protein in the woman's urine.

PIH affects about 6 per cent of primigravidae, and 4 per cent of multigravidae, but if it is detected and treated early complications are avoided. If the disease progresses, protein may appear in the woman's urine (which is why a urine specimen is tested at each antenatal visit). When this occurs the fetus is at some risk of dying. Further progression of the disease may cause serious complications such as convulsions or 'fits' and the death of the baby may result. This condition is called 'eclampsia'. The expectant mother can understand, therefore, the insistence made by the doctor for regular antenatal visits, when the blood pressure is estimated, oedema looked for, and the urine examined for protein. She can also appreciate why she must follow her doctor's instructions implicitly should a rise in blood pressure or other signs of PIH occur. The instructions may be simple, such as restricting the diet, particularly the amount of salt added to the food she eats, and by making sure that she rests more, as this improves the quantity of blood flowing to her placenta. Sometimes the doctor may ask her to be admitted to hospital, even when she feels she is quite well. In hospital she may be given drugs, and the doctors and nurses will observe her blood pressure very closely, her 'fluid balance' (that is, the amount of fluids drunk against the quantity of urine passed), and the well-being of her baby. This is done in several ways, as discussed later.

The aims of managing of PIH are to control the height of the blood pressure and to make sure that the baby is healthy and is growing normally (see p. 318). If either or both aims fail to occur, the doctor will induce labour (see p. 323) or perform a caesarean section. These measures are taken when it is felt that the danger to the baby is greater inside the uterus than if it were born and cared for in a special intensive neonatal care nursery.

Obviously if a way of preventing the onset of PIH could be found it would be valuable. Unfortunately all the suggestions made so far, from manipulating the diet to doing complex tests have proved useless. Recently a new method is being tested. This is to ask women to take small doses of aspirin each day. The results of the trial which is being conducted in several countries are promising.

'Essential hypertension' is the other form of hypertension and affects about 3 per cent of pregnant women. The name implies that doctors do not know the cause of the illness. Women who have essential hypertension in pregnancy require special care and may have to spend some of the time in hospital. This is because in 50 per cent of the women the blood pressure rises, and in about 25 per cent, protein appears in the urine. If this happens the baby is at risk of dying. The management of 'essential hypertension' then becomes the same as that of PIH.

Bleeding in the second half of pregnancy

Bleeding from the birth canal occurs in the second half of pregnancy in about 3 per cent of women. Usually they are women who have previously delivered children, and primigravidae uncommonly develop this complication. If an expectant mother bleeds sufficiently to soil a sanitary pad, or to make a large stain on her clothes or her bed sheets, she should call her doctor at once. He may visit her in her house, or he may insist that she go into hospital immediately where he will examine her.

Bleeding in the second half of pregnancy is called 'antepartum haemorrhage'. Apart from the few cases due to local conditions of the cervix, there are two main causes, which were first distinguished in 1775 by Dr Edward Rigby in Norwich. At that time maternity care was conducted by untrained midwives, and they attended the woman only when she was in labour. If labour failed to progress, or was abnormal, the midwives called in the doctor. Because of the current ideas of modesty at that time, he usually had to make his diagnosis without a pelvic examination, or if he performed one, he did it under a sheet! Considering the difficulties, Rigby made a remarkably clear distinction between bleeding that was *inevitable* because the placenta was filling the lower part of the uterus in front of the baby, and the bleeding which ocurred *accidentally* because a portion of the placenta separated from its bed on the wall of the uterus.

Today the two types, the inevitable bleeding due to a *placenta praevia*, and the accidental bleeding of *abruptio placentae*, still require to be distinguished because treatment is different. The usual way of making the diagnosis is to take an ultrasound picture of the woman's abdomen. This will identify the position of the placenta clearly. An expectant mother who is diagnosed as having a placenta praevia remains in hospital until the pregnancy has reached the end of the 37th week. This is called 'expectant treatment', and is used so that the baby may grow in the uterus rather than having to cope with life in a premature nursery.

A problem in diagnosing placenta praevia has arisen because most women have an ultrasound picture taken at about the 20th week of pregnancy. In about 5 per cent of women a placenta praevia is found. In nearly all cases the placenta 'moves up' during the next 10 weeks and is no longer in the lower part of the uterus. For this reason if the 20 week ultrasound shows a placenta praevia, a second ultrasound picture must be taken after the 30th week of pregnancy to confirm or reject the diagnosis.

During the expectant treatment the woman may have episodes of bleeding which usually settle but occasionally necessitate delivering a preterm baby by caesarean section. About the 37th or 38th week a decision is made by the doctor whether it is safer for the expectant mother to be delivered normally or by caesarean section; 4 patients in every 10 can deliver normally, and 6 in every 10 who have a placenta praevia require to be delivered by caesarean section.

Abruptio placentae, the other main condition which causes bleeding in the second half of pregnancy, is of two kinds. In most cases the amount of separation of the placenta is slight, and the pregnancy can safely continue. In a few cases – no more than one-quarter of all – the amount that the placenta separates is greater. In these cases the expectant mother may lose a good deal of blood. Because of this, the doctor gives blood transfusions and brings on labour by breaking the bag of waters or performs a caesarean section, if the baby is alive. Unfortunately, in the severe forms very few babies are alive.

Diabetes mellitus

Diabetes, which usually needs insulin to control it, affects about 1 pregnant woman in every 500, and gestational diabetes affects about 2 per cent of pregnant women. As I mentioned on page 157, screening for gestational diabetes is now commonly performed. Both forms of diabetes (especially true diabetes) may lead to the death of the baby either in the uterus or after birth, unless the woman eats an appropriate diet and often is given insulin. In pregnancy, diabetes tends to get worse, as the blood sugar levels rise and more insulin is required. Diabetes is associated with an increased chance that the woman will develop pregnancy-induced hypertension, or have a baby which has congenital defects.

These problems can largely be avoided if a diabetic woman controls her blood sugar carefully with insulin injections before she decides to become pregnant. A test measuring a substance called glycated haemoglobin is made to establish if it is within the normal range before she becomes pregnant. In early pregnancy (about the 12th week) an ultrasound examination is made to see if the baby is growing normally. If it is not, the chance that it has a congenital defect is about 80 per cent, and other tests are made.

In pregnancy the woman attends regularly for antenatal care, preferably at a pregnancy diabetes clinic, and monitors her blood sugar levels at home. She is regularly advised about her diet by a dietician. If the control she obtains of her diabetes is good and she does not get pregnancy-induced hypertension, she may wait for labour to start spontaneously. However, some doctors prefer to induce labour at about the 37th week or to do a caesarean section.

Women who have gestational diabetes have fewer problems but require meticulous care during pregnancy. They also need to be followed up as 10 per cent of the women will have developed diabetes 10 years after the pregnancy, and 40 per cent in 20 years.

Heart disease

Better nutrition and better hygiene have reduced the number of pregnant women who have rheumatic heart disease, but some of them and women who have congenital heart lesions become pregnant. About 1 in every 300 pregnant women will be found to have heart disease. This is why the doctor listens to a woman's heart at the first antenatal visit. If he hears a suspicious heart murmur, he may send the woman to see a cardiologist who will make tests to determine the damage to the heart.

Most women with heart disease have no problems during pregnancy provided that they do not become anaemic, and rest each day. The woman should make frequent visits to her doctor, and should eat a balanced diet so that her weight gain is controlled. If she becomes breathless she should contact her obstetrician or cardiologist. Childbirth is usually uncomplicated, but the obstetrician may discuss with her the need to help the baby's birth with forceps.

Prolonged pregnancy

Most pregnant women have given birth by the end of the 42nd week after the last menstrual period. About 8 per cent of pregnant women have not given birth by this date and are considered to have a prolonged pregnancy (also called postdatism). If the woman has a complication of the pregnancy, such as high blood pressure, or is over the age of 35 and it is her first pregnancy, her doctor may discuss with her the need to deliver her baby quickly. In other cases the woman may choose to have the labour induced (see p. 323), provided that her cervix is soft or may prefer to continue the pregnancy and let labour start spontaneously.

If she chooses the latter, she will be asked to make daily fetal movement counts (page 319) and will probably have ultrasound examinations to make sure that the amniotic fluid is not decreasing in quantity. If the fetal counts become abnormal or the amniotic fluid becomes scanty, her doctor will probably suggest that the baby should be delivered.

Rhesus iso-immunization

Experiments in the 1940s showed that all humans can be divided into two classes: those whose blood is Rhesus positive and those whose blood is Rhesus negative. The name Rhesus is obtained from the Rhesus monkey as all Rhesus monkeys are Rhesus positive and have the Rhesus antigen attached to their red blood cells. In human populations about 85 per cent of Europeans and North Americans have Rhesus positive blood and 15 per cent have Rhesus negative blood. Among Chinese women or men Rhesus negative blood is almost never found.

If a Rhesus negative person is given Rhesus positive blood, the Rhesus antigen provokes the person receiving the blood to form anti-Rhesus antibodies. If a second Rhesus positive blood transfusion is given, the antibodies seek out and stick to the Rhesus negative blood cells and 'explode them' causing anaemia. This is called Rhesus iso-immunization. And Rhesus iso-immunization is important in pregnancy.

A woman marries a man not because of his blood group, but because he is attractive to her, or has qualities which appeal to her, in short, because she is in love with him. Since 85 per cent of people are Rhesus positive and 15 per cent Rhesus negative, the odds are that in 10 per cent of marriages the wife will be Rhesus negative and the husband Rhesus positive. At some stage, quite naturally, they decide to have a baby. Because it inherits half of its genes from its father, it may be Rhesus positive or it may be Rhesus negative. If it is Rhesus negative, no problem arises; but if it is Rhesus positive, problems may occur with a later pregnancy, although the first baby will not be affected. During the pregnancy, the Rhesus positive baby grows happily in its mother's womb, but off and on in late pregnancy tiny numbers of its Rhesus positive red blood cells may seep across the placenta and enter the mother's bloodstream, where they are destroyed. At delivery, however, much larger amounts of fetal blood get into the mother's bloodstream. The amount may be too great to be destroyed immediately, and the surviving cells are recognized as being foreign invaders which have Rhesus positive badges on them! The mother's defence system goes into action and special commando cells, called immuno-competent cells, manufacture the destroying substance (the anti-Rhesus antibody) which attaches itself to the foreign Rhesus positive cells, coats their surface, clumps them and literally blows them apart.

The mother's defence system, once stimulated, remains ever on the alert should any further Rhesus positive cells enter her body.

The couple decide to have another child. Again it inherits half its genes from its father, and again it may be Rhesus positive. If it is, a strange thing now happens. The anti-Rh antibody, which the mother's immuno-competent cells have continued to manufacture, circulates through her bloodstream, and because of its peculiar shape is able to pass through the placenta and enter the bloodstream of the fetus. This does not happen in very early pregnancy, but becomes more and more likely as pregnancy advances. In the bloodstream it meets the baby's normal Rhesus positive red blood cells, and coats them so that they burst. The burst red cells release a substance called bilirubin, which accumulates in the baby's blood and some of it is excreted into the amniotic sac in the baby's urine. If many of its red blood cells are destroyed, the baby becomes progressively so anaemic that it is bloated and dies. If fewer red blood cells are destroyed, the baby remains alive but is born anaemic and jaundiced from the accumulation of bilirubin in its blood.

Once these facts had been discovered, it was possible to find out first, if the Rhesus negative mother had been stimulated to manufacture antibodies by doing a test on her blood; and second, to determine how badly the baby was likely to be affected, by taking a sample of the amniotic fluid and estimating the amount of bilirubin in it. This test on the amniotic fluid was done first at about the 24th week of pregnancy, and repeated once or twice more. Before the 24th week of pregnancy, testing the amniotic fluid is not very helpful. If the fetus is thought to be in danger of becoming severely anaemic before that time, a sample of the fetal blood is taken from the umbilical cord using a fine needle under ultrasound control. The object of all these tests was to find out when it was more dangerous for the baby to be inside the uterus than to be born. Once born, its damaged blood could be replaced in an 'exchange transfusion' of Rhesus negative blood, which the antibodies could not attack since the red cells had no antigen on their surface. The transfused blood kept the baby alive while such antibodies as remained slowly decayed over the following weeks. Some babies needed further 'topping-up' transfusions, but by six weeks of life, they were all well. None of the antibodies the mother had transferred to them remained, and their Rhesus problem was over. Using these methods of care, most Rhesus affected babies now survive, but a few still die in the uterus. These are the babies which are severely affected at a stage when they would die if they were born. Medical science has found a way of treating these small babies in the womb. Under ultrasound guidance, a needle is introduced through the mother's abdomen and the wall of her uterus, into the amniotic sac and then into a blood vessel of the umbilical cord as it enters the baby's body. A blood transfusion of Rhesus negative blood is given through the needle. This corrects the baby's severe anaemia and enables it to grow in the uterus. A second transfusion may be needed.

Today, the Rhesus problem can almost be eliminated. It has been found that most Rhesus negative women become immunized during the process of childbirth. This is because Rhesus positive blood from the baby gets into the mother's blood in small amounts during childbirth. Once in her blood, the fetal blood cells initiate the sequence of events described earlier. Scientists have found that if Rhesus negative women, who have not yet started to make antibodies, are given an injection of a special substance, they will not be immunized. The special substance is an immunoglobulin and it is made in the blood of Rhesus negative volunteers. The anti-Rhesus immunoglobulin seeks the baby's Rhesus positive red cells in the mother's blood and coats them (before destroying them) so that they are unable to 'sensitize' the mother to make the anti-Rhesus antibody.

The amount required is determined by taking a sample of the mother's blood and measuring the number of fetal blood cells in the sample. This is called the Kleihauer technique.

At birth the baby's blood is tested to find out if it is Rhesus positive or negative. If the baby is Rhesus positive and the mother has no anti-Rhesus antibodies in her blood she is given an injection of the immunoglobulin within 72 hours of the birth. The injection is also given to Rhesus negative women following a spontaneous or an induced abortion; and prior to attempting to 'turn' a breech baby.

This procedure has virtually eliminated the Rhesus problem, although a few women become sensitized during pregnancy. Research suggests that soon these women may also be protected against Rhesus iso-immunization.

Rubella (German measles)

The careful observations by Dr Gregg in Sydney in 1941 first brought to our attention the dangers of rubella in the first half of pregnancy. Rubella (German measles) is caused by a virus which can cross the placenta and infect the baby. It is a peculiar virus, as it prefers to grow in tissue which is just forming. Before the 10th week of pregnancy it has a wonderful opportunity, for the heart, the ears, and the skull of the fetus are forming at this time. If the virus gets into the tissue, the heart may be damaged, the hearing impaired, the eyes may develop cataracts, and the skull may not expand. Because of these serious complications affectings more than half the babies, many doctors believe that a therapeutic abortion should be performed if a woman develops rubella in the first 12 weeks of pregnancy.

Some pregnant women come into contact with a case of rubella, either in their own family or in a neighbour's. Until very recently it was the custom to give them an injection of 'gamma globulin', which was painful, but which was said to protect the fetus from the virus. It is now known that the injections of 'gamma globulin' are of no value in protecting the babies.

It would be sad if nothing more could be said, but it can. A test has now been developed which will tell if a patient has had rubella, and once you have had rubella, you are protected for all time. A specimen of the person's blood is taken and the test made. In Australia, the USA and probably in most other countries, it has been found that more than 85 per cent of women have had rubella before they reach the age of 16. The other 15 per cent have not had rubella, but a vaccine is available which will give these women a mild attack of rubella. They will not know that they have had rubella, but they will be protected.

Testing to tell if a woman has had rubella is rather expensive, and because of this the vaccine is now being offered to all schoolgirls when they reach the age of 12. But since many women do not know if they have had rubella, it is expected that they will be tested if they wish. The most suitable time for testing to see if a woman has had rubella is when she decides to marry, or just before she decides to have a baby. If her test is positive, she knows that her baby is in no danger of being damaged by the rubella virus. If she decides that she will have the injection, she must take precautions to avoid becoming pregnant for two months after the injection. After that time she will have become protected against rubella, and there is no chance of her baby's being damaged by the rubella virus.

Because of the chance that a few women will not be immune to rubella, and will be infected when they become pregnant, in the USA, Sweden, and Britain from 1989, a rubella injection is given in childhood. The Americans and the Swedes give a combined measles, mumps and rubella injection when the baby is 15 to 18 months old and a further injection when the child is 12 years old. This programme should eliminate all rubella-induced deafness and the other consequences of the fetus being infected by the rubella virus.

Herpes in pregnancy

Genital herpes is discussed on page 357 and you may care to read that

303

section first. In pregnancy the virus may cross the placental 'barrier' to infect the fetus. This is more likely in a first attack than in recurrent infections. Overall the risk is low: only 1 fetus per 1000 being infected. The risk is greater during childbirth, particularly if the mother has developed a recurrence or is shedding the virus from her cervix.

These findings suggest: (1) A woman with a *history* of genital herpes needs have no anxiety that her baby will be infected and may expect to be delivered vaginally, unless a recurrence of the infection or a new infection occurs during the pregnancy. (2) If a first infection or a recurrence of genital herpes occurs during the pregnancy, but has healed by the time labour starts, the woman may give birth vaginally. (3) If herpetic ulcers are present when the membranes rupture or labour starts, a caesarean section should be performed to avoid the risk that the baby will acquire a herpetic infection during the passage through the birth canal. The strategy of taking endocervical swabs for viral culture every 2 weeks from the 34th week of pregnancy in these women can be abandoned as positive swabs do not predict the risk of the infant being exposed to herpes infection during birth.

Age and obstetric performance

Examination of the records from very large numbers of pregnancies in many countries has been made to see if age has any effect, good or otherwise, on obstetric performance. There has been surprising agreement that the least complications in pregnancy and during childbirth are found if the mother has been well nourished from childhood, has some knowledge of what happens in pregnancy, is more than 155cm (61in) tall, not overweight nor emaciated, and aged between 18 and 30! Of course, this does not mean that younger or older mothers, fat or excessively thin mothers, or short women do not perform well. They do, but there is a greater chance that complications will arise.

The teenaged mother

There has been concern, particularly in the USA, Britain and Australia, about the increasing number of teenaged mothers, particularly those under the age of 17 who are unmarried. In Eastern countries, it is normal for marriage to take place soon after puberty, and for consummation of the marriage to occur either then or, as with Hindus, two to three years later, so that teenaged pregnancies are not unusual. There is nothing to suggest that the teenaged mother is in any way disadvantaged in pregnancy, provided that she seeks antenatal care as early as possible. In a study of teenaged mothers which we have conducted in Sydney, we found that if the girl received antenatal check-ups, she had only a slightly greater chance of developing pregnancy-induced hypertension than her older sisters and was a bit more likely to become anaemic. The duration of labour was not increased; in fact labour seemed easier, and the average birth-weight of her baby was not different from that of her older sisters, nor was there any increased risk that her baby would be born dead or die soon after birth. If the girl did not attend the antenatal clinic until late in pregnancy, as happened with many of the unmarried teenaged mothers, we found that there was twice the chance that she would develop pregnancy-induced hypertension or become anaemic; and although the duration and conduct of labour was not altered, she had double the risk of losing her baby.

The importance of these observations is that every teenaged girl who becomes pregnant, whether she is married or not, should seek antenatal care as early as possible. She need not be worried that the doctors and nurses will condemn her for getting pregnant – they will not; and they will be happy that she has had the sense to come along so that her pregnancy and labour may be made as easy as possible. Often an unmarried girl has many problems to face, and most maternity hospitals have a staff of qualified social workers who can advise and reassure her, can give her confidence, and talk to her with kindness and wisdom.

The older primigravida

About 10 per cent of women, usually of the higher socio-economic groups, delay becoming pregnant until they are more than 35 years old. Such a patient is called an 'older primigravida', rather than the previous term 'elderly primigravida', which is somewhat insulting to the expectant mother! The older primigravida may develop more complications in pregnancy than her younger sister, and because of this she should obtain antenatal care as early as possible in pregnancy so that any complications can be diagnosed and treated quickly.

An older primigravida has three times the risk of developing pregnancy-induced hypertension, and a slightly greater chance of having a breech baby or a twin pregnancy than her younger sister. Labour in the older primigravida tends to last rather longer than among her younger primigravid sisters, and her baby's birth needs to be helped by forceps or caesarean section more frequently. This is because of the concern of the obstetrician that the baby is particularly precious as a further pregnancy is less likely to occur. Because of the concern, the caesarean section rate is about 20 per cent, and the forceps rate about 10 per cent. The decision to perform an operative delivery by caesarean section or by forceps should only be made after the doctor has explained the reasons and obtained the woman's agreement.

The grande multigravida

This term was first used in Dublin to describe those women who have had at least four previous pregnancies. These mothers are more likely to have complications in pregnancy and labour than women who have had fewer children, and the risk is greater if the mother is aged 35 or more. Unfortunately, this is the patient who most frequently neglects to obtain antenatal care. If she does seek antenatal care, the chance of a complication occurring in pregnancy or labour is greatly reduced. She is more likely to develop bleeding in pregnancy, and pregnancy-induced hypertension is a little more frequent. Although she may deliver a bigger baby, labour is usually quite rapid. However, she has a risk of bleeding after delivery unless action is taken.

These findings emphasize the importance of regular antenatal visits, and delivery in a well-equipped hospital under the care of a well-trained doctor.

CHAPTER 18

The Baby in Pregnancy

Most babies reach the time of birth head-down and consequently are born head-first, but about 3 per cent decide to be breeches. This poses certain problems for the baby, the parents and the doctor. In about one pregnancy in every 90, the mother has a multiple pregnancy, usually twins. Twins also pose problems. These problems will be discussed later in this chapter.

A few women (about 5 in every 100) go into labour prematurely, that is their baby is born before the 37th week of pregnancy, while in another 2 or 3 per cent the baby fails to grow in the uterus as quickly as expected, and is underweight when it is born. Both premature (pre-term) and growth-retarded babies may have medical problems and need special care.

Another problem which affects between one and three babies in every 100 born is that the baby has a congenital malformation. The birth of a congenitally abnormal baby can cause much distress to the parents.

All these babies, and babies of mothers who develop high blood pressure in pregnancy, who are diabetic, have anaemia or heart disease or go over their expected date of childbirth, need monitoring. Today sophisticated methods of monitoring 'at risk' babies are available.

Breech babies

In the middle of pregnancy, because the fetus is small and the amniotic sac relatively large, the baby tends to move around a good deal. At this time about 40 per cent of babies present with their bottom nearest the mother's pelvis. These are called breech presentations. By the 28th week, the percentage has dropped to 15; by the 34th week to 6; and by the 40th week less than 4 per cent of babies still present by the breech.

The reason is that as the pregnancy advances, there is more room for the baby's legs in the upper part of the uterus, and the baby gets into the most comfortable position! Most of the babies which remain as breech presentations have their legs straight, the feet under the chin (Fig. 18/1).

In the past breech babies often died during delivery, but today with skilled attention and teamwork by the obstetrician, the anaesthetist and the nurses, these problems have been overcome. However, if the expectant mother still has a breech presentation when the pregnancy has reached 34 weeks' gestation, the doctor may try to 'turn' the baby. This is a simple manipulation, and is not painful, so the expectant

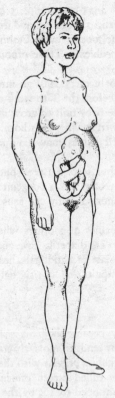

FIG. 18/1 The breech baby.

mother does not need an anaesthetic. Many doctors give a muscle-relaxing injection before attempting to turn the baby, and most check on the baby's heart (using ultrasound) before and after the manipulation. The doctor is very gentle as he attempts to do the 'external version', and if the baby does not turn easily, he does not persist (Fig. 18/2). Before the manipulation, the mother should be sure that her bowels and bladder are empty and that she is relaxed. If the doctor fails to turn the baby, he will probably ask the mother to have an x-ray to make sure that the pelvic bones and the cavity of the pelvis have a normal shape. A few obstetricians who fail to turn the baby without anaesthetizing the expectant mother make a further attempt after giving her a general anaesthetic. When this is done, the woman may feel some slight abdominal discomfort and tenderness for a few days but, generally, the procedure is not followed by much pain.

Most breech babies are born easily, after a labour which is no longer or more difficult than if the baby was 'head-down', or more correctly was a cephalic, or vertex, presentation. But in certain cases, particularly if the baby is very small or very large a caesarean section is usually performed.

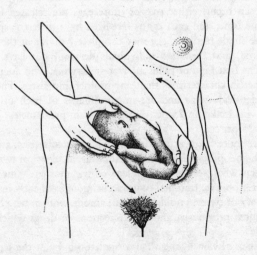

FIG. 18/2 Turning a breech baby.

The reason in the case of small babies (less than 1500g or 32 weeks' gestation) is that the doctor may be anxious that the baby's soft head will be damaged during a vaginal delivery. A large baby (more than 4000g) obviously makes the birth difficult. More caesarean sections are being made to deliver breech babies. In some centres the rate is over 65 per cent of all breech births. A woman has a right to discuss the way her baby will be delivered with her doctor, and he has a duty to explain his reasons if he decides on a caesarean section.

If the woman and her doctor agree that a vaginal delivery is appropriate, the mother whose baby remains as a breech need have no anxiety, and when her baby is born she will see that its head has a beautiful round shape. When the baby lies as a cephalic presentation, its head is often temporarily distorted for a few hours after birth. It is of no consequence to the baby, and the shape becomes normal very rapidly.

Multiple pregnancy

It is quite normal for most mammals to have a multiple pregnancy or litter. The human female usually has only a single baby in each pregnancy, but 1 pregnancy in 90 is a twin pregnancy; 1 pregnancy in 90 × 90 is a triplet pregnancy; and quadruplets occur once in 90 × 90 × 90 pregnancies. There are two ways in which a multiple pregnancy can occur: either two or more eggs are released from the ovary at one time, and each egg is fertilized by a different spermatozoan, or the single fertilized egg may completely divide at the stage of the blastocyst, and then *two* individuals develop, but have a single placenta. The first kind of twins are fraternal twins, who are no closer to each other in chracteristics than any brother and sister. The second kind are identical twins and are mirror images of each other. The fraternal twins make up 75 per cent of all twin pregnancies, identical twins only 25 per cent.

Twins are more frequent in African and Asian countries, and this is due to the higher proportion of fraternal twins, as identical twins occur equally often whatever the race or age of the mother. Among Caucasians, or Europeans, fraternal twins occur more frequently in families with a history of twins, in older women, among women who have had several children previously, and after injections of drugs which induce ovulation.

Each twin is always lighter than a singleton baby at the same stage of pregnancy, although, of course, the combined weight of the twins is greater than that of the singleton. Because of this, twins tend to be underweight at birth. As well, the size of the twins can vary very considerably. The difference between them is greater when they are identical twins, as one of them is greedy and takes the greater part of the nourishment which arrives through the placenta. Inside the womb, the twins lie side by side. In late pregnancy, it has been shown that in 45 per cent of cases both lie with their heads over the mother's pelvis; in 25 per cent the leading twin has its head down, and the other twin is a breech; in 10 per cent the breech leads, and in 10 per cent both are breeches (Fig. 18/3).

The doctor may suspect twins when he finds that the uterus is larger than he anticipated, calculated from the date of the last period. There are other causes for the undue enlargement of the womb, but twins is the most common cause. It is possible he will be able to feel both babies, but this is unusual before the 28th week of pregnancy, by which time the expectant mother may herself suspect that she has twins. If

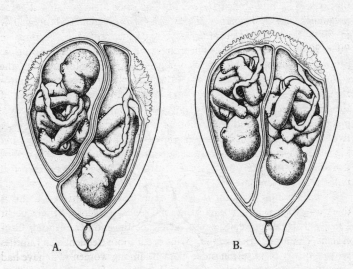

FIG. 18/3 Twins.
(a) Fraternal twins from the chance fertilization of two ova.
(b) Identical twins, from the fertilization of a single ovum and its later division into two identical embryos.

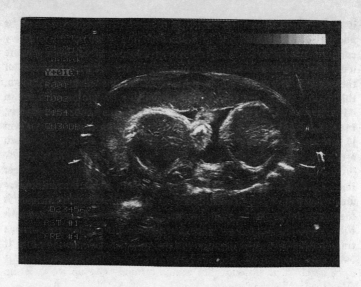

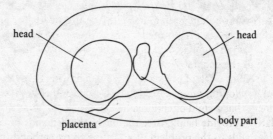

FIG. 18/4   Twins seen by ultrasound.

the doctor is uncertain, he will arrange for an ultrasound picture (Fig. 18/4) which will show the two babies and their position in the uterus.

A multiple pregnancy is a little more risky than a single pregnancy, but provided the exptectant mother attends regularly for antenatal care, the risk is small. A raised blood pressure (pregnancy-induced hypertension) occurs more frequently, as does anaemia. Many doctors prevent anaemia by giving the expectant mother iron tablets with a tiny amount of folic acid added, from about the 30th week of pregnancy. In late pregnancy, twins usually impose more discomfort on the expectant mother than does a single infant. Her abdomen feels heavier, she has more backache, and swelling of her ankles and legs is quite common. It has also been found that twin pregnancies tend to end prematurely, and about one-quarter of twin babies are delivered by the 36th week. This premature rate can be reduced considerably with good antenatal care and if the mother rests for a good deal of the time from the 32nd week. She does not need to be in hospital if she can rest at home, unless she develops a raised blood pressure when she will need to be admitted to hospital. She should certainly give up work, if she can afford to, by the 28th week.

Contrary to popular belief, labour in a twin pregnancy lasts no longer than in a single pregnancy, but the delivery of one or both of the twins may have to be aided by the doctor. There is often an interval of about 10 minutes between the birth of the twins, but no doctor today would allow an interval as long as the 65 days which was reported some years ago.

The knowledge that a woman has a multiple pregnancy often has a considerable psychological effect on the woman and on her partner. First, there is the problem of the 'vanishing' twin. If an ultrasound examination made in the first quarter of pregnancy reveals twins, in a few cases a second ultrasound made in the third quarter of pregnancy, shows that one has disappeared. This is because that twin had an inadequate blood supply, died and withered away. This is obviously distressing to the couple.

After the 20th week of pregnancy a woman bearing twins has a higher chance of developing complications which require admission to hospital. If she already has a child or children her absence from home may require that relatives provide help. After the birth, the demands of caring for two babies adds to the problem of adjusting to parenthood (page 253) and usually means that the couple have little time to be with each other to enhance their general and their sexual relationship. If these issues are thought about during pregnancy and arrangements made to reduce the 'stress', their impact is less. Fortunately, in many communities there are 'multiple pregnancy self-help groups' whose resources can be tapped by the woman and her partner.

Finally, an old myth should be demolished: twins are not less fertile than singletons when in their turn they marry.

Premature childbirth

About 1 woman in every 15 will deliver her baby before the 37th week of pregnancy. In some cases the birth occurs early, often by caesarean section, because the mother has an illness which may affect the baby's well-being. In most cases this is a worsening of a pregnancy-induced hypertension (p. 295). In a few cases the baby has to be delivered because of antepartum haemorrhage (p. 297). If a woman has a multiple pregnancy premature birth is more likely than if she had only one baby. But of the 7 per cent of women who give birth prematurely (more correctly preterm), in nearly half no reason can be found. As small babies, whether they are premature or have grown slowly in the uterus, are more likely to die than mature babies; it would be wonderful if the reason why women go into premature labour was known. In spite of much research the reason remains obscure.

A woman usually becomes aware that she may be in premature labour if she starts getting regular painful uterine contractions which increase in pregnancy. She may also notice a 'show' (p. 228) or her membranes may rupture, leading to a gush of water from her vagina. If any of these events occurs, she should contact her obstetrician and will probably be asked to go into hospital.

In hospital she will be examined to check the size of the baby and where he is lying in the uterus, and whether her cervix is showing any opening. Her general health will be checked, particular attention being paid to her blood pressure.

In most cases a nurse will 'monitor' the frequency and strength of the uterine contractions, or a monitor will be attached to her abdomen. The monitor is an electronic device which is attached to the woman's abdomen by a wide belt. It records the uterine contractions on a piece of specially printed moving paper.

Of all women admitted in threatened premature labour, further examination shows that 2 out of 3 are not in labour. The uterine activity is not progressive and childbirth is not imminent. But if the woman is in true premature labour, what can be done?

The answer to this question depends on where the woman is, how much her pregnancy has advanced, and if the membranes have ruptured.

If she is in a small hospital which does not have a neonatal intensive care nursery, she will probably be transferred. If she is in such a hospital and her pregnancy is less than 35 weeks advanced, the staff may try to suppress labour by giving drugs. Before they do the obstetrician should explain to the parents what is proposed so that they can help make the decision. Between 35 and 37 weeks of pregnancy some doctors use drugs and some wait for nature to decide. This is because there is as yet no real evidence that the drugs work. Currently drugs called beta-agonists are given intravenously in a drip. The dose has to be adjusted so that the side-effects are controlled, but the uterus stops contracting. The side-effects are a pounding heart, a rapid pulse and a flushed feeling. The most that can be said is that a few days may be gained by using the drugs. This may enable the doctors to give the mother injections of cortisone which help mature the baby's lungs and reduce the chance of his developing breathing problems (respiratory distress).

If the membranes have ruptured, the effect of the drugs is even less, but some obstetricians try to suppress labour using them to gain a little time for the baby in the controlled environment of the uterus.

Congenital malformations

If 1000 women become pregnant and the pregnancy is diagnosed early, 150 may expect to abort (or miscarry) spontaneously in the first 20 weeks. Careful examination of the aborted fetuses shows that nearly half have been expelled by nature because the chromosomes were not the proper number or the baby was deformed in some way.

A few women carrying babies with abnormal chromosomes, or with some other inherited congenital defect (which is usually one of metabolic function, the baby lacking the ability to make some special enzyme) fail to abort spontaneously. The pregnancy continues but a congenitally deformed baby is born. The most common congenital defect due to abnormal chromosomes is Down's syndrome. This affects 1 baby in every 1500 born to women under the age of 30, but the incidence rises to 1 baby in 300 if the expectant mother is over the age of 35. Down's syndrome used to be called mongolism, and the child affected by Down's syndrome is mentally retarded. Scientists have found that two forms of chromosome abnormality can cause Down's

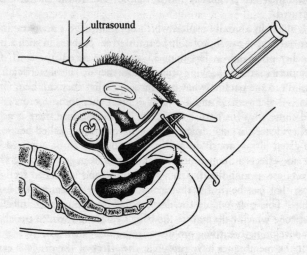

ultrasound

FIG. 18/5   Chorionic villus samplings.

syndrome, and if the baby has one of them there is a high chance that a subsequent baby will also be affected.

Today, a mother who has previously had an affected baby or who is over the age of 35, can find out early in her pregnancy whether or not her baby will have Down's syndrome in one of two ways. The first way, *chorionic villus sampling* (CVS) is done when the pregnancy is about 8 weeks advanced. A flexible needle is inserted through the woman's cervix. It is then pushed further in, under ultrasonic guidance, until the tip is just inside the edge of the placenta (Fig. 18/5). A syringe is attached to the needle and some of the placental tissue, called chorionic villi, is sucked out. This tissue is analysed. A chromosome count is made to detect or exclude Down's syndrome. The answer is obtained in 2 or 3 days.

Chorionic villus sampling is also being used to detect some rare abnormalities which affect the metabolic process of the fetus and infant. CVS is painless and leads to only a 1 per cent increase in miscarriage. The second method is to wait until the pregnancy has advanced to 16 weeks and to perform an *amniocentesis*. In this test a narrow needle is inserted into the uterus, through the woman's abdominal wall and a sample of amniotic fluid is removed. The fluid contains cells shed by the fetus. The cells can be grown in specially equipped laboratories and chromosomal examinations can be made. The growth or culture of the cells takes about 20 days.

If the expectant mother is found to have a baby affected by Down's syndrome she can choose either to have the baby, or to have an abortion induced. If the diagnosis is made by CVS, the fetus and placenta can be removed by a suction curette. If the diagnosis has been made by amniocentesis, a prostaglandin infusion has to be used as I describe on page 324.

Other congenital abnormalities occur which are not due to abnormal chromosomes or inherited abnormal metabolic processes. At present we do not know why they occur. One important group includes those due to abnormalities of the spine or skull. These are called neural tube defects and affect about 4 babies in every 1000 born. But, oddly, the incidence varies in different countries – in some the rate is 10 in every 1000, in others it is only 2 in every 1000. A woman who has had a baby with a spina bifida (the spinal column defect) or an anencephalic baby (the skull defect) has twice the chance of having another affected baby compared with other women.

It is possible to find out if the next baby will be similarly affected. At about the 16th week of pregnancy, an ultrasound picture is made. This may identify a defective baby and will outline the position of the placenta. The doctor then introduces a thin needle into the amniotic sac through the woman's abdominal wall and a sample of amniotic fluid is removed. It is tested for a substance called alphafetoprotein. If large amounts of alphafetoprotein are found, the baby has a 99 per cent chance of having a neural tube defect. The mother and her partner are counselled and may choose to have the pregnancy terminated by giving an injection of prostaglandin into her uterus.

In some countries, all pregnant women are now being 'screened' to determine if they have a baby with a neural tube defect (either a spina bifida or an anencephalic baby).

Blood is taken about 16 weeks after the last menstrual period and the level of alphafetoprotein is measured. If it is raised, the test is repeated after the period of pregnancy has been checked and twins excluded. A second raised level suggests that the baby may have a defect. An ultrasound examination is made and then, if necessary, an amniotic fluid sample is taken and alphafetoprotein measured. If this is raised the mother has a defective baby and has to decide if she wants the pregnancy terminated using prostaglandin, after discussion with and explanation by her doctor.

A study made with the collaboration of many hospitals has shown that if a woman eats a diet rich in folic acid and probably takes folic acid tablets (2–4mg a day) from the time she decides to become pregnant, she will have a reduced chance of having a baby affected by a neural tube defect. (This finding applies particularly to a woman who has previously had an affected baby.)

Foods which contain folic acid are green leafy vegetables such as cabbage, sprouts, and broccoli. Lettuce, nuts and frozen peas are also good sources. The problem is that you have to eat a good deal of these foods, to obtain the extra folic acid and if you choose vegetables they should be eaten raw or only lightly cooked as the vitamin dissolves in boiling water. For this reason folic acid supplements may be the best way of increasing your folic acid intake.

Monitoring an 'at risk' baby in pregnancy

Since the whole purpose of good antenatal care and careful observation during labour is to make sure that you have a live and healthy baby, and are as healthy, or healthier, after your pregnancy than you were before it, doctors have become increasingly aware that in some pregnancies a greater risk of losing the baby is present. These pregnancies include those in which bleeding occurs in the second half of pregnancy, or pregnancy-induced hypertension develops; women aged 30 or more who become pregnant for the first time; women who previously have given birth to a stillborn or a deformed child; women whose pregnancy has been prolonged for more than 42 weeks; women who have diabetes, high blood pressure or kidney disease; and women with a Rhesus problem. If a mother-to-be has, or develops, any of these conditions, or other rare ones, her baby is at greater risk of dying before birth, of being born prematurely or of dying during labour. In other cases the baby is diagnosed as growing too slowly (being growth retarded). The clinical diagnosis may be confirmed by ultrasound.

Modern technology has made it possible to monitor the health of the 'at risk' baby. Older methods such as measuring the level of the hormone oestriol in the woman's urine or blood have been superseded.

At present several complementary methods are available. These are: (1) fetal movement counts; (2) cardiotocography; (3) serial ultrasound; and (4) fetal blood flow.

Fetal movement counts: Most mothers know that their baby moves or 'kicks' many times during the day. Babies have periods of activity and periods of rest, but move at least 100 times in a 24-hour period. Research has shown that if the baby moves more than 10 times a day it is probably healthy. (A 'run' of rapid movementts counts as one movement.)

Women are asked to record their baby's movements, either over a period of an hour twice or three times a day, or for a single longer period. Once 10 'kicks' have been counted the mother stops for that day. If she detects fewer than 10 movements she notifies her doctor or the hospital.

Cardiotocography: This means that the baby's heart rate is recorded electronically by a machine, and this is related to the uterine contractions. The baby's heart forms patterns on the cardiotocograph and these can be interpreted as indicating that all is well, or otherwise. Special pads are placed on the mother's abdomen to record the baby's heart and leads from the pads go to the machine. The test is made twice or three times a week if the woman is an out-patient and often daily if she is required to be in hospital.

Serial ultrasound: There have been many advances in the precision of ultrasound to measure the growth of the baby, but the method does not seem as popular as fetal kick counts and cardiotocography.

Fetal blood flow: A new technique to determine fetal well-being is to measure the velocity of the blood flowing through the umbilical arteries or the baby's aorta using ultrasound. Experience with the test shows that its main value is as a 'screening test'. If the blood flow is normal the baby can continue to live in the uterus; if the test is abnormal one of the other tests is made to find more about the baby's condition.

The purpose of the monitoring is to help the doctor decide, after discussion with the parents, whether it is safe to let the pregnancy continue, or whether it is in the best interests of the baby to deliver him either by inducing labour or by doing a caesarean section.

Monitoring an 'at risk' baby during childbirth

If a woman with a 'high risk' pregnancy is permitted to go into labour, either spontaneously or after induction of labour, her baby is at greater risk during labour than that of a normal or low risk woman.

Increasingly such women give birth in maternity units which have an array of electronic equipment, a special nursery for small babies and highly trained staff who are ready to rescue the baby by delivering it quickly should problems arise unexpectedly. The electronic equipment which has been developed helps the doctor to reach a decision and also detects early which baby may be in jeopardy.

Two pieces of equipment are useful. The first is the cardiotocograph (which in labour is also referred to as the fetal heart monitor). As I have mentioned, this apparatus electronically measures the fetal heart rate and determines the strength and frequency of the uterine contractions. The information is translated into a visual continuously moving graph. By studying the patterns on the graph, the medical attendants can make sure that the baby is well and that the uterine contractions are occurring at the correct strength and the best intervals for the baby to get all the oxygen he needs. If the doctor detects an abnormal pattern, he may decide to deliver the baby at once, depending on the stage labour has reached, or he may use the second piece of equipment. This machine measures the acidity of the baby's blood. A small sample of blood is taken from the baby's scalp as it presses into the mother's vagina. This blood is then put into the machine and its acidity is measured with great accuracy. If the scalp blood of the baby is very acid, the baby is in danger of dying, and the doctor can rescue it from the danger. If the blood is not acid then the baby is safe, and labour may continue.

Perinatal death (stillbirths and infant deaths)

Of 100 pregnancies which reach the half-way mark of 20 weeks, fewer than 2 will result in the birth of a dead baby (a stillbirth) or in the death of the baby in the first month of life. The reasons why babies die in this way are rather complex. In over 30 per cent the cause is unknown, although most of the babies are born either premature or weighing less than expected for the time of birth. About 15 per cent of the deaths occur because of an antepartum haemorrhage (see p. 297), and a similar number are malformed babies. Nearly 6 per cent occur because of pregnancy-induced hypertension and about the same number because of disease in the mother.

The loss of a baby at this time is deeply distressing to the mother and to the father, but the deaths of these babies (called perinatal deaths) have been reduced remarkably in the past 50 years. Fifty years ago, 60 babies in every 100 born were stillborn or died in the first month of life. Today fewer than 12 in every 1000 born are lost in this way in developed countries.

The usual, and quite normal, reaction to a perinatal death by the parents is one of emptiness, restlessness and physical exhaustion: in short a sense of bereavement. Many women believe, quite wrongly, that the baby has died because of something they did, or did not do during their pregnancy. Some women feel a sense of failure: that by losing the baby they have failed their families or themselves.

A woman who loses her baby in this way need feel no shame or anxiety about her grief: it is as strong as that following the death of an older child or spouse.

Grief over the loss of a baby follows the same pattern as grief following the loss of any loved person. At first the mother, and often the father, feel numb. After a few days the reaction changes. The mother wants to know why the baby died. Some mothers become angry, others feel guilty that the baby may have died because of something the mother did or did not do. Other mothers become depressed, and this may last for months.

The reaction can be reduced if the woman has someone knowledgeable to talk to, usually her doctor. In the words of an editorial in the *British Medical Journal*, 'a willing ear tolerant of confusion and anger is probably more important than tonics or sedatives.' A Woman who has had the misfortune to give birth to a stillborn baby or whose baby died in the first month of life, has the right to expect that her doctor will try to explain to her and her partner clearly and simply the cause of the death, if it is known, and to tell her what she can expect in her next pregnancy. Both the doctor and the other medical attendants should show sympathy but not condescension to the mother; should answer her questions fully and unemotionally, and should offer her support, as should her husband and relatives, until her sense of bereavement diminishes.

A photograph of the baby may help her to adjust and the couple should have the opportunity of holding their dead baby if they wish to do so. In these ways they may overcome a troublesome, unhappy period.

To put perinatal deaths into perspective, remember that of every 100 pregnancies which reach the 20th week, 98 will end with the birth of a live baby which will survive.

CHAPTER 19

Obstetric Operations

Most pregnant women could deliver their baby by themselves, but in all cultures in history women in childbirth have been attended and helped by a 'doula' or more recently by a trained midwife. The fashion to hire an obstetrician or a general practitioner who has had obstetric training is recent. Trained attendants have reduced the danger of damage to or death of mother and baby, but have also led to an increase in interventions. These interventions are made either to reduce the chance of the mother becoming seriously ill or to deliver the baby before it is damaged or dies in the uterus. The interventions are obstetric operations, and include induction of labour, forceps delivery and caesarean section.

Induction of labour

For several reasons, such as pregnancy-induced hypertension, haemorrhage in pregnancy, Rhesus iso-immunization or pregnancy which has become prolonged to more than 42 weeks, the obstetrician may decide that it is best to induce labour. The usual way in which this is done is to rupture or 'cut' the bag of waters just inside the cervix. The procedure is quite painless, although rather inelegant. The expectant mother is put on an obstetric bed with her feet in stirrups (Fig. 19/1). The vulva is cleaned, antiseptic lubricant is poured into the vagina, and the doctor makes a pelvic examination. In this, he feels the cervix and notes whether it is soft or not, and how wide open it is. If it is 'suitable', that is soft and at least one finger dilated, he will go ahead and rupture the membranes. This is done with a small instrument, which tears a hole in the bag so that the water runs out. The procedure is called 'surgical induction of labour', or amniotomy. The mother can feel the warm amniotic fluid running down her vagina.

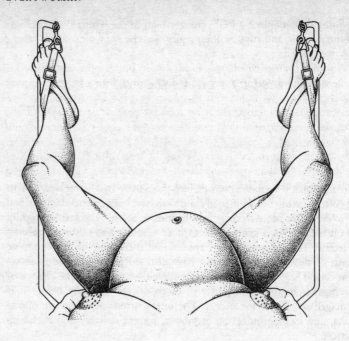

Fig. 19/1   The position in which the mother is placed for certain obstetric manipulations.

Labour usually starts quite quickly, and the doctor may encourage it to start by setting up a drip into an arm vein of the mother, and carefully running in a drug (oxytocin), which stimulates the uterus to contract.

Recently many doctors have begun to use the substance, prostaglandin E_2 in place of oxytocin. PGE_2 can be given as a vaginal tablet or as a gel which comes in a syringe and can be 'injected' high up in the vagina. PGE_2 softens the tissues of the cervix and makes the uterus contract. After having PGE_2 placed in her vagina, the baby's heart is monitored for about 30 minutes. After this the woman can return to her room and walk about until labour starts. If labour has not started in 6 hours a further amount of gel or a tablet is placed in the vagina. Using PGE_2 over 90 per cent of women go into labour.

Some doctors place a PGE_2 pessary high in the woman's vagina late in the evening and rupture the membranes the next morning if labour has not started.

Another change which was fashionable (but is now less so) is for some doctors to perform surgical induction on most of their pregnant patients. I have written about this on page 238. The woman and the doctor agree that labour will be induced near or at the end of the pregnancy on a special day, provided that the cervix is 'suitable' and the baby's head is 'engaged' in the pelvis. If the doctor has a number of pregnant women, he induces labour by surgical induction on all of them early on that day, and starts an intravenous drip containing oxytocin at once. The idea is that all his patients will have their babies during the afternoon or the evening of the same day, which is convenient for the woman and for the doctor, who can rearrange his schedule. If you support this attitude you can choose a doctor who uses this method. But for the safety of the baby it is essential to know that he is not premature and that he has grown sufficiently in the uterus to have the best chance of being healthy after birth. There are now tests which can be made to find out if the fetus is mature or not.

Fetal maturity and the L–S ratio

By convention a baby weighing less than 2500g at birth, or born before the end of the 36th week, is said to be premature or 'preterm'. The definition is not very exact because some babies grow slowly in the womb, and are mature but below the 'normal' birthweight, while others are small because the pregnancy has been shortened and they have been born prematurely.

The first group are called dysmature or growth retarded babies. This implies that the baby has lacked nourishment in the womb, usually because the mother developed pregnancy-induced hypertension or had some other disease which reduces the transfer of nourishment across the placenta so the baby's growth is retarded. These babies are mature as far as their ability to adjust to life is concerned, provided that they receive proper care.

The second group of low birth-weight babies are genuinely premature. For one reason or another, pregnancy does not last 40 weeks but is curtailed, labour starting before the 37th week. These babies are less well able to adjust to life as their vital processes have not become properly mature.

Because doctors induce labour in some normal women for convenience, it is important to be sure before doing so that the baby is mature.

Information that the baby is premature is also important when the doctor has to induce labour or do a caesarean section before the end of pregnancy because the baby is 'at risk' of dying in the mother's uterus (see p. 318). It is very important for you and your doctor to know the maturity of your baby and in this you and the laboratory can help.

The easiest way of knowing how much your pregnancy has advanced is for you to have kept a calendar of the dates of your menstrual periods, and to have visited your doctor beteween the 6th and 10th weeks of pregnancy. A pelvic examination at this time enables the doctor to estimate the duration of the pregnancy accurately by detecting the size of the uterus. Later in pregnancy he can refer back to this information.

Many doctors now recommend that their pregnant patients have an ultrasound examination made at about the 12th week, or between the 16th and 20th weeks of pregnancy, as this examination provides a very accurate method of estimating when the baby will be due (Fig. 19/2). If a woman has irregular menstrual periods and has failed to keep a menstrual calendar, ultrasound is even more helpful.

Some women fail to attend for antenatal care until late in pregnancy, and in other cases the doctor may wish to know whether the baby's lungs are sufficiently mature for him to live if he has to be delivered. The maturity of the baby's lungs is tested by taking a sample of the amniotic fluid. A narrow needle is pushed through the abdominal skin and muscles and into the uterus. The doctor takes care to avoid pushing the needle through the placenta and often has an ultrasound picture made first to find out where the placenta is. When the needle enters the amniotic sac, a sample of about 10ml of fluid is taken and sent to the laboratory, where two substances produced in the fetal lungs are measured. They are called lecithin and sphingomyelin. As the baby's lungs become mature, more lecithin is secreted and its quantity rises in the amniotic flud. When there is twice as much lecithin as spingomyelin in the sample, the baby's lungs are sufficiently mature for him to have little or no trouble in breathing after birth. But if the quantity of lecithin compared with that of sphingomyelin is less than twice as much (in other words if the lecithin:sphingomyelin ratio is less than 2), the baby has an increased chance of getting a lung disorder called hyaline membrane disease which can make its survival uncertain.

You can understand from this that if you choose to have your baby by the 'elective induction' of labour you may need to have the amniotic

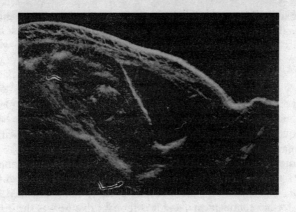

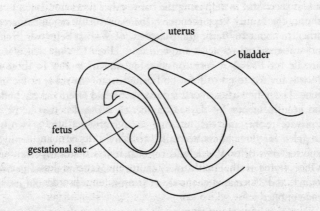

FIG. 19/2 Ultrasound picture of twelve-week fetus. Drawing shows relevant points.

fluid test (called amniocentesis) made to estimate your baby's maturity before the surgical induction.

Forceps delivery

In July 1569 – over 400 years ago – a family of Huguenot refugees called Chamberlen fled from France and arrived in England. One son, Peter, was about 6 years old, and two more sons were to be born subsequently in England, one of them also being called Peter. Although this may not have led to confusion within the family, it has led to confusion of medical historians, for both Peters became doctors, and one of them invented a secret instrument for the help of women in labour. The elder Peter had a dramatic rise to fame, attended Queen Anne for her confinements, and it is thought that he was the inventor. The Chamberlens kept their secret most successfully, and it is said that when asked to help in a difficult labour, one of them would arrive at the bedside, sit in front of the patient, and have a sheet stretched from the abdomen of the patient and tied round his neck. In the obscurity of the sheet, he would draw a bundle from the pocket of his coat, and manipulations were seen to move the sheet; but the secret instrument was never glimpsed. It was in fact the first obstetric forceps.

Chamberlen's forceps were like a pair of outsize sugar tongs, made of metal and covered with leather. He introduced them into the vagina, applied them to the sides of the baby's head, and pulled. Sometimes he was successful in delivering the baby, other times not. But successful or not, the family kept the secret for over 100 years, son succeeding father. In about 1670, the grand-nephew of the first Peter was in charge, and was tempted to sell his instrument. Hugh Chamberlen offered it for sale for £1000, a very considerable sum of money in those days. He was invited to go to Paris and demonstrate the value of his instrument. The patient chosen was a dwarf, who had severe rickets, and who had been in labour for days. Chamberlen demanded that he be given a private room, and that no one should observe him at work. He struggled for three hours but failed to deliver the patient, as might be expected. His offer of sale was rejected, but six months later he was in Paris trying again. Finally, in 1728, the male Chamberlen line became extinct, and 30 years later the secret instrument was sold and its design made public.

Since that time many changes in the design of the obstetric forceps have made it a precision-tooled, correctly constructed instrument. Over the years, too, the indications in which the forceps are needed, and for which they can be used with safety, have been identified. Doctors who proposed to practise obstetrics learn how to handle the instrument, or more correctly the instruments, for today each blade of the forceps is separate. Each blade is inserted into the vagina separately, so that it lies over the side of the baby's head, and once both are in position, the handles of the blades are crossed and joined together at a lock (Fig. 19/3). In this way the least possible damage is done to the mother or the baby.

The percentage of mothers on whom forceps are used to effect delivery of the baby varies. In Asia about 4 per cent, in Britain about 8 per cent and in Australia about 10 per cent of the mothers are delivered by forceps, while in the USA the rate exceeds 30 per cent. This is because women in labour in America are sedated, often heavily, or are given an anaesthetic so that they are unable to help in pushing the baby into the world. It is a matter of custom, but even in the USA most

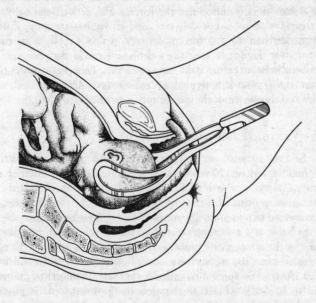

FIG. 19/3 The obstetric forceps. The mother has received a local anaesthetic, and the forceps fit snugly along the sides of the baby's head, like sugar tongs fit along a lump of sugar.

obstetricians are realizing that the more natural childbirth is made, the better it is for mother and for baby.

If forceps are required, the mother can be assured that the operation will be quite painless. Either a local anaesthetic is given, or else an injection is administered into her spine, called an epidural anaesthetic. The forceps are only inserted into her vagina when the anaesthetic has taken effect. The baby may be born with red marks along the sides of its face corresponding to the shape of the forceps blades. The mother can rest assured that the marks will disappear rapidly.

'Taking the baby with instruments' is still regarded as a serious step by many expectant mothers. Years ago it was, but today with skilled doctors and well-made precision instruments, forceps deliveries are safe. By far the majority of forceps deliveries are made to help the head of the baby over the mother's perineum. This is called a low forceps delivery. In a few cases the baby's head may fail to advance in the second stage of labour, despite strong contractions and good 'pushes' by the mother. If the second stage lasts for more than one and a half hours, the doctor usually introduces the forceps and delivers the baby. This is termed a 'mid-forceps delivery', and it requires far more skill and experience than the low forceps delivery, which is really quite easy. It is usual for the doctor to make a deliberate cut in the perineum with a pair of scissors before delivering the baby. This prevents the tissues from tearing, and it is termed an 'episiotomy'. After the birth of the baby and the placenta, the episiotomy is stitched (see p. 233).

The Ventouse (vacuum extractor)

In the last 30 year, an instrument has been developed which was originally invented 120 years ago by a famous Scottish obstetrician, Sir James Simpson, who also first used anaesthesia in childbirth. The instrument consists of a flat cup, about 7.5cm (3in) in diameter. This is connected to a vacuum apparatus. The cup is pushed against the head of the baby, and a vacuum created, so that it is held firmly against the scalp by the atmospheric pressure. The doctor then pulls on the tubing which connects the cup to the vacuum bottle, and the baby is delivered (Fig. 19/4). The apparatus, called a *ventouse*, is simple to use, and is said to have the advantage that less of the instrument is physically introduced into the vagina than when forceps are used. Because of this, damage to the mother's tissues is less likely to occur.

It does not really seem to make much difference in most cases whether

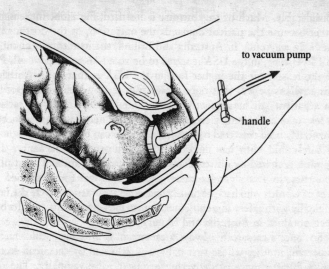

to vacuum pump

handle

FIG. 19/4 The 'vacuum extractor'. In place of forceps, a small suction cup may be applied to the baby's head, a vacuum created and the baby delivered by pulling on the cup.

forceps or a ventouse is used to deliver a baby which is delayed on its journey into the world.

Caesarean section

The operation of caesarean section has nothing to do with Julius Caesar. The word derives from the Latin *caedere*, to cut, for that is what is done. If for some reason the baby cannot be born through the birth-canal, an incision is made in the lower part of the abdominal wall and through the lower part of the uterus. The child is removed through the incisions, which are then carefully repaired with stitches. In the past most mothers were given a general anaesthetic and only woke up after the operation was complete. In recent years, increasing numbers of women are choosing to have a caesarean section performed under epidural anaesthesia. This type of anaesthetic is, in general, safer for the baby and enables the mother (and often the father of the child) to witness its birth and to cuddle it soon after it has been born.

In the past 30 years, the incidence of caesarean section has increased considerably. Much of this increase is justified; but some inexcusable, either because the patient demands the operation, or the doctor takes the 'easy way out'. In Australia and Britain, the incidence is about 10 to 15 per cent; in the USA it seems to be about 16 to 20 per cent. Part of the reason for the higher rate in the USA is that most American obstetricians believe that once a caesarean section has been performed on a patient, all subsequent deliveries should be by caesarean section. A few take a different view, and believe that many women who have previously been delivered by caesarean section can be delivered vaginally as safely and with less discomfort in a subsequent pregnancy. This opinion is shared by obstetricians in Australia, Britain and most other countries. In a very careful study in Britain, it was found that 45 per cent of women who had previously had a caesarean section were delivered vaginally with safety in a subsequent pregnancy, and similar results have been obtained in Australia and Malaysia.

So 'once a caesarean, always a caesarean' is no longer valid, and an expectant mother whose first baby was delivered by caesarean section has a 50:50 chance of delivering her next baby vaginally. The only stipulation upon which all obstetricians agree is that a patient who has previously had a caesarean section must be looked after by a specialist obstetrician, and have her baby in a properly equipped hospital.

Caesarean section is a safe procedure today. Most obstetricians give the mother antibiotics to reduce the risk of infection. The risk of dying after a caesarean section is about 1 in 2500 caesareans, and if the caesarean is done electively, rather than as an emergency, the risk of dying is about 1 in 11 000 which is no greater than the risk of dying after a vaginal birth.

Retained placenta – manual removal

You will remember that normally the placenta (afterbirth) is expelled within a few minutes of the birth of your baby, especially when the doctor has given you an injection of ergometrine as the baby was being born. Occasionally, perhaps once or twice in every 100 deliveries, the afterbirth is retained in the uterus. Often it will be expelled after a 15-minute interval but in some cases, particularly if bleeding occurs, the doctor may decide to remove it. The woman is given an anaesthetic and the doctor introduces his hand, very gently, into her uterus and eases the placenta from its attachments. The procedure is quite safe, painless and in no way affects the mother's progress in the lying-in period, or her ability to have another child.

CHAPTER 20

The Things that Happen
to Women

During life it is inevitable that a woman will have her share of anxiety, of illness, of strain, as well as her share of satisfaction and happiness. But because she is biologically different from man, she may develop conditions unique to woman. Many of these are minor, but require attention. In most instances a woman should consult her doctor, but as doctors are busy people and all too often do not explain adequately to the patient the nature of the condition from which she is suffering, she often remains anxious. This chapter attempts to redress this, and to give a woman the chance of understanding herself better. There is no doubt that fear of the unknown is a potent factor in aggravating disease, and insight into the nature of a disorder is a major step to its cure. For convenience, the conditions which may affect a woman in her reproductive years are considered in as alphabetical an order as is practicable.

Cervical 'erosion' (cervical eversion)

As noted previously, the lining of the vagina is built up of layers of cells, rather like a wall is built up of bricks, and the same arrangement of cells covers the cervix where it pokes into the upper part of the vagina. However, a sudden change occurs at the edge of the canal leading through the cervix. The cells which line this are a single layer thick. They are large and very active in secreting mucus so that the woman may complain of a vaginal discharge. During puberty, and again in a first pregnancy, the exact position of the change from the flat wall-like cells of the vaginal part of the cervix to the tall single mucus-secreting cells of the cervical canal moves, and in many women it moves outward. This means that the tall cells now appear around the entrance to the canal to look like lips (Fig. 20/1). The same effect can be obtained if

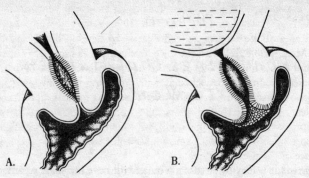

FIG. 20/1   The junction between the lining cells of the cervical canal and those of the cervix move in pregnancy.

you close your mouth and draw in your lips. Your mouth now appears as a slit ringed by pink skin. If you now pout your lips, your mouth is ringed by red lip mucous membrane.

In the past, the 'pouting' of the cells of the cervical canal was called an 'erosion' or an 'ulcer' because doctors believed it was abnormal. And, of course, it is *not* an ulcer. The treatment of the 'ulcer' was to burn it by applying a cautery stick or by using an electric cautery. It is now known that such treatment is usually unnecessary, and indeed is only needed if at childbirth the mouth of the cervical canal is torn or damaged. However, even in these cases treatment should be withheld for at least six months after childbirth, as the 'pouting' often disappears. If the discharge persists for more than 6 months, treatment may be needed. The cervix is treated using laser, electrocautery or by freezing (cryocautery). 'Stick' cautery is no longer used. The treatment can be given in the doctor's office, but may be done in hospital under an anaesthetic.

After laser treatment, cautery or cryosurgery of the cervix, the woman will notice that she has an increased quantity of vaginal discharge, often dirty-looking with streaks of blood in the first few days. The discharge is due to the burned area being shed as the cells beneath it make a new lining and push off the old one. The discharge may last for 4 to 6 weeks, but this is normal. At the end of this time, the doctor usually wants to see the patient once again, so that he may inspect the cervix to see how well it has healed.

Depression

At all ages of life women are more likely to develop depression than men. Most people feel miserable or have the blues at some stage of their life, and this is normal. Depression or melancholia is less common, but can be serious. In the USA, twice as many women as men have an episode of depression sometime in their life. The reasons for this difference are not clear. It may be that in our culture women are permitted to show emotion and have changes in mood, whilst men are not and consequently are more likely to deal with emotional problems by anger, aggression, violence or the use of alcohol.

Depression seems to be more common in some families, which suggests that some cases of depression have a genetic cause. In some causes the hidden antecedent is physical or sexual abuse during childhood or adolescence. Depression is not due to hormonal changes in a woman's body and is not more common at puberty or during the menopausal years, but a break up of a relationship or a bereavement may be a precipitating factor.

People who have clinical depression feel miserable or hopeless for most of the day, as if they were under a black cloud, and the sadness is worse in the morning. They lose interest or pleasure in all or most activities. Often they wake early in the morning (at least two hours before their usual waking time). They lose their appetite and may lose weight. They have less energy and less sexual desire. They may have episodes of irritability or agitation for no apparent reason.

If a woman feels that she has clinical depression she should seek help. This may merely mean being able to talk to a professional about her problem or it may mean that she should take antidepressant drugs for a period of time. In some cases of severe depression, electroconvulsive therapy may be the only way to cure the depression.

Enlargement of the womb

The most common cause of enlargement of the womb is pregnancy! But sometimes the womb is enlarged by a muscle tumour, or by a tumour called an adenomyoma.

The muscle tumours are called myomata or 'fibroids'. For some unknown reason, one or more of the muscle fibres which make up the uterus start developing, and quite soon a few small pea-sized tumours appear deep in the muscle wall of the uterus. At this stage no one can detect them, but as the months or years pass – for they grow very slowly – the tumours become the size of a golf ball, a tennis ball or even of a grapefruit. By this time the patient can feel a lump in her abdomen, or if the tumour has grown inwards and distorted the shape of the cavity of the uterus, she may have heavier or irregular menstrual perods. Usually she goes to her doctor, who performs a pelvic examination and can tell from this if there is a single fibroid, or if the womb is misshapen and enlarged by several fibroid tumours. It is unusual for a woman who has children early in life to develop fibroids, and the tumours are more likely to occur in women who have never had a baby or who have delayed childbirth until after the age of 30. This has led to the saying that 'fibroids develop in a disappointed womb'. The tumours are very common, and more than 20 per cent of women have fibroids in their womb. In many cases no treatment is required, as the tumour is not causing any symptoms, but in the few women who have symptoms, treatment is needed. The treatment chosen depends upon the patient's age and her desire to have further children.

If a young woman, who is anxious to have children, is found to have fibroids which are causing symptoms, the doctor can often operate to remove the fibroids and leave the uterus. It is a bit like a complicated shelling of peas, and although there is a slight chance that the fibroids may grow again, the chances of pregnancy are good. In an older woman, or a woman who wants no further children, the operation chosen is usually that of hysterectomy, in which the womb is removed.

The second kind of muscle tumour is called an adenomyoma. This leads to a smooth enlargement of the uterus. It is not malignant, and is a form of endometriosis.

In a few women hormone imbalance, leading to an excess production of oestrogen, may cause an enlargement of the uterus over a period of time. The hormone imbalance may be caused by the emotions, but this has never been proved. Often the woman has heavy menstrual periods. Often this leads the doctor to suggest a hysterectomy. Hysterectomy may be the right treatment, but often, although the bleeding ceases, the emotional problems remain. It is important to try hormones first to see if they will relieve the symptoms, before deciding on hysterectomy.

Endometriosis

Endometriosis is a strange disorder which, more commonly, affects women who have chosen not to have children, or who are infertile. The term means that pieces of the lining of the womb (the endometrium) either form small nests (or cysts) in the muscle of the womb (which will, of course, then become bigger), in the ovaries, or in other parts of the pelvis. These nests of endometrium act like miniature wombs, and at the time of menstruation a tiny amount of bleeding occurs. Since the blood cannot escape, the cyst is stretched and becomes painful. The woman complains of menstrual pain, which increases during menstruation and is worse on the last day. If a cyst has formed in the pelvis behind the womb, as sometimes happens, sexual intercourse can be painful when the man's penis is moving deeply inside the vagina. Because of menstrual pain, painful sexual intercourse, or failure to become pregnant, the woman attends her doctor. In the past the only treatment was surgery, but today hormone treatment using drugs like those contained in the Pill can cure the condition, and enable the patient to conceive if she so wishes. A new drug called danazol is more effective than the Pill, but in the dose needed to cure endometriosis it causes amenorrhoea and has some side-effects, such as muscle cramps and acne which affect about one woman in every seven taking danazol. A new treatment using a synthetic hormone related to the gonadotrophic releasing hormone (see p. 28) has been developed. The woman sniffs a quantity of the hormone four times a day or has a monthly injection of a long acting form of the hormone. The hormone suppresses the ability of the ovaries to make oestrogen, so that the woman becomes 'menopausal'. Her periods cease and she may get hot flushes. Deprived of the stimulus to grow provided by oestrogen the endometriotic patches shrivel and heal. Some women need surgery, but often all the gynaecologist has to do is to make a tiny incision below the umbilicus and introduce an instrument, called a laparoscope, so that he can see the extent of the disease. This minor operation is done under anaesthesia. Once the doctor knows how much the endometriosis has involved the genital organs, he can decide if surgery or hormone treatment is best, or if both are needed. If the doctor decides that surgery is required and the endometriotic cysts are not too big, they can be vaporized with a laser, using a laparoscope to see. The hospital stay after laser treatment is only 1 to 2 days. If the cysts are big or there are many adhesions, the doctor may have to make a cut in the lower abdomen and operate through it, which means a longer hospital stay.

Hirsutism (hairiness)

The amount of body hair varies between different races, for example Chinese generally have very little body hair, while Southern Europeans tend to have more body hair than Northern Europeans.

Some women have increased body hair and this may cause great concern, especially if the hair grows on the upper lip, on the legs or the breasts. The concern is that the hair, growing in an inappropriate place for a woman, makes her feel and look less feminine.

A few women with excess or inappropriately placed body hair also develop signs of de-feminization. Their clitoris enlarges; their scalp hair recedes and their voice deepens. These women require investigation as they may have a tumour which needs to be removed by surgery.

Most hirsute women do not have these additional changes and do not have a tumour. Their increased body hair is due to an increased sensitivity by their hair follicles to the small amounts of male hormone which circulates in their blood, or to an increase in the amount of the hormone in their circulation.

Cosmetic aids and reassurance are all that many women request, but for the others, drugs are now available which will reduce the excessive hair. One of these drugs is a diuretic drug, called spironolactone. Another is a drug which opposes the male hormone. It is called cyproterone, which is taken for 10 days each month, together with an oestrogen. (It is available as a pill.) It takes about 3 months for the excessive hair to cease growing and the drug is taken for an additional 6 months.

Heart Disease

Heart disease is a common cause of death in middle-aged men, 3 men in every 1000 aged 40 to 69 die each year from a heart attack. Women have about one-third the risk of developing coronary heart disease and of dying from a heart attack, but more women seem to be developing heart disease. Information from Australia (which is similar to that expected from Britain and the USA) is that, as far as can be estimated, 3 women in every 1000 aged 40 to 49 will have a non-fatal heart attack each year and one woman in every 3000 will die from a heart attack. Women aged 50 to 59 have an increased risk: 7 women in every 1000 will have a non-fatal heart attack each year, and 1 in every 1000 will die from a heart attack. The risk is increased amongst middle-aged women who are obese, particularly if more fat is deposited in their 'stomach' than on their hips. The risk is also increased if a woman smokes cigarettes, has a high blood pressure, and avoids exercise.

The risk of developing heart disease is reduced if middle-aged women eat a prudent diet (low in fat and sugars); if obese women reduce their weight, take regular enjoyable exercise (a half hours brisk walk three times a week is probably sufficient) and stop smoking. There is new information that if a woman stops smoking cigarettes, her risk of having a heart attack due to smoking declines soon after she ceases to smoke, and is dissipated after 2 or 3 years.

Hysterectomy

One of the most common surgical operations performed on women is removal of the womb, or hysterectomy. In fact, many doctors believe that the operation is done too often for too little reason. By the age of 55, 1 American woman in 3, 1 Australian woman in 4 and 1 British woman in 5 will have had a hysterectomy, although with the new treatment described on page 345, the numbers are falling. In most cases a well-performed hysterectomy can cure a patient who was previously miserable. But, even so, the operation is still done too often, for too little reason, and without explaining to the woman its effects. Unfortunately, if the operation is performed for a trivial reason and without proper counselling, a number of women develop depression, which may last for 2 years or more. Recent studies indicate that most of these women were depressed (as judged by a special test) before the operation, and the hysterectomy aggravated the depression so that it became obvious to others. The severity and the duration of depression would be reduced (and hysterectomy sometimes avoided) if the woman, who is advised to have the operation, had the opportunity to talk to a counsellor before the operation. Some gynaecologists are able to talk with women: some are not. In some instances it would be more appropriate to talk with a psychiatrist or a psychologist. It is a woman's right and a doctor's duty to tell you what is wrong with your uterus and why you need the operation. You should not feel that you are wasting the doctor's time, nor that you are asking stupid questions. You should not feel ashamed about asking *any* questions and you should expect an answer in clear language that you can understand. It is also helpful to ask for a pamphlet or a book about hysterectomy. Some women believe that they have to have the operation because of some earlier sexual activity, such as masturbation or a previous abortion, or an extramarital affair, and the operation is a punishment. This, of course, is not so. Other women believe, falsely, that without a uterus a woman is no longer a proper woman. This too is untrue.

Hysterectomy does not make a woman sexually mutilated and undesired; it does not shorten or narrow her vagina so that sexual intercourse is impossible, painful or potentially dangerous. Provided that the gynaecologist is skilful, the only after-effects of hysterectomy are that you have no more menstrual periods and pregnancy cannot possibly occur. All the other fears, anxieties and unhappiness connected with the operation occur because a woman has not had the chance to talk, properly and openly, with her doctor.

Myths associated with hysterectomy

'AFTER HYSTERECTOMY I SHALL BECOME OLD, UNFEMININE AND UNDESIRABLE.' This is untrue. A woman is sexually desirable because of her character and personality. She is feminine because of the way she has been brought up and because of the female sex hormones which are secreted by her ovaries. It is usual, if a woman is under the age of 45, and often whatever her age, to leave her ovaries in place, so that they can continue to function. And if they need to be removed, oestrogen hormone tablets can be taken to replace those lost. But talk with your doctor.

'AFTER HYSTERECTOMY I WON'T WANT OR ENJOY SEX ANY MORE.' This is untrue. Your enjoyment of sex does not depend on the presence of your uterus, but on the presence of a good, communicating relationship with your partner. The operation does not shorten or narrow your vagina; in fact, if anything it is longer, as you can see in Fig. 20/2. When the womb is removed the vagina has to be cut and then stitched again at its upper end, and the cervix no longer projects into it. Once the cut has healed properly, which takes between 4 and 6 weeks, you can start enjoying sexual intercourse once again; before that time you can enjoy mutual pleasuring, including digital or oral stimulation of your clitoris (see p. 3).

'AFTER HYSTERECTOMY WOMEN BECOME FAT.' This is untrue. Hysterectomy is not followed by obesity, unless the woman takes no exercise after the operation and spends her time eating. If she does this, of course she will get fat.

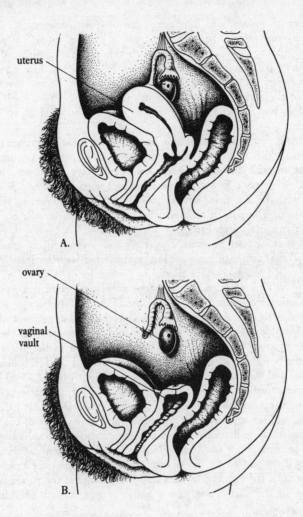

FIG. 20/2   The length of the vagina shown in A is not shortened by hysterectomy shown in B.

Irritable bowel

A number of women who have symptoms of 'pelvic congestion' also have a disorder referred to as the 'irritable or irritated bowel'. It also is called 'spastic colon'. A woman with this disorder complains of intermittent pain in her abdomen on the left side and low down. Some sufferers also complain of painful intercourse. Recent investigations in England show that one woman in 7 aged 20 to 60 complains of irritable bowel, but only one or two in every hundred go to see a doctor.

The main complaint in irritable bowel is abdominal pain, usually left sided, which is relieved when the bowels are opened. A woman who has irritable bowel may feel nauseated, have heartburn, feel 'bloated' or 'gaseous' in her abdomen and pass wind excessively. Some women with the complaint have episodes of diarrhoea alternating with constipation. The pain is relieved when she opens her bowels but it returns, particularly after eating.

The condition can be quite disturbing and investigations usually show nothing, although some women are infected with an intestinal parasite called giardia, which should be looked for in a specimen of the motions. This is because if it is present there is a specific treatment. In most cases, treatment is rather unsatisfactory, mainly because it is a psychosomatic disorder. Recent research has shown that patients who have an irritable colon often have a disturbance in the speed with which food moves along their gut, and as well the tension in the affected part of the bowel is increased. The speed of transit of the faeces along the bowel and the tension within the colon can both be regulated by the simple expedient of cutting down sugar and eating coarse bran. If a woman eats wholemeal instead of white bread she needs to eat less bran, and for most women an additional 2 tablespoons of coarse bran eaten daily will relieve the pain and regulate the bowel habits. Because her bowels are not conditioned to 'roughage' she should start by taking 2 teaspoons each day of coarse bran and increase the amount each day until she gets regular soft bulky motions and the pain goes. You can eat the bran alone, like a horse, or mix it with breakfast cereal or yoghurt.

Patients who do not 'get better' in spite of treatment are often depressed or have 'anxiety'. They should seek counselling or explore the cause of the underlying psychological problem.

Menstrual disorders

Because of the complicated control of menstruation which was described in Chapter 4, and because of the impact of the emotions upon the controlling area in the brain, it can be readily understood that from time to time during a woman's life menstrual disorders may occur. These are, in general, of three kinds: the menstrual periods may occur less frequently, or cease altogether; they may occur regularly but be very heavy; or they may become quite irregular in time of onset, in their duration and in the amount of blood lost. These irregularities are more usual before the age of 20 and after the age of 35, but may occur at any time during the reproductive years. Furthermore, many women find that the character of their menstrual period alters during the reproductive years. Often the periods become heavier for a while after childbirth, and as the age of 40 is approached.

The three patterns of menstrual irregularity need further discussion because many women become very anxious when the periods are not 'normal'.

Less frequent periods or no periods (amenorrhoea)

Less frequent menstrual periods and amenorrhoea may be caused by many conditions. Amenorrhoea occurs when the hormone relationships between the hypothalamus, the pituitary gland and the ovaries is disturbed (see p. 23). In some cases this is due to an emotional upset (such as leaving home or the loss of a loved person). In some cases it is due to pregnancy. In some cases it is caused by excessive exercise or by strict dieting – women who train for a marathon run often stop menstruating, as do women who starve themselves. In some cases amenorrhoea is due to a tumour of the pituitary gland or to a disturbance of the thyroid gland. In some cases it occurs while a woman is taking the Pill or after stopping taking the Pill.

As many cases are due to an emotional upset, it is usual to wait until 6 months have passed before starting investigations (except for a pregnancy test), as most women will start menstruating again by that time. If a woman has less frequent periods occurring over a period of 6 months, or if she has amenorrhoea, she should seek help from a doctor. Infrequent periods are generally of no concern and what a woman needs is to be reassured that she is normal. This can be done once the doctor has made an examination. Treatment using hormones is not indicated, and many women, once they have been reassured, may prefer to have less frequent periods!

If a woman has amenorrhoea, the doctor should exclude pregnancy, check if she has lost weight or has an eating disorder, and find out if she is taking the Pill. If she is pregnant she will have to decide whether or not she wants the baby, while if she is taking the Pill she need not be concerned that she has no periods, as menstruation has no real function. If she has an eating disorder she should be referred for treatment.

However, if the amenorrhoea persists for 9 months or more it is wise for a woman to be seen by a specialist so that he can find out why she is not menstruating. The doctor will do a general and a vaginal examination and will arrange for some blood tests to measure the levels of certain hormones. With this information he can assess whether the amenorrhoea is not due to disease (and usually it is not), and provided the woman does not want to become pregnant, there is no indication for giving hormones to produce a menstrual bleed. It is better to remain without periods.

Heavy regular periods (menorrhagia)

The pattern of a woman's periods may change so that they become excessively heavy and often last for longer than previously, although their regularity is unchanged. In some women, the problem is aggravated by clots being expelled during menstruation and the woman feels heavy and exhausted.

If the pattern does not revert to normal quickly she should see a doctor. He will examine her generally, making sure she has not become anaemic or has high blood pressure, and also vaginally to be sure that she has not developed a 'fibroid' (see p. 335) or a tumour of her ovary. In many cases he will also recommend that the woman has a diagnostic curettage performed. In this minor operation, the lining of the womb is 'cleaned' off ('scraped' is too strong a verb!) and looked at under the microscope so that the doctor can choose the correct treatment. The operation is performed under an anaesthetic, and the woman need not spend more than a few hours in hospital and certainly does not need to suffer the indignity of having her pubic hair shaved off. Although the operation is loosely called a 'D and C', the proper term, which stresses the fact that it is done *to make a diagnosis*, is a 'diagnostic curettage'.

Recently some doctors have replaced the 'D and C' and use a

hysteroscope (rather like a small telescope) to look inside the cavity of the uterus so that they can detect a thickened lining or a polyp or a fibroid, and to treat the problem accordingly.

Not all women with heavy regular periods need a diagnostic curettage, but if a woman is aged 40 or more it is usual to do it to make quite sure that no cancer of the womb is present.

The choice of treatment should be a matter for discussion with the doctor. Most women will be cured if progestogen hormones are given; or one of the newer anti-prostaglandin drugs. Only if these medications fail to relieve the heavy menstruation need surgery be considered. There are two choices: endometrial ablation, and hysterectomy.

Endometrial ablation means that the lining of the uterus is removed using an electrically heated roller ball which burns the endometrium and prevents it regrowing. Other methods are to vaporize the endometrium using a laser or a method of radiofrequency-induced heat. The operation is done after a hysteroscope has been introduced into the uterus through the cervix, and the uterus filled with a liquid, so that the surgeon can see exactly what he or she is doing. The instrument used to perform the ablation of the endometrium is introduced into the uterus through the cervix so there is no cut. The operation may be performed under general or local anaesthesia, depending on the woman's wishes, and she does not need to stay in hospital for more than a day. She may have some uterine cramps for a day or two after the operation but that is all. About 85 per cent of women have no periods or light periods after the operation, but 15 per cent are not relieved and can choose to have a further 'endometrial ablation' or to have a hysterectomy.

Until endometrial ablation was developed, hysterectomy was the method used to treat menorrhagia in women who had tried hormones which had failed to relieve the heavy periods or who had chosen not to use hormones. Many doctors – and many women – prefer hysterectomy. Hysterectomy is discussed on page 339.

Some women do not want a surgical treatment. They have a further choice, particularly if hormones have failed to stop the heavy periods and the woman wishes to keep her fertility. This treatment means that she has to sniff a brain hormone (called a gonadotrophin releasing hormone, analogue of GnRH) 4 times a day or have an implant every month. GnRH suppresses all ovarian activity and consequently the periods cease. Unfortunately most of the women get 'menopausal' symptoms, but these can be treated (see page 383).

Irregular bleeding

If a woman has episodes of bleeding which are irregular in duration, in amount and occur unpredictably, it is inconvenient, disturbing and produces anxiety. She should see her doctor who will examine her and must perform a diagnostic curettage, usually at a time when the woman is not bleeding, so that the most information can be obtained.

This is important as in some cases the irregular bleeding is caused by a cancer of the lining of the womb. If the curettage shows that there is a cancer, treatment is for the doctor to perform a hysterectomy. If there is no cancer the woman may choose one of the treatments mentioned in the previous section. Which treatment is best for the woman can only be decided after full discussion between the woman and her gynaecologist, who has spoken with her family doctor, as he knows her family circumstances, which may be important in making a decision.

Menstrual cramps (dysmenorrhoea). See page 34.

Obesity

In the past 75 years, almost for the first time in history, women living in the richer nations of the developed world are under strong pressure to be slim, or if fat to lose weight. The public perception, encouraged by the media, particularly television, is that to be attractive, desirable and successful a woman should be slim.

Investigations made in many countries show that women of all ages, but especially women under the age of 25, perceive their body to be larger than it really is.

Because of this concern about body weight and shape, an enormous variety of drugs (mostly ineffective, except over the first few weeks), drugs, regimens, exercise programmes, massages and hydrotherapy appear in books and magazines. These profit the promoters, but do much less for the participants.

The first thing to remember is that there is no 'ideal' body weight. There is a preferred body-weight range. It is preferred because if your weight lies in this range you are less likely to develop high blood pressure, diabetes and some other illnesses.

You can determine if your weight lies in this preferred weight range

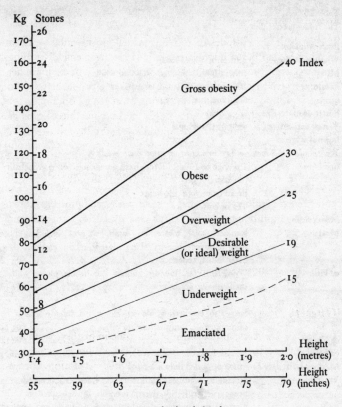

FIG. 20/3   Weight/height² index.

by calculating your body mass index (or BMI). The BMI is obtained by dividing your weight in kilograms by your height in metres squared. The results of these calculations are shown in Figure 20/3.

If your BMI lies in the 19–24.9 range, it is in the preferred range for health and appearance; if it lies in the 25–29.9 range you are overweight and may consider losing weight by increasing your exercise and choosing a weight-reducing diet. If your BMI is 30 or more you are obese. Obesity occurs when over a period of time you ingest more energy than you expend. In Western societies between 5 and 7 per cent of adult women are obese.

Table 20/1
The Addenbrooks diet

Daily Allowance

Wholegrain bread:	3 slices of 50g (1½oz)
Milk:	either 600ml skimmed or 300ml whole
Potato:	100g (3½oz) boiled, 1 large baked
or:	60g (2oz) rice
Butter or margarine:	15g (½oz)
Water, tea, coffee, mineral water:	unlimited amounts

You should eat 3 meals a day: breakfast and two main meals

Breakfast:	1 orange or 100ml (3½oz) fresh orange juice or ½ grapefruit (no added sugar)
	Bread from your allowance
	Tea or coffee

Main meals

Meat:	lean beef (steak, mince), lean lamb, lean pork (including chops if fat removed), poultry (skin removed), rabbit, game. Liver, heart, tongue 60g (2oz)
or Fish:	*White fish:* cod, flounder, halibut, lemon, sole, plaice, whiting, shell fish ....90g (3oz) or
	Fatty fish: eel, herring, bloater, kipper, mackerel, pilchards, salmon, trout, sardines (discard oil)..................60g (2oz)
or Cheese:	....60g (2oz)
or Eggs:	....(65g) 2

Meat and fish may be grilled or boiled only not fried

Vegetables:	asparagus, cabbage, cauliflower, celery, lettuce, cucumber, beans (runner, french, dwarf) broccoli, Brussels sprouts, marrow, mushrooms, spinach, courgettes – unlimited amounts or:
	peas, beans (butter, haricot, red, baked), carrots, leeks, parsnips, pumpkin, swedes, squash, turnips 50g (1½oz)
Fruit:	Apples, oranges, grapefruit, peaches, pears, plums (all soft fruits) or melon 100g (3½oz)

You must not take any of the following:

alcohol	jams, honey	milk shakes
sugar	canned fruit	soft drinks, cordials
sweets, chocolate	pastries and puddings	sauces

As long as you keep within your allowances you can devise your own meals to suit your own circumstances

This diet provides:

Energy	1200Kcals (5040kJ)		Carbohydrate	172g
Protein	78g		Fibre	36g
Fat	19g			

Some people are more likely to become obese. If your parents are fat you have a greater chance of becoming obese.

Obesity is a health hazard! Middle-aged obese women are more likely to develop diabetes and have a three fold chance of developing heart disease compared with women whose weight is in the normal range.

If you wish to lose weight you can do this, but it isn't easy. 'Gimmicky', 'crash' and other diets do not work. You will only lose weight and keep to your chosen weight if you have the discipline, self-control and the persistence to keep to your diet. Drugs do not really help except for a few women over a short period of time. They should only be taken after obtaining advice from a doctor.

A weight-reducing diet which has proved helpful is to be found in Table 20/1. This diet is easy to adhere to and enables you to eat much the same foods as your family and friends. Problems may arise when eating out but they are not major. Rather than refuse the food you are offered, take a smaller portion, and try to eat less on the two days before the dinner party.

There is no instant method of losing weight. It takes time and discipline. If a woman is 6kg (14lb) overweight, for example, she can calculate that 5kg of this is due to excess fat and perhaps 1kg to water retention. Five kilogrammes of fat contain about 50 000 calories. The normal, averagely-active woman needs about 2100 calories a day, and the suggested diet only gives her 1200 calories a day, so that each day she burns up 900 calories from her stored fat. To lose 50 000 calories will take 12 weeks. There is no instant cure! The recommended diet will enable a woman to lose just under 0.4kg (1lb) a week, but she will have to accept that in some weeks she will lose less than in others, because at certain times of the month, usually in a week before menstruation, a woman often retains water. So do not weigh yourself more than once a week.

If you want more information you may care to obtain the book I have written with Suzanne Abraham called *Eating Disorders – The Facts*, 3rd edn, 1992).

Ovaries – removal

The removal of a woman's ovaries by surgery when she is younger than 45 years is followed by very severe 'menopausal symptoms'. These can be very distressing. In the past, unfortunately, many ovaries were removed unnecessarily by surgeons who had not had a proper training in gynaecology. A gynaecologist who has to operate on a young woman because of pelvic disease will use all his skill to preserve her ovaries. This is possible, even if the ovaries are enlarged by cysts. The cysts can be carefully dissected out of the ovaries, leaving enough ovarian tissue to reconstruct an ovary which functions well. Very occasionally a woman younger than 45 years develops ovarian cancer. In this disease it is essential that both ovaries are removed, but treatment with small tablets of oestrogen hormone, given by mouth, will reduce or eliminate menopausal symptoms.

Ovulation pain and bleeding

A number of women develop abdominal pain, which lasts for a few hours and which occurs at the time of ovulation fairly consistently. In a few women a small amount of bleeding occurs. If the pain is uncomfortable analgesics such as aspirin will relieve it. Alternatively, if the woman suppresses ovulation by taking the Pill the pain will be relieved.

Pelvic inflammatory disease (PID)

This is the name for the condition of pelvic infection. It may follow non-gonococcal genital infection, gonorrhoea, an induced abortion, a spontaneous abortion or some other infection. If the infection is marked the woman complains of pain in her lower abdomen, sometimes pain on intercourse and sometimes she develops a smelly vaginal discharge. The diagnosis may be obvious, but for accuracy an examination of the woman's pelvis through a laparoscope is valuable. The procedure is discussed on page 90. It is a minor procedure and prevents the diagnosis of pelvic inflammatory disease being made when, in reality, it was not present. Investigations in Sweden and the USA show that a clinical diagnosis of PID was wrong 1 time in every 5.

Many cases of PID are so mild that the woman does not go to a doctor and receive treatment and PID becomes chronic. The inflammation may cause damage to the Fallopian tubes and make the woman sterile. In these cases the illness is diagnosed unexpectedly during investigations for infertility. When pelvic inflammatory disease is diagnosed, treatment is given. The woman is prescribed antibiotics. If the infection is severe she will be very ill and needs to be in hospital. In this case the drugs are given into a vein. In milder cases the antibiotics may be taken by mouth. Women who have PID usually need to take the antibiotics for at least 10 days, although after 4 or 5 days they have no symptoms. Failure to complete the course of antibiotics may cause residual infection and sterility.

Pelvic pain

Pain deep inside the pelvis or in the lower abdomen, which is 'nagging', or 'stabbing' or 'burning', and which occurs at irregular unpredictable intervals, affects a number of women. As the pain may be due to pelvic infection, endometriosis or an ovarian cyst, the doctor usually looks inside the woman's abdomen using a laparoscope. If no abnormality is found after examining the woman, the diagnosis is made that she has psychosomatic chronic pelvic pain. The woman needs considerable reassurance that she has no disease in her pelvis; and help so that she may learn to adjust to accept the recurrent episodes of chronic pelvic pain. Medications have not proved of much help but a recent suggestion that the woman take doses of a hormone called Provera for 3 months may be of some value.

If all these methods fail and the pain is incapacitating, the woman may choose to have a hysterectomy and the removal of her ovaries. This is a drastic solution, and should only be considered after much thought and consultations with a doctor. After the operation many women find that the pain has ceased and that they can lead a normal (including sexual) life. Other women find that the pelvic pain continues.

Of course the woman should take hormone replacement treatment as discussed on p. 384.

Periodic 'bloating'

A number of women complain that periodically they develop 'bloating'. When an attack starts, the woman finds her face and hands are puffy when she wakes up; she may be irritable or depressed, and under some domestic or occupational stress. As the day goes on she finds that her belly becomes distended, and by evening her ankles are swollen. The attack may last only one day or persist for a few days, when constipation seems to be likely, and then disappear only to recur again unexpectedly. Some women find that the 'bloating' is worse in hot weather and, in some, it occurs just before a menstrual period, when it can be confused with the premenstrual syndrome, although usually the weight gain is greater, exceeding 1.5kg (or 3½lb).

The cause is that, for some unknown reason, fluid 'leaks' out of the circulation into the tissues. It is difficult to know how to treat the disorder. First, a woman should know that the irritability and depression are caused by the fluid retention and should make sure that her sexual partner or her family are aware of this. She needs sympathy not hostility. Second, diuretics should be avoided. Third, if she is constipated she should not use laxatives but increase her bran intake. Fourth, she should stop smoking, as nicotine seems to aggravate the problem.

Perimenstrual syndrome (menstrual distress)

Women with this syndrome complain of symptoms occurring within 2 days of the onset of menstruation, the earlier part of the menstrual cycle being symptom-free. The symptoms vary in character and severity in different cycles. The most common mood symptoms are: lassitude, fatigue and lethargy. The most common physical symptoms are: abdominal discomfort or bloating, a feeling of pelvic pressure, headaches and menstrual cramps (dysmenorrhoea). In some women the menstrual flow is altered, the periods either becoming more frequent or heavier. It was originally thought that the symptoms were due to pelvic (broad ligament) varicose veins which became congested in the perimenstrual period. This is why menstrual distress used to be called 'pelvic congestion'. It is now known that these are not the cause. The symptoms usually cease within 24 hours to 48 hours after the onset of menstruation. Treatment, when required, is to prescribe analgesics for headache, and mefenamic acid (or one of the other non-steroidal anti-inflammatory drugs) for the other symptoms, particularly menstrual cramps.

Premenstrual syndrome (premenstrual tension; PMT)

Most women notice changes in mood, or develop physical symptoms at some time during the 2 weeks preceding menstruation. The changes are usually minor and do not disturb the woman's life to any significant degree. In about 25 per cent of women the mood and physical changes are of sufficient magnitude to reduce the woman's feeling of well-being and to cause a deterioration in her interpersonal relationships. These women have the premenstrual syndrome (PMS). In the premenstrual syndrome the changes in mood and the development of physical symptoms occur between 12 and 5 days before menstruation and are relieved within 48 hours of the onset of menstruation. The symptoms may vary in character and severity between menstrual cycles, but are always cyclic – a symptom-free period intervening between each premenstrual episode. The common symptoms are shown in Table 20/2.

PMS appears to be more common in women aged 30 to 45 and may become evident following childbirth or a disturbing life-event.

Although PMS affects many women the cause of the syndrome remains unknown. Some doctors believe that there is a deficiency in progesterone; others that brain transmitting substances are involved. No theory has been proved and it is clear that psychological and emotional factors may influence a woman's perception of her premenstrual symptoms. Recently it has been found that if the normal fluctuating level of oestrogen can be flattened out, the symptoms disappear. This can be achieved in a few women, if she takes the Pill or by removing the woman's uterus and her ovaries, but clearly this approach is not practical except in rare circumstances. However it does offer hope for a new, less mutilating treatment which is being researched.

Because of this it is difficult to be sure if any of the many medications prescribed have any real value. Many women with PMS, and their doctors, find it helpful if the woman identifies the three most severe mood symptoms and the three most severe physical symptoms, and makes a chart, listing the severity of each symptom (on a scale of 0 to 3) each day, for at least two menstrual cycles. During this time previously taken medication should be avoided. This exercise enables

Table 20/2
Symptoms of premenstrual syndrome

Mood (emotional)	Physical
Irritability	Abdominal bloating
Anxiety	Abdominal discomfort, tenderness or pain
Nervous tension	Breast swelling, tenderness or pain
Depression (feeling sad)	Feeling of weight gain
Lethargy, exhaustion, mood swings, aggression, panic attacks	Oedema (swelling)
	Headache
	Backache
Confusion	Nausea
Craving for sweet foods	

the doctor to identify the problem more clearly, and helps the patient gain insight into her condition.

Of the many treatments suggested for PMS, few have been studied in a properly designed trial. The medications suggested include:

- vitamin B_6 (pyridoxine) up to 200mg a day
- diuretics, including spironolactone
- evening primrose oil capsules
- progesterone (vaginal suppositories) 200–800mg daily
- dydrogesterone 10mg twice daily
- bromocriptine 2.5mg twice daily (which may help breast symptoms, but has no effect on the remainder)
- mefenamic acid 250mg 4 times a day

The drugs are usually prescribed from 2 days before symptoms are complained about (judged from the menstrual cycle diary) until menstruation starts.

Careful studies have shown that Vitamin B_6 (pyridoxine), diuretics, evening primrose oil capsules, progesterone vaginal suppositories, and dydrogesterone are no more effective than sugar pills (placebo) in relieving the symptoms of PMS. Bromocriptine relieves the breast symptoms in some women, but is associated with nausea, and mefenamic acid only helps a few women and then not consistently.

As all the medications available are ineffective, research continues to try to find new treatments. Until such a treatment is found, a study reported in 1990 suggests that exercise taken regularly may help reduce the symptoms.

Prolapse

If the tissues which support the vagina and uterus are abnormally stretched during childbirth, or if a tear of the perineum is not repaired, the woman may later experience symptoms of prolapse, or what is often called a 'fallen womb'. The prolapse may involve a weakness of the front wall of the vagina – called a *cystocele*; a weakness of the back wall of the vagina, usually associated with damage also to the tissues between the vagina and the rectum – called a *rectocele*; or a weakness of the supports of the womb, which is a *uterine prolapse*.

The weakness of the front vaginal wall – or cystocele – may make a bulge or lump which can be felt just inside the vagina or at its entrance when the patient strains. Unless it is associated with bladder symptoms such as frequency of urination, infection of the urine (as shown by laboratory tests) or unless it is very marked, surgery is not required. The weakness of the back vaginal wall – or recto-cele – particularly if there is also an unrepaired tear of the perineum, makes the entrance to the vagina larger, and a lump may be felt there on straining. Once again, unless it causes symptoms, treatment is not really required.

The *prolapse* of the womb itself only needs treatment if the cervix projects from the vagina, or if the symptoms of 'something falling out' become annoying. The womb normally 'drops' a little down the vagina when the pressure in the abdomen is increased, as in straining to open the bowels, and the cervix may be felt just inside the vaginal entrance. So long as the tissues have good tone and a good blood supply, the minor degree of prolapse does not worry most women; but after the menopause the blood supply is reduced and the tissues become less flexible, so that the prolapse becomes more obvious and symptoms begin. Prolapse of the womb does not cause backache, despite what is believed.

Once a 'prolapse' causes symptoms, treatment is generally surgical. However today, with better obstetric care, severe prolapse is less common, and the big operations of the past are less often required. Since many patients who have small degrees of prolapse do not need treatment at all, the decision to operate should only be made by an experienced gynaecologist.

'Retroversion' of the uterus

Normally the uterus lies bent forward at an angle of nearly 90° to that of the vagina, and it is able to rotate about an axis at the level of the cervix (Fig. 20/4). As the bladder fills, it pushes the uterus up and backwards, and if a woman lies on her back her uterus may 'tilt backwards'. In 10 per cent of women the uterus is normally tilted backwards. The condition is called 'retroversion', and it can occur from time to time in women whose uterus normally lies bent forwards, or anteverted. In the past an amazing variety of gynaecological disorders were attributed to retroversion of the uterus; these included backache, sterility, vaginal discharge, pelvic pain, headaches, constipation, diminished sexual desire, frequency of urination and 'wind'! The many operations devised to 'correct' the retroversion made the doctors rich, but did little to cure the patient's symptoms which, although temporarily relieved, returned after a while. Retroversion is often called 'twisting'

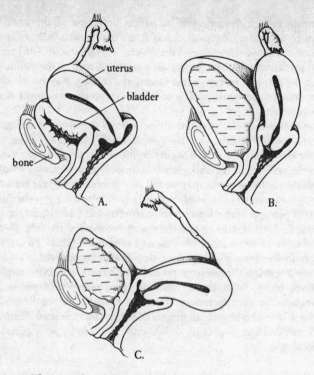

FIG. 20/4 The 'normal' and 'retroverted' uterus, showing (A) how the uterus normally lies in the pelvis; (B) how it may move when the bladder fills and (C) a 'retroverted' uterus.

of the womb by doctors who try to explain the condition to their patients. This is a bad term, for a twisted womb implies a dangerous condition which needs careful surgery for correction, when all that has happened is that the uterus has *tilted* backwards, a quite normal event.

It is now known that unless the womb is *fixed* in the retroverted position by infection or endometriosis, it is of no importance that it is retroverted, as it causes none of the symptoms attributed to it, and there is no need for an operation or the use of supporting 'pessaries' which were once popular.

Sexually transmitted disease (STD)

It is a sad commentary that although more men than women acquire a sexually transmitted disease, women tend to suffer from more adverse affects, particularly becoming sterile. Until recently the diseases were called 'venereal diseases', but the term has been replaced as more diseases have been found to be exclusively or predominantly transmitted during sexual intercourse.

The most common STDs today are genital herpes, genital warts, non-gonococcal genital infection, gonorrhoea, syphilis and the minor vaginal infections, trichomoniasis and candidosis. Recently AIDS has been added to the list.

The sexually transmitted diseases would be eliminated if a man and a woman only had one sexual partner. The chance of catching an STD increases if either one of the couple has or has had sexual intercourse with several partners. As many people choose this type of sexual behaviour, the STDs continue to spread. One way of reducing the spread is for a man to use a condom every time he has sex, if either of the sexual partners is unsure about the previous sexual behaviours of the other.

With this introduction the individual STDs will be considered.

Genital herpes

Genital herpes is caused by a virus, which is a close relative of the herpes virus which causes cold sores on the lips and nose. To distinguish the two, the virus which usually causes genital herpes is called *Herpes virus, type 2, or HSV2*. HSV2 is transmitted by sexual intercourse with a person who has active herpes infection. The herpes virus which affects the lips (HSV1) may also infect the genitals if oral sex takes place with a person who has herpes blisters on his or her lips.

The first herpes attack tends to be more severe than subsequent attacks, should they occur. At first the person experiences a 'burning' feeling on her labia. This is followed by itching, and a crop of small blisters appears, which rapidly crust. They take about 7 days to heal. During the time the blisters are present and for 5 days after they have healed, virus is shed and a sexual partner may be infected. During the first attack the person begins to make antibodies to the virus which circulate in her blood and offer some protection against further attacks.

357

However, HSV1 and HSV2 invade the nerves which supply the affected area and move down them to lodge near where the nerve enters the spinal cord. In an unknown proportion of women, following stress or menstruation or for some other reason, the virus is reactivated. When this happens it tracks along the nerve back to the same area of the skin and a recurrent attack of herpes blisters appears. Most women only have two attacks, but in some repeated attacks occur.

There is no cure for herpes, although work is taking place to develop a vaccine. Nor is there any specific treatment, although many have been suggested; but if you put gentian violet on the ulcers you will obtain some relief and you will probably need some form of pain relief, and an anaesthetic ointment to apply to your vulva.

A drug called acyclovir (Zovirax) reduces the severity of the symptoms of a first attack if it is given early enough. Its main place is for women who have recurrent attacks most months of the year. If these women take acyclovir every day (usually a dose of 400mg twice a day is enough), the frequency of the attacks is reduced from 10 to 12 attacks a year to one attack a year. As the years pass the attacks tend to become less frequent and often cease. The saying that 'herpes, unlike love, lasts forever' is not true!

Sometimes genital herpes occurs during pregnancy. The problem is discussed on pages 303–4.

Genital warts

Warts may occur on the genitalia, usually on the tissues surrounding the vaginal entrance or in the vagina. They tend to form clusters and vary in size from pin-heads to a 'cauliflower' appearance. They are caused by a virus, are sexually transmitted, and may be so small as to escape notice. Recently there has been much concern about the wart virus as it has been found that it is a factor in the development of cancer of the cervix (see p. 374). The virus may infect any part of the lower genital tract, and then spread to infect the cervix or it may infect the cervix directly. There are several strains of the wart virus and at least two of these seem to be the ones which may alter the cells of the cervix so that the later development of cancer may occur.

It is fortunate that the virus alters the appearance of the cells which cover the cervix, as the changes can be detected by the Pap smear. If the cervix is treated at this stage cancer will be prevented in most cases.

All women who are sexually active, or have been sexually active should have Pap smears made at regular (1- to 3-year) intervals. This is particulary important if you (or your partner) have or have had several partners. If you form a new sexual relationship and do not know your new partner's sexual history you should insist that he wears a condom until he has been checked for warts on his penis. These may be so small as to be almost invisible, but if a cloth soaked in vinegar is placed around his penis, white areas may appear indicating possible wart virus infection.

Warts on the external genitals can be treated by applying a substance called podophyllin (0.5 per cent in ethanol) to the warts twice daily for 3 days. As podophyllin burns normal tissues, the solution must be put only on the warts themselves. The warts usually dry up and drop off after a week. Warts are found in the vagina or on the cervix and should be treated by a doctor a laser, or by freezing or burning them.

Wart infection of the cervix is discussed further on p. 375.

Non-gonococcal genital infection

This sexually transmitted infection is now about three times as common as gonorrhoea and as serious. In most cases it is caused by an organism called chlamydia. Most men, and a few women, infected with chlamydia develop a discharge from the urethra which settles after a couple of weeks. This is called non-gonococcal urethritis. Unfortunately for women chlamydia often infects the woman's cervix rather than her urethra and causes no symptoms. But the infection may spread upwards, infecting the woman's uterus and often infecting her Fallopian tubes. This is called pelvic inflammatory disease and unless treated may make the woman sterile – unable to have children.

Studies in several western countries, using a blood test, show that about 15 to 30 per cent of sexually active people show evidence of previous chlamydial infection. Although this finding is interesting, it is more important to know how many people have '*active*' chlamydial infection. In women this is tested for by taking a swab from the cells lining the cervical canal and growing the organism in a culture. This test has shown that between 1 and 5 per cent of women aged 15 to 29 have chlamydial infection of their cervical canal and could infect a sexual partner, or lead to pelvic inflammatory disease. A woman who has several sexual partners or whose partner admits that he has had other sexual partners, would be wise to consider having the test made, as antibiotic treatment will cure the infection and prevent it being transferred to a sexual partner.

Chlamydial infection can be controlled if you have safe sex. This means that you avoid having several sexual partners, and if you don't know your partner's sexual history, insist that he uses a condom.

A test for chlamydia is now available and, once it is diagnosed, treatment with antibiotics guarantees a cure.

Gonorrhoea

Gonorrhoea occurs more frequently than syphilis, and in the USA alone it is believed that over 5 million people are infected each year. In a man the disease is diagnosed easily. Within 3 to 5 days of intercourse with an infected woman, or an infected homosexual man, he notices a creamy, purulent discharge from his urethra and finds it hurts him to pass urine. In a woman the same symptoms may occur, then the diagnosis is easy. It is made by taking a specimen of the urethral discharge and looking at it through a microscope after staining the specimen with special dyes. *But over 70 per cent of women who are infected with gonorrhoea have no symptoms.* They act as a 'silent reservoir' for the disease and can transmit gonorrhoea to other men if they are sexually active. The infected man may then infect other women or men. And so it goes on.

Gonorrohoea has more serious consequences for a woman than for a man. The disease may infect the Bartholin glands at the entrance to her vagina which can swell up forming an abscess. Occasionally, the gonococcus spreads upwards through the uterus to infect the oviducts. This usually occurs during menstruation. Infection of the oviducts is called salpingitis. It is painful, as the oviducts become swollen with pus. And unfortunately if treatment is not given quickly the oviducts may be so damaged that they become kinked and blocked so that the woman can never become pregnant.

Luckily the treatment of gonorrhoea is effective, provided the person seeks help early on in the disease. Penicillin is effective in killing the gonococcus, and its killing power is increased if another drug, called probenecid, is taken at the same time. The usual treatment is for the woman (or the man) to take 2 tablets of probenecid and to be given an injection of penicillin. She then takes tablets of probenecid 6, 12 and 18 hours later, when she is given a second penicillin injection, and continues to take probenecid every 6 hours for another 2 days.

(An alternative treatment is to take a single large dose of penicillin by mouth and to take probenecid as described.) A week later, even if she feels well, she must go back for further tests to be made to be sure that she is cured. The tests are repeated each week for 2 more weeks.

Because of the number of women who have 'silent gonorrhoea', a woman who has 3 or more sexual partners over a short period of time would be wise to have smears taken to make sure that none of them has infected her with gonorrhoea. Tiny cottonwool sticks, 'Cotton-buds', are used to take a smear from her urethra and from her cervix. It is a painless procedure.

Syphilis

Syphilis is a serious condition, and is often hard to detect in a woman. Usually within 14 to 28 days, but sometimes as long as 90 days after sexual intercourse with an infected man, a small sore appears on one of the lips of the vulva (the labia). It is relatively painless, but the labia may become swollen and tender. Usually the sore persists for a few weeks, unless treatment is given, and then disappears. Unfortunately in some infected women the sore, or chancre, may not develop on the labium, but upon the cervix where it is undetected, and only when a faint pink, spotty rash appears on her chest, back and arms does the woman seek medical advice. The rash, if due to syphilis, persists for several weeks, so that a rash which appears and fades over a few days is not due to the disease. However, if a woman develops a pink, spotty rash which lasts for more than 10 days, and if she has had sexual intercourse with more than one man, or even with a man she knows well, it would be wise for her to have a blood test done.

Syphilis carries two dangers to a woman unless it is treated. The immediate danger is that when she becomes pregnant, her baby is very likely to develop syphilis while still in the womb; the long-term damage is that untreated syphilis causes damage to the nervous system and may lead to madness.

Neither of these two disasters need occur if treatment is obtained early. Syphilis is completely curable if it is treated early in the course of the disease and the infected person follows the directions exactly. Penicillin is given daily by injection for 10 to 14 days. Following treatment, blood tests for syphilis are made each month for 6 months, and again at 9 and 12 months. If all the tests are negative the person is cured. If the tests become positive a further course of penicillin injections is given.

HIV and AIDS

This new and frightening disease is caused by a virus, called the human immunodeficiency virus or HIV. HIV is usually transmitted during sexual intercourse, but may spread if drug addicts use the same needle for mainlining. A few cases have occurred following a blood transfusion.

In Central Africa and parts of Asia, it has been estimated that the AIDS virus has infected up to 30 per cent of the population, and is spread by having sex with prostitutes. In Western societies, most AIDS victims are homosexual men or drug addicts.

The word AIDS is derived from the *a*cquired *i*mmune *d*eficiency *s*yndrome. The term means that a person infected by HIV is more likely to develop severe, often fatal, infections which a non-infected person could 'shake off' relatively easily.

Usually a person infected with HIV feels well and has no symptoms at first (although a blood test for the HIV shows positive within 2 months of being infected) they can infect a sexual partner. After about 5 years those infected with HIV will develop a chronic illness. The illness makes the glands swell, produces fevers, and the person feels tired and often depressed.

This is called 'second stage AIDS' or the AIDS Related Complex. The person who has it either gets better or develops full-blown AIDS in the next 3 years. If that happens he or she has a 70 per cent chance of dying from a severe pneumonia, some other severe infection or special kind of cancer, usually within a year.

AIDS is not exclusively a 'homosexual disease'. The virus is passed from person to person only in blood or in semen. You cannot get AIDS from casual contact. You cannot get AIDS from shaking hands, hugging or socially kissing an infected person. The virus is not transmitted if an infected person sneezes or coughs at you. You cannot get AIDS from sharing crockery, cutlery, towels or bed linen. You cannot get AIDS if you swim in a place where an AIDS victim has swum. You cannot get AIDS from toilets, telephones or household furniture. You cannot get AIDS from non-sexual body contacts.

Although research is taking place no vaccine is available to prevent

AIDS, nor is there any effective treatment. This means that the only way to control the spread of AIDS is to avoid drug addiction and sharing needles and to practise 'safe sex'. This means having few or only one partner, and using condoms when you do not know about your partner's sexual behaviour.

('Trouble with the water') Urinary incontinence

A singularly distressing complaint, which most often occurs after the age of 40, is an 'irritable bladder'. This is not the medical term, and the condition is more properly called 'urgency incontinence', but in fact the patient complains of an 'irritable bladder'. In most cases the woman finds that she gets the urge to empty her bladder at very frequent intervals, and the urge may be stimulated by coughing, jolting in a bus or car, or something of that nature. Once she begins to urinate, she has to go on until her bladder is empty, but because she passes urine so frequently, she only voids a small amount of urine each time. Occasionally an irritable bladder is due to some disorder such as infection, but in most cases it is due to an emotional upset which shows itself in this way. The doctor will have to make tests to decide what is the cause, as only then can he give treatment. This is always medical, and surgery is not needed.

There is another kind of urination trouble which may inconvenience a woman. In this a tiny amount of urine escapes and soils the underclothes when the patient strains, coughs or laughs. The woman may be young or old, but has usually given birth to one or more children. The condition is called 'stress incontinence' because the loss of urine occurs after a stress or strain. It can occur whether the bladder is full or apparently empty. The doctor has to differentiate this condition very carefully from urgency incontinence, because the more annoying forms of stress incontinence require surgical treatment. The lesser forms, when the loss of urine only occurs occasionally, can be treated by the patients doing exercises to strengthen the muscles which support the vagina and the urethra – the short tube connecting the bladder to the outside. The exercises consist of tightening the muscle of the 'tail' without using the abdominal muscles. I describe this as 'trying to make the anus, or back-passage opening, touch the mouth'. A woman can do these exercises in any free moment, and should aim at doing them at least one hundred times a day (see below).

If the doctor is in any doubt whether the woman has urgency

incontinence or stress incontinence he may refer her to a urodynamic clinic for special tests. The tests are painless but may be a bit embarrassing. In the first test the woman wears a sanitary pad and drinks 500ml of water. She then walks about or climbs stairs, for example. The pad is removed and weighed one hour later and the amount of urine in it is measured. The second test is more complicated. The woman may have an ultrasound picture taken from an instrument the size of a thin sausage placed in her vagina. As well, she has a tube inserted into her bladder and the bladder filled with water. She then passes the urine sitting on a special collecting toilet. The tube in her bladder records many important things which enables her doctor to make a diagnosis about the cause of her incontinence.

Pelvic Floor exercises

The muscles of the pelvic floor support the bladder, the vagina and the rectum. As a woman grows older the pelvic floor muscles may become weaker, which increases the chance that she will become incontinent. The pelvic floor exercises are designed to help strengthen the muscles. They are not difficult to learn, but if a woman has a problem her doctor or a physiotherapist can help her.

1. Sit or stand comfortably and squeeze the muscles around the back passage as if you were trying to control diarrhoea. Hold the squeeze for the slow count of five, then relax.
2. If you prefer you can insert a finger into your vagina and tighten the muscles so that your finger is squeezed. Hold the squeeze for the slow count of five.
3. Repeat the exercise four times slowly, and then four times rapidly, holding the squeeze only for the count of two.
4. Do the exercise any time you like during the day – while watching TV, preparing a meal, resting. Try to do the sequence of exercises about every hour.

The woman should do the pelvic floor exercises in any free moment and aim to do them at least one hundred times a day.

Recently 'vaginal cones' have been suggested as an alternative to pelvic floor exercises. The cones come in sets of five and each weighs a bit more than its predecessor although all are the same size. The woman inserts the vaginal cone and uses her pelvic floor muscles to keep it in for a period of time. Over the next weeks she inserts heavier vaginal cones. The success of vaginal cones is claimed to be equal to that of pelvic floor exercises. As an additional treatment, women who have passed the menopause may choose to take oestrogen tablets. Oestrogen improves the tone of the vagina and the surrounding muscles and helps to reduce the incontinence.

About 30 per cent of women who have stress incontinence and who are prepared to persist with these treatments for a few months are relieved or cured of their incontinence.

Women who have more severe and disabling incontinence usually require special tests to differentiate between the types of incontinence. The tests are painless, although some women are rather embarrassed as they have to urinate during the tests.

Urinary tract infection

The urinary tract starts at the kidney, continues as a tube (the ureter) between the kidney and the bladder, expands as the bladder and then goes on as a tube (the urethra) between the bladder and the outside. Infection of the urinary tract is usually due to the spread of bacteria from the outside up along the urethra to infect the bladder (called 'cystitis'), and then in most cases up the ureter to infect the kidney (called 'pyelonephritis'). Because a woman has a shorter urethra than a man, she is more likely to develop infection of the bladder. Luckily, in most cases this is of no importance as the bladder itself kills the bacteria, so that the urine is sterile, but it appears that about 5 per cent of girls and women harbour active bacteria in their bladders. These bacteria may cause infection at any time, but especially during the first weeks of marriage ('honeymoon cystitis'), and in pregnancy. It is thought that the movement of the penis against the urethra and bladder which occurs in sexual intercourse stimulates the bacteria to grow, and in pregnancy the urine tends to stagnate in the bladder.

The symptoms of urinary tract infection are frequency of urination and painful urination especially towards the end of voiding. If infection has involved the kidney, backache in the kidney area, fever and chills develop.

If a woman develops these symptoms, she should consult a doctor. Her urine will be examined for bacteria and if infection is present the doctor will prescribe treatment. Untreated urinary tract infection can lead to kidney damage.

POSTCOITAL CYSTITIS. An unpleasant form of cystitis sometimes begins during a period of frequent sexual intercourse. Usually this clears with treatment but some women have the misfortune to develop cystitis every time they have coitus. This, in turn, prevents any enjoyment because the woman knows it will be followed, within 36 hours, by frequencey of urination and pain.

The cause of postcoital cystitis is due to bacteria which live in the urethra being massaged back up into the bladder by the movement of the man's penis in the woman's vagina. (If you look at Figs. 1/4 or 20/2 you can see how close the urethra is to the vagina.) Once inside the bladder, bacteria are usually killed by secretions of the cells which line the bladder, but in some women this does not occur. Instead the bacteria thrive, doubling their number every half hour. The result is cystitis.

Doctors have tried many drugs in an attempt to cure this distressing complaint, but with indifferent success. A woman has found an answer which seems to be more successful. It is quite simple. If you suffer from postcoital cystitis, all you have to do is to empty your bladder completely within half an hour of sexual intercourse. You will do this more easily if you drink three or four glasses of water immediately after intercourse. Should this simple method not cure you, you should obtain some tablets of the drug, nitrofurantoin, from your doctor, and take one 50mg tablet each night, in addition to emptying your bladder in the way I have suggested. In addition, women who have postcoital cystitis, which is also called '*the urethral syndrome*', should avoid using soap when washing their genital area.

Vaginal discharges

In several investigations it has been found that the most common reason for a woman to see a doctor is that she has a vaginal discharge. Vaginal discharges are of several kinds, some requiring treatment and others being perfectly normal and of no importance. To understand them it must be remembered that the vagina, like the uterus, is part of the genital tract, and that the tissues which make up the tract are very strongly influenced by the female sex hormones, oestrogen and progesterone. Oestrogen stimulates the tissues to mature, and progesterone further develops them. This is most obvious in pregnancy, but changes occur in the lining tissues of the vagina, the cervix, as well as the uterus during each menstrual cycle. The changes caused by oestrogen make the cells lining the cervix secrete a thin, slightly sticky mucus, and this is most marked midway between the periods. The cells which make up the lining of the vagina are arranged rather like bricks making up a wall. The top cells are thin and large. These top cells are constantly shed into the vagina, rather like leaves falling off a tree; in fact, they are said to 'exfoliate' which means just that. In the vagina they are acted upon by the helpful bacteria which normally live there, to produce a weak acid. This acid – called lactic acid – prevents dangerous bacteria from growing in the vagina. The vaginal cells and the cervical mucus add to the vaginal discharge. As well, some fluid seeps between the cells of the vaginal wall to join the secretions in the vagina. This seepage is increased during sexual excitement, during anxiety, when sexual frustration occurs, or if the woman is ill or emotionally upset.

It can be seen that the quantity of the normal vaginal secretions can vary very considerably and still be quite normal, just as the quantity of secretions in the mouth (the saliva) varies very considerably. The secretions not only keep the vagina moist, which is desirable, but keep it clean. However, from time to time the increased secretions may stain the woman's panties and cause her concern. Usually, if the discharge is not irritating, it is of little importance and treatment is not required. Indeed, in certain conditions, such as when taking some kinds of oral contraceptive, an increased vaginal discharge may be expected to occur. However, if the amount of the discharge is annoying, the woman should consult her doctor. He will take a swab sample of the discharge and look at it under the microscope before prescribing treatment. This non-irritant vaginal discharge, which may or may not have an odour, is called leukorrhoea – or the 'whites' – but it is bad to give it a name, as it immediately becomes something abnormal in most people's minds, whereas in fact it is quite normal.

Irritating vaginal discharges

If the discharge causes itching and pain in the vagina and around its opening in the vulva, the condition is generally due to some disease and certainly requires investigation. Three main kinds of disorder can cause the trouble.

These are candidosis (also called monilia and thrush), trichomoniasis and 'amine' vaginosis.

● *Candidosis:* This is the most common cause of vaginal itch. The infection often involves the vulva as well, which itches intolerably. The fungus burrows into the cells which line the vagina and the cells of the skin of the vulva. In some women the fungus burrows into the deeper layers of cells where it may lie dormant until reactivated for some reason. The superficial infected cells are shed into the vagina causing the thick discharge. Candida probably gets into the vagina from fungal infection of the intestinal tract, but may be spread by sexual intercourse.

About 15 per cent of women are infected, but the symptoms of vaginal discharge and itchiness occur in only 3 to 5 per cent.

Candida albicans grows more readily if the environment contains glucose. Candidosis is more common in pregnancy or if the woman has diabetes. But fungal infection can occur in other women.

The vaginal discharge varies in amount as does the itchiness. In some cases the woman's sexual partner is infected and has an itchy penis, particularly the glans.

The diagnosis is made by examining a specimen of the discharge under a microscope, when the branching threads of the fungus may be seen. However, if they are not seen, a vaginal swab should be sent to a laboratory.

In 90 per cent of cases treatment is easy. The woman is given antifungal tablets or creams (usually imidazoles) to place in her vagina for one night or three nights depending on her wishes and her doctor's advice. There are several varieties of imidazoles available, but none is more or less effective than any other. If the woman prefers she can take an antifungal drug, called ketoconazole, by mouth twice a day for 5 days. If her vulva skin is itchy she may request an antifungal ointment to rub into the itchy area.

The problem is with the 5 per cent of women who get repeated attacks of candidal vulvo-vaginitis. The attacks may occur as often as every second month and may be very incapacitating. The use of oral ketoconazole in small doses each day for six months cures many of these women.

As the fungus grows more rapidly in a moist warm environment, the woman should not wear tight pantyhose, choosing cotton panties

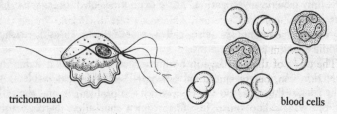

trichomonad   blood cells

FIG. 20/5   Trichomonads seen under the microscope.

or none at all. It is also believed that, to avoid possible reinfection of the vulva from the bowel, women should pay attention to hygiene, wiping themselves backwards after opening their bowels.

● *Trichomoniasis:* This vaginal infection occurs when a tiny living organism (called a trichomonad) gets in the vagina, usually following sexual intercourse with an infected man. Trichomoniasis infects about 1 woman in 10 some time during her sexually active years. The organism is the size of a white blood cell and has 'feelers' and a powerful tail (Fig. 20/5).

In most women it lives quietly in the velvet-like lining of the vagina and causes no symptoms; in most men it lives quietly in the urinary tract tube within the penis. But in some women, for some unknown reason, it causes a severe vaginal and vulval itch. The diagnosis is made after the doctor has taken a specimen from the vagina and looked at it under a microscope, when the organism can be seen wriggling about, its tail thrashing. Treatment is easy and effective. Tablets of metronidazole (Flagyl) are taken three times a day for 7 to 10 days or a single large dose of tinidazole (Fasigyn) may be preferred. Since the sexual partner often harbours the trichomonads without knowing it, treatment should be given to him as well as to the woman.

People taking either metronidazole or tinidazole should avoid drinking alcohol as the drugs have an antabuse effect.

● *Amine Vaginosis:* The third cause of a vaginal discharge is due to infection by an organism called *gardnerella* interacting with anaerobic bacilli which normally live in the vagina. The discharge is thin in texture, has a strong 'fishy' smell and is dirty-grey in colour. It is called 'amine vaginosis' because amines are produced which cause the fishy smell. Amine vaginosis responds to treatment with metronidazole or tinidazole.

Not uncommonly an irritating vaginal discharge occurs and investigations, including examination of the discharge in a laboratory, fail to show any infection. Some of the women have repeated episodes of the irritating vaginal discharge and sometimes feel discomfort inside the vagina. All the tests made by the doctor on the discharge are negative, but the problem persists.

The cause of the discharge in both groups of women is not due to local infection, but to emotional causes, either anxiety, depression, a poor relationship or some other psychological problem. If the woman is prepared to talk about the problem with a counsellor, the discharge usually ceases.

Vaginal odours

The vagina is self-cleansing, but some women notice that there may be a 'smell'. It is quite normal for the vulva and vagina to have a faint 'odour', just as does the penis, and in general it is quite unnoticeable to other people. However, some women *imagine* that the vaginal odour can be detected by all the passers-by. This is not true and, in fact, if a woman baths each day, the odour will be undetectable. But the belief of a 'vaginal odour' is encouraged by manufacturers who sell deodorants for 'personal, intimate, feminine freshness', or to give the woman 'day-long protection and a new sense of feminine security'. These sales gimmicks work by making a woman who does not use deodorants feel less feminine and less secure, and appeal to her need for hygiene. In fact, a deodorant works by adding a different smell – usually a perfume – which vanishes in a short time, but inspires the belief that it persists. In general, then, a girl or woman who baths or showers each day has no need for vaginal deodorants, but if she wants to spend her money on these unnecessary gimmicks, they are readily, if fairly expensively, available.

Vaginal douching

The use of the vaginal douche for purposes of feminine 'hygiene', to 'remove odour', and immediately after sexual intercourse is a pecul-iarly American habit, which in recent years has waned in popularity. The idea that the vagina needed washing out was based on false premises, and was connected with the American obsession for personal cleanliness. While it is reasonable and proper to wash the body, including the vulva, daily to remove the accumulated secretions of the sweat glands, the logic of washing out the vagina is less certain. The vagina is 'self-cleansing' because of lactobacilli bacteria which normally live in it. These bacteria produce lactic acid and hydrogen peroxide which kill most bugs which enter the vagina and cause vaginal discharges. Douching alters the environment of the vagina and may permit growth of organisms such as candida, gardnerella and trichomonads. The conclusion must be that there is in general no need for a woman to use vaginal douches, and in fact there is every reason to avoid them.

Vulval itchiness

The skin of the vulval area is particularly sensitive to stimuli, and an itching vulva is a fairly common complaint. If the itch is sufficiently annoying for the woman to seek medical help, she will require proper investigation, as a vulval itch has several causes. Most commonly it is due to vaginal infection (especially candidosis, which also may infect the vulval skin), or to a vaginal discharge. Because of this, vaginal swabs should be taken and sent to the laboratory in all cases of vulval itchiness. Sometimes it is due to a general disease, such as diabetes or general skin conditions; but in a fairly large number of cases, the itch is an outward sign of an inward frustration, usually of a sexual nature. The itch makes the woman scratch, especially at night; scratching irritates the vulval skin, which causes further itchiness, which causes further scratching, and so on. After careful investigation, the doctor can make a diagnosis and can offer treatment. In this, three things need to be known: first, treatment is medical not surgical; second, the longer the woman has had the itch before seeking help, the longer it takes to cure; third, if any cause is found it needs proper treatment, and the patient cannot hope for instant cure. She must be patient and rely upon her doctor.

Vulval pain

A few women suffer from pain at the entrance to the vagina, which is made worse when the woman has sexual intercourse and may be so severe as to prevent her having sex. Cracks may appear in the tissues. The other causes of vulval itchiness have to be excluded before a diagnosis can be made. The condition is called vulvo vestibulitis. Unfortunately the cause is unknown and treatment unsatisfactory, but sometimes ointments containing testosterone help.

CHAPTER 21

An Ounce of Prevention

As most of the diseases which previously killed people in infancy, childhood and adolescence have come under control, the cancers which afflict older people have come under increasing investigation and study. Calculations have been made which show that a woman has a 7 per cent chance of developing cancer of the breast; a 2.7 per cent chance of developing a cancer of the gut; a 2.3 per cent chance of developing cancer of the cervix of the uterus; and a 2 per cent chance of developing a cancer of the body of the uterus. This means that of every 100 females born, 5 will develop cancer of the breast, and 4 will develop cancer of the uterus at some time before death. Apart from cancer of the gut, cancers of the genital organs (in which I include the breast) are the most common cancers found in women.

The only sure way to control cancer and to prevent it from killing its host, is to detect it before it has grown very far. Women are luckier than men in this respect, for the breasts and the uterus are relatively easily accessible for examination, provided the patient attends for regular periodic check-ups.

The American Cancer Association, in an admirable series of booklets, emphasizes the imortance of early detection of cancer, and advises women to consult their doctor immediately if any of the following symptoms or signs appear.

1. Any sore that does not heal quickly, especially about the mouth.
2. Any unusual bleeding or discharge from any natural body opening.
3. Any painless lump, especially in the breasts, lips, tongue or soft tissues.
4. Any persistent indigestion or unexplained weight loss.
5. Any persistent hoarseness or cough or difficulty in swallowing.
6. Any unexplained change in normal bowel habits.

This advice is sensible and timely, and if women followed it, would lead to a reduction in the deaths which occur from cancer. The three signs which may indicate a cancer of the breast or genital tract are: (1) any painless lump in the breast, (2) any unusual bleeding or discharge from the vagina, and (3) a sore or ulcer on the vulva which does not heal quickly. Only by early detection and proper treatment can the fatal outcome of the cancer be prevented. An ounce of prevention is far more valuable than a pound of attempted cure!

Cancer of the breast

The earliest sign of cancer of the breast is a small, rounded painless lump. Only one lump in every five found in the breast is due to cancer, but every lump is suspect. Many women are comfortable about examining their breasts each month (in the week after menstruation if the woman has not reached the menopause); some women have their breasts examined each year by a doctor. These methods have some value in detecting breast lumps early, but are not as effective as mammography. Mammography is a method of breast examination, using a very small dose of x-rays, which is not dangerous to the woman.

In order to obtain a good image, the woman's breasts have to be compressed slightly, which may feel uncomfortable, but only a few women feel it's painful. The compression lasts only a few seconds while the x-ray picture is taken.

Most medical authorities, including those in Australia, Canada, Britain and the USA now recommend that mammography should be performed at intervals of 1 to 3 years on the breasts of all women aged 45 or more and on women of all ages who are at risk of developing breast cancer. You are 'at higher risk' if anyone in your family has had a breast cancer, especially if this occurred before the age of 40, if you have never been pregnant or have had your first baby after you were 30, if your periods started before the age of 12 or if you menstruated after the age of 50, or if a previous mammogram showed abnormalities. You should also ask for a mammogram if you have very lumpy breasts as these may prevent your doctor from examining them properly.

In Britain, for example, studies show that 95 per cent of women who have a mammogram do not have breast cancer; 5 per cent need further investigation, and 1 per cent will be found to have cancer. A woman who is referred for further investigation will be very worried that she may have breast cancer, and should ask for counselling, explanation and support during the interval between the mammography and the investigations. This interval should be made as short as possible.

The good news is that if the lump proves to be cancer, the cancer is usually at such an early stage that it can be treated and cured.

In 1986 a Consensus conference on the treatment of breast cancer was held in London. The main recommendations of the conference may help women who develop breast cancer be aware of current thought. A careful study of 75 000 women with early breast cancer reported in 1991, confirmed the recommendations and added some additional ones. The recommendations are that:

- A woman should generally have the opportunity to discuss her treatment with the surgeon if a sample (biopsy) of a lump in the breast shows that she has cancer. The practice of taking a biopsy and going straight on to remove the breast without the patient having a chance to discuss her treatment with the surgeon is rarely justified.
- There is no evidence that removal of the entire breast (mastectomy) will prolong the woman's life any more than if the surgeon takes out just the lump and some surrounding tissue – although local recurrence is more likely after less extensive surgery.
- Women live longer if they either have their ovaries removed, start taking tamoxifen, a drug which opposes oestrogen in the body, or are given drugs which selectively kill cancer cells (cytotoxic drugs) over a 6 month period after surgery, or choose both treatments.
- Women over 50 survive longer if they are given cytotoxic drugs over a 6 month period and tamoxifen for a period of 2 years.
- Doctors generally underestimate the amount of information that patients want. Women who want to take part in decisions about their treatment should be able to do so.
- Following treatment, doctors should be aware of the possibility of problems, such as depression and anxiety, which can be successfully treated.

Cancer of uterine cervix

It is unfortunate that by the time cancer of the cervix is visible to the naked eye, it is so far advanced that no matter what treatment is given, 1 woman in every 5 will be dead within 5 years.

Cancer develops in the cells which cover the cervix. This takes a relatively long time. Before the cells become cancerous they undergo changes in their appearance. The 'warning changes' indicate that a cancer may develop unless treatment is given. They do not say that the woman has cancer. The warning changes can be detected by smears made from the cervix called Pap smears, because Dr Papanicolaou, who worked in New York, first pointed out that early cancer cells of the cervix were less sticky than normal cells, and were shed (or exfoliated) more readily into the vagina. To take the specimen the doctor inserts a small instrument, called a speculum, into the vagina and looks at the cervix. He then takes a 'scraping' from the cervix using a wooden spatula, similar to that used for depressing the tongue when he wants to look down the throat. He also takes a sample from the upper vagina, and from the canal of the cervix. The whole procedure is quite painless, and the doctor takes the opportunity to do a pelvic examination at the same time to be sure that there is nothing wrong with the uterus or the ovaries.

The woman should make sure that her doctor phones or writes to her giving her the result of the tests even if only normal cells are found. This information is important to know as a normal result reassures the woman, and warning cells are an indication for further tests.

There is evidence that cancer of the cervix is related in some way to sexual intercourse. A likely cause has recently been found. Many women who have 'abnormal cells', detected by the Pap smear, have been found to have been infected by the human wart virus (HPV). HPV is the virus which causes genital warts. Although HPV is often sexually transmitted, it may also be present in women who have not been sexually active and in women and their husbands who have not had any other sexual partner. In some cases the infection may have occurred years before it is detected. The risk of infection is greater among women who have had several sexual partners (or whose partner has or has had several sexual partners), is at greater risk of developing cervical cancer. The cancer may take some years to develop or may occur rapidly.

It is becoming clear that many women and men are infected with the wart virus and only a few women develop cervical cancer, so something else must interact with the virus in women who develop cervical cancer. What that something is is not known at present, although smoking is believed to be a factor.

There are two ways of reducing the chance of developing cervical cancer, and both should be considered to reinforce each other. The first is to limit your sexual partners to one only. If you have several sexual partners you may have been infected with the wart virus. The second way is if you don't know about your partner's sexual behaviour, to insist he uses a condom until he has been cleared of having genital wart infection.

On the other hand if you or your regular partner have been diagnosed as having HPV, you do not need to use condoms as you will probably both have been infected.

The second way is to have Pap smears at regular intervals. Two Pap smears should be made in the first year after starting sexual intercourse. If you or your partner have several sexual relationships you should then have a Pap smear taken each year. In other instances a Pap smear every 3 years is sufficient.

Any campaign to eliminate cancer of the cervix must include an attempt to get every woman in the area – especially the poor – to have a pelvic examination and cervical smears performed at regular intervals.

The Pap smear is looked at down a microscope by a trained technician and 'abnormal' smears are checked by a qualified doctor. Of every 1000 smears examined, about 20 will show 'abnormal' cells, and 3 of these will be really worrying. If 'abnormal' cells are found, a further smear is done, and if this is abnormal a specimen is taken from the cervix. This specimen may be taken with a tiny biopsy punch, after looking at the cervix with a special magnifying instrument called a colposcope. If this instrument is used, the patient does not need an anaesthetic, and the whole procedure can be done without admitting her to hospital.

If the appearance of the cervix, viewed through the colposcope is abnormal or the biopsy shows precancerous cells, treatment is given. Treatment is to burn, freeze or vaporize the cells using a laser. The last method seems the most successful and the least inconveniencing. After burning (cauterization) and freezing, the woman has a smelly vaginal discharge which may persist for up to 4 weeks.

In some cases the colposcopic findings indicate a need for more extensive treatment. The woman is admitted to hospital so that a larger piece of her cervix can be removed. It is like coring an apple and is called conization. The cervix is then stitched and heals easily.

If the biopsy or the cone shows early cancer, treatment is essential.

Usually if the patient wants to have more children, the cone is sufficient treatment, but if she has completed her family, a hysterectomy is performed. In either case, she will have to continue to attend her doctor after the operation at regular intervals, for further cervical smears. If the tissues show more advanced cancer – and only a very few do – the woman will have to have a much more extensive regimen of radiation therapy or surgery.

Only by regular pelvic examintions and cervical smears will cancer of the cervix be eliminated. Every woman should therefore make sure that she has this simple, painless test done at regular intervals from the time of her first pregnancy or the age of 25, whichever is the earlier, to the age of 65 or later.

Cancer of the endometrium

The endometrium is the lining of the womb, and cancer can develop in it. It is sometimes called cancer of the body of the uterus. Endometrial cancer occurs nearly as frequently as cancer of the cervix, but affects women who are rather older, usually aged between 50 and 60. In recent years an increase in endometrial cancer has been observed. The increase is thought to be due, in part, to the practice of doctors prescribing oestrogen tablets to menopausal women for periods of one or more years. Recent research shows that the possible cancer-promoting effects of oestrogen can be reversed if the hormone progestogen is also taken for 12 days each month.

Unfortunately 'smear' tests do not readily detect cancer of the body of the uterus, and consequently the doctor has to rely on symptoms. Any woman who develops irregular bleeding after the age of 35 should see her doctor. The bleeding is most likely to be due to hormonal changes, but it may be the first sign of cancer of the womb. An even more sinister sign is bleeding which occurs *after* the menopause. However scanty the bleeding is, the woman must see her doctor at once so that he can arrange for a diagnostic curettage if he thinks this is necessary. Luckily cancer of the body of the womb grows very slowly, so that if the woman follows this advice, it is generally curable.

Cancer of the ovaries

About 5 per cent of all cancers which develop in women are cancers of the ovaries, and these account for 10 per cent of cancers of the genital tract. In all cases the first sign is enlargement of the ovary, which can be detected on pelvic examination; but 95 per cent of ovarian enlargement is non-cancerous, and only 5 per cent of the enlargements are due to cancer. Cancer is more likely to occur after the age of 40, and particularly likely after the menopause.

Since the growth is silent and slow, the disease is difficult to detect, and the only way is for women aged 40 and over to have periodic pelvic examinations to detect ovarian enlargements. The finding of an enlarged ovary at this age is an indication for surgery, so that the tumour may be removed and examined under the microscope.

Cancer of the vulva

This is a relatively rare form of cancer found principally in old women and preceded by a vulval itch, usually of long duration. Any elderly woman who has an itchy vulva which persists should seek medical attention. In order to exclude early cancer of the vulval skin, the doctor may need to take tiny pieces of skin. The procedure is done under a local anaesthetic and does not disturb the patient.

CHAPTER 22

Not the End of Life

At a time which is quite variable and individual for a woman, the remaining egg follicles in the ovary (numbering about 8000) begin to disappear. This strange and unexplained event occurs some time between the 45th and 55th year of life. The changes are not abrupt, and there is a gradual transition from the normal ovarian activity of the reproductive years, to the relatively inactive ovary of the menopausal years.

The first change in the sequence of events which culminates in the cessation of menstruation, or the menopause, is that the egg follicles in the ovary become increasingly less sensitive to stimulation by the hormones of the pituitary. In addition, there is a change in the quantity of the two pituitary hormones – FSH and LH – which have stimulated the growth of some follicles each month since adolescence. These two changes mean that fewer egg follicles are stimulated and consequently reduced, but variable, amounts of oestrogen are released during each menstrual cycle. For this reason the lining of the uterus is less satisfactorily stimulated, and the menstrual flow becomes less regular and predictable. The quantity of the blood lost gets less, and the interval between the menstrual periods is usually increased. The co-ordinated control of menstruation, which has been so effective since adolescence, is getting out of gear, as the controlling hormone-secreting glands 'unwind' into a quieter phase of life.

As the months pass fewer egg follicles are stimulated and the amount of oestrogen secreted by them diminishes still further, until eventually the menstrual periods cease altogether. The menopause has arrived.

Of course, the sequence may not be so smooth. Some women develop heavy bleeding episodes, as sudden surges of oestrogen occur, followed by long intervals when the menstrual periods are absent. For this is a time of hormonal turbulence, only slightly less than that which occurred at puberty. The whole period of change is more properly called the climacteric, or 'change of life', while the ceasing of menstrual periods is called the menopause; but the term menopause is commonly used for both events.

The changes in the body

All the changes which occur are due to altered hormone secretion, and result from a fall in oestrogen, an absence of progesterone, and a rise in pituitary hormones. It used to be thought that oestrogen ceased to be produced after the menopause, but now it is known that some continues to be secreted well into old age, but of course the quantity is small.

The main changes which occur in the body of the menopausal woman are due to the diminished secretion of oestrogen. Because oestrogen is most active on the tissues which make up the female genital tract and on the breasts, these are most affected. But because of the continuing but variable amounts of oestrogen secreted, the degree to which they are affected is quite variable.

In the few years before the menopause, the breasts often increase in size as extra fat is deposited; but after the climacteric, this fat is reabsorbed, the gland tissue decreases and the nipples get smaller. These changes take place slowly, but by the age of 70 the breasts are usually flattened and tend to droop. In the same slow manner the utuerus, the oviducts and the ovaries become smaller and inactive. The lining wall of the vagina becomes thinner and more easily irritated as the years pass, but this is less likely to occur if sexual intercourse continues to take place. The tissues which surround and support the vagina and the muscles of the floor of the pelvis tend to become flabby, and to lose their elasticity, so that some degree of prolapse may occur. This may be of the front or back wall of the vagina, so that a bulge or lump appears at the vulva when the woman strains; or it may be of the uterus itself, the cervix projecting through the vaginal entrance. The prolapse may look more serious than it really is, because the main lips of the vulva – the labia majora – decrease in size at this time of life. Only a few cases of prolapse give discomfort and need surgery. Most can be left alone. Once again, these changes take place slowly over the years.

Menopausal symptoms

The change of life is a period when a woman has to adjust psychologically to an altered life-style. The adjustment is less difficult if she has a sympathetic relating partner, but there is still a need to adjust.

During the menopause many women complain of a number of symptoms. It is difficult to determine which of these symptoms are due to the changing hormones, especially the decline of oestrogen, and which are psychologically induced because of the need to adjust.

Objectivity is not helped by the spate of articles in newspapers and women's magazines and by the relatively paternalistic attitude of some doctors.

Five surveys, which avoid methodological defects, have been made of well women and the symptoms that they experienced during the menopause. These surveys show that only three of the many symptoms complained about by women are due to declining levels of oestrogen. The symptoms are: irregular menstruation, hot flushes and vaginal dryness or burning. Women approaching the menopause have three patterns of menstruation. First, the periods continue regularly and then suddenly cease. Second, the periods become less frequent, the intervals becoming longer, until they cease. Third, the periods become irregular. Sometimes they are heavy, sometimes light and the interval between periods is quite unpredictable. Women who have this menstrual pattern should visit a doctor, who may suggest a curettage to make quite sure that the lining of the uterus is normal, and so that treatment may be prescribed.

Hot flushes are noticed by at least three-quarters of menopausal women and in half of them they are severe enough to cause physical upset. A hot flush (or flash) is a sudden intense feeling of heat which sweeps over the body, a blush spreading over the face and neck. A flush lasts only a few moments and then disappears, but they tend to recur many times during the day and may be accompanied by tingling sensations, which sweep over the body. If the hot flush occurs at night it may be associated with sweating, and then insomnia. Hot flushes tend to be triggered by excitement. They vary in intensity and in frequency and recur over months or years. In one survey 65 per cent of women said that they had had hot flushes for more than two years.

Vaginal dryness and burning are not so common but are reported by a number of menopausal women. They are noticed particularly when sexual intercourse is attempted. Lubrication fails to occur properly. Women who have sexual intercourse regularly are less likely to complain of vaginal dryness than women who only have sex at long intervals.

If a woman has hot flushes of such severity to be distressing, treatment is available. Usually, hormone tablets of oestrogen are given, as we shall discuss in a moment.

Oestrogen will also cure a woman who has a painful dry vagina, and in this case it is usual for the doctor to prescribe a vaginal cream which contains oestrogen.

The other symptoms often attributed to declining hormones, which include depression, irritability, headaches, palpitations, dry skin, frequency of passing urine and mental 'imbalance', are no more common at the time of the menopause than at other times of life. They are not due to hormone lack, but occur because of the need to adjust to being menopausal.

These symptoms do not respond to oestrogen tablets, but other treatment is available for some of them. All of them are less distressing if a woman going through the change can talk about her feelings to a sympathetic listener.

Psychological changes

Just as the waxing turbulent tides of hormones and the need to adapt to new ways made puberty and adolescence a difficult time, some women find that the waning tides of hormones and the need to adapt to them make the menopause a difficult time. It is very difficult for doctors to decide if the symptoms of depression, fatigue and insomnia are due to hormonal changes, or to a deep emotional disturbance as the woman looks around and does not like what she sees. Her children are growing up, or have already left the family home; her youthful hopes and desires have dissipated into a routine 'suburban' life; her husband appears to have found other interests, leaving her increasingly alone; her friends have similar problems, and constantly complain about them. She sees these changes, she feels that she has missed something, often a great deal, of what she had imagined life had to offer, and she has to adjust to the strange symptoms of the menopause – or strange to her at any rate. The peculiar irregularity of her periods may subconsciously increase the anxiety that her physical and sexual attractions are waning. She is becoming old, and thinks she is rejected; she has reached the 'end of life'. These vividly felt emotions are, of course, only temporary. Psychiatrists have discovered that many women at the menopause pass through three phases before becoming adjusted to their new life. The first is one in which feelings of anxiety and turmoil are most evident. Usually this period is fairly short and merges into a period which may last months, when irritability, depression and other mood changes are common, and the woman feels rejected by everyone. Nothing is right. In time this phase merges into a phase of readjustment, when all the misery of the previous months seems like a bad dream.

What to do at the climacteric

The first thing for a woman to remember is that the strange feelings which she has are temporary, and that adjustment will come in due course. Women who have interests outside the home find it easier to adjust; but women whose outlook is confined to the house, the back-yard, the immediate neighbours and the television set often have problems.

Careful investigations in the USA and in Britain have shown that about two-thirds of women pass through the 'change of life' without any trouble, or with only a little upset. The remaining one-third need help. Help is available from the family doctor, who knows about the woman and her background. He is particularly well suited to offer sympathetic understanding and the reassurance which is so often needed. The doctor will be able to explain that the symptoms of hot flushes, a dry vagina will be relieved if the woman chooses to take the hormone oestrogen, to replace that which her ovaries no longer makes. Oestrogen will also delay the onset of osteoporosis (page 388), it has a protective effect against having a heart attack, and may improve the woman's feeling of well-being. The doctor should explain that oestrogen will not rejuvenate the skin, make the hair glisten, put a blush on the cheeks or a sparkle in the eye of the menopausal woman. She can do all these things by her attitude to the 'change of life', and by realizing that it is a *change* and not the end of life. Unfortunately some doctors are not aware of the benefits of oestrogen and tend to prescribe tranquillizers and antidepressants for women who have menopausal problems. As the evidence is that oestrogen is so beneficial, it is sad that fewer than 10 per cent of menopausal women choose to take the hormone for the first 10 years after the menopause, when its benefit are maximal.

The dose of oestrogen required to control the number of hot flushes differs, and most doctors try to use the smallest dose needed to regulate them in that particular woman. To help the doctor, she may be asked to make a 'hot flush count'. She counts the number of hot flushes she gets each day, and the doctor increases or decreases the dose of oestrogen so that she gets no more than three hot flushes a day. This is 'tailoring' the drug to the patient, and is the best way of controlling the symptoms.

Unfortunately, oestrogen has one side effect which causes concern. This is that it may cause the lining of the uterus (the endometrium) to grow and possibly become cancerous in 6 women in every 1000. Fortunately this side effect can be prevented if a woman who has not had a hysterectomy takes the hormone, progestogen, for 12 days each month.

With this treatment the woman may expect to have a bleed during the last two days of the progestogen tablets or after she has finished taking them. If she bleeds during the first 10 days of taking the tablets the dose is too small, and needs to be increased. The treatment is called hormone replacement treatment or HRT. Another side effect whilst the woman takes progestogen is that she may develop premenstrual-like symptoms.

There are several regimens for HRT. In the first the woman takes oestrogen in the smallest dose which prevents the symptoms for 21 days, and also takes a progestogen for the last 12 days. She takes no hormones for the next 7 days when she may have a small uterine bleed. She repeats the course again each month. During the hormone-free weeks, the hot flushes may return. This has led many doctors to prescribe oestrogen continuously. In this regimen the woman takes the progestogen tablets for the first 12–14 days each month.

Many women resent having a 'period' after their menopause. A new treatment is being tested which may relieve women of this annoyance. This is for the woman to take both hormones in a combined pill, every day. If the method proves successful and safe it may become popular amongst menopausal women.

How long should a woman take oestrogen?

In the past 30 years much discussion and controversy has taken place about the need for women to continue to take oestrogen into old age. Those doctors who believe in oestrogen claim that a daily tablet of oestrogen keeps a woman younger, more feminine, protects her against heart attacks and retards the changes which occur in her vagina so that sex continues to be pleasurable. There is no evidence that a daily dose of oestrogen keeps a woman younger but it may protect her against a heart attack. There is strong evidence that a daily dose of oestrogen, taken for 5 to 10 years after the menopause, helps to protect her against osteoporosis (see p. 388). Small doses of oestrogen also help a woman whose vagina feels 'burning' and for whom sexual intercourse is painful.

At least six different oestrogen preparations are available to treat 'menopausal' women. Three main forms are available: the semi-synthetic forms, such as ethinyl oestradiol; that derived from the urine of pregnant mares (equine oestrogen or Premarin); and those which are changed in the body in a natural way.

The so-called 'natural' oestrogens includes piperazine oestrone (Harmogen, Ogen) micronized oestradiol (Estace), oestradiol valerate (Progynova) and oestriol (Ovestrin). It was believed that the natural oestrogens were safer as they carried a lesser risk of blood clotting and had fewer side effects, but this is doubtful.

Some women, particularly if they have had a hysterectomy, may choose to have injections of a long-acting oestrogen every six months.

Recently a new way of giving oestrogen has been developed and seems a good idea. If tablets of oestrogen are taken by mouth, the oestrogen is absorbed from the gut and reaches the liver. In the liver it induces the production of certain enzymes which may be disadvantageous. In the new method a small patch of plastic containing oestrogen is stuck to the skin on the abdomen or between the buttocks. The oestrogen is absorbed through the skin, into the bloodstream and only a small amount passes through the liver. The patch is changed every 3 days or so.

A new hormome preparation called Livial which is taken each day may supersede many of the existing treatments. In the first 3 months of using Livial, the woman may get unexpected small bleeds (especially if she is in the first year after her menopause) which can be annoying. If the woman waits to start using Livial for one year after the menopause, and uses one of the other treatments taken before that time, the bleeding episodes are less likely to occur. Livial effectively relieves menopausal symptoms, prevents periodic bleeding and does not stimulate the endometrium or alter blood lipids to any significant degree. It protects the woman against heart attacks and against osteoporosis as effectively as oestrogen.

If the woman has a painful vagina, oestrogen cream can be placed in it. The oestrogen stops the pain and makes the vagina more comfortable.

Postmenopausal bleeding

In the years after the menopause, a few women notice that they have a scanty, or more profuse, bloody discharge coming from the vagina. This is an urgent reason for going to consult their doctor. The bleeding may be unimportant, due to the use of oestrogens (which can cause bleeding), or to a vaginal irritation, but in some cases it is caused by cancer of the womb. It is essential to see the doctor as soon as possible after bleeding is discovered. The doctor may ask the woman to have a transvaginal ultrasound picture taken of her uterus. This is done by inserting a probe about the size of a sausage into her vagina and taking the picture of the uterus through her vagina. It is painless. The idea is to determine the thickness of the endometrium. If it is thin cancer is very unlikely to be present. Alternatively the doctor may wish to do a diagnostic curettage and take a cervical smear, so that he may be quite certain that cancer is not present.

Getting fat

A woman's weight depends on three things: the disposition of fatness she has inherited from her parents; the amount of food and drink she consumes; and the amount of energy she uses for her activities. She cannot alter her disposition to fatness (and most people tend to put on a little weight as the years go by), but she can control the other two factors. If she obtains more energy from food and drink than she uses in her daily tasks, the excess will be converted into fat and stored. At the time of the 'change of life' women tend to eat more and to do less, so that their weight increases. Women can avoid excessive weight gain during and after the menopause if they are careful about what they eat, and remember to keep on exercising themselves. This does not mean that the woman needs to do special exercises, although these often help, but that she gardens, goes for walks, plays golf or swims, depending on her inclinations. There is a tendency for women at this time of life to do less housework than formerly, as there is less to do now the family is grown up and helps; to go to more morning tea or coffee parties; to eat cakes more often; and in general to sit around, sometimes thinking, sometimes just sitting. This inertness is a great contributor to the weight gain which occurs at the 'change of life'. It can be avoided if a woman puts her mind to it. Obesity is discussed in Chapter 21.

Heart disease during and after the menopause

Women in the premenopausal years have about 20 times less chance of having a heart attack compared with men. After the menopause the difference is considerably reduced. This suggests that oestrogen may protect a woman against a heart attack. Evidence is accumulating that oestrogen taken daily in the years after the menopause has this effect. However it must be stressed that taking oestrogen is only one of the preventative measures a woman may adopt to reduce her chance of having a heart attack. The chance of having a heart attack is reduced considerably if a woman takes exercise regularly, does not smoke cigarettes, keeps her weight within the desirable range (see p. 347), and eats a prudent diet.

Exercise: It has been shown in several studies that exercise is important in reducing the chance of heart attack and has the additional benefit of helping a woman reduce her weight. The exercise must be enjoyable or the person will not persist. It should be taken for about 30 minutes three times a week. You can choose the exercise you like best, which may be walking briskly, jogging or some other weight bearing exercise which puts your heart rate up and makes you a bit breathless.

A prudent diet: A prudent diet is one in which the person eats much less saturated fat and sugar and more complex carbohydrates, vegetables and fruits.

Reducing dietary fat: You should eat fewer processed meats like sausages; choose lean beef (or cut off the fat) or lamb; eat chicken, but not the skin; and eat fish at least once a week. You should not fry the meat or fish, but grill or casserole it. If you need a cooking oil, choose sunflower or safflower seed or olive oil rather than dripping, lard or beef fat. Olive oil which is used by many people living in the Mediterranean seems to have a protective effect, as do cold water fish such as herrings, salmon, trout and mackerel.

It is better to eat a polyunsaturated margarine rather than butter, but if you prefer butter spread it thinly. You should also eat cakes, pastries and confectionary only occasionally as they contain hidden fat.

Reducing sugar: It is better to eat complex carbohydrates, such as wholemeal bread or pasta, than sugar and other 'refined carbohydrates'.

You can reduce your sugar intake by cutting down (or stopping) the sugar you add to your tea or coffee. If you like breakfast cereals avoid the 'sugared' ones, and try not to put sugar on the cereal in the breakfast bowl! If you like fruit juices and cordials or canned fruit eat them only sparingly.

Adding fibre to your diet: Eat wholegrain bread rather than white bread, and try and eat green vegetables and fresh fruit, including the skins of apples and stone fruit.

There are many books which will help you eat a prudent diet and still enjoy the tastes, textures and flavours of food.

Checking your blood cholesterol: High levels of cholesterol in the blood increase the risk of a heart attack. These levels can be reduced to safer levels by choosing a prudent diet. If this doesn't work, certain drugs are now available which will reduce the cholesterol level.

Finally, let me repeat: don't smoke. A recent scientific study from the USA showed that smoking more than 15 cigarettes a day doubles the risk of a heart attack, and smoking more than 25 cigarettes a day increased the risk five-fold compared with non-smokers. Smoking is the main reason for heart disease in middle-aged women.

Osteoporosis

As people grow older they begin to lose bone and their bones become brittle. Women lose bone more rapidly than men, particularly in the 5 to 10 years after the menopause. The thinning of the bones is called osteoporosis. Osteoporosis has become a major health problem.

Bone is not static: it is dynamic, constantly being made, remodelled and destroyed by special bone cells. Up to about the age of 25 you make more bone than you lose, so your bones become stronger and thicker. You have two kinds of bones. Your spine, the pelvic bones and the jaw, and the ends of long bones are formed of an interlocking meshwork of tiny spicules of bone, the so-called spongy bone, covered by a thin (but strong) shell, the cortex. The long bones of your body – your arms and legs – are different. They have a thick compact outer layer (the cortex) and a hollow inside, usually filled with bone marrow. The bones are strong and rigid because calcium impregnates them.

From about the age of 25 no new bone is added and in women, from about the age of 45, bone begins to be lost. At first the loss is slow, about 0.5 per cent of the total bone mass being lost each year. But with the menopause, the rate of loss increases to between 2 and 5 per cent of the total mass each year. This goes on for between 5 and 10 years. In these years more bone is lost from the long bones so fractures of he wrist and hips are most likely to occur. Bone is also being lost slowly from the 'spongy' bones of the spine, and small fractures causing backache may occur.

The larger the 'bone bank' before loss starts, the less is the risk of osteoporosis. From this it follows that calcium intake in the form of food (Table 22/1) should be encouraged in young women, who should take in 800–1000mg of calcium each day.

Men are largely spared the effects of this bone loss. First, because they have a larger bone mass to start with, and second, because they produce the male sex hormone, testosterone, which helps to prevent bone loss.

The female sex hormone, oestrogen, also helps to prevent bone loss, but of course, after the menopause only a little oestrogen is produced. This is the reason for the greater bone loss which occurs in the years just after the menopause.

After the age of 70, the pattern of bone loss alters. Now women and men lose bone at a similar rate. Slowly the strength of the bone is reduced. Fractures of the hips become more common, and in some people one or more of the vertebrae which make up the spine collapses. Backache may become a problem, and some women (and fewer men) develop a 'dowager's hump'.

Prevention of osteoporosis

Osteoporosis, at least before the age of 70, largely can be prevented if you are prepared to co-operate. The most effective preventive agent is to take oestrogen (and progestogen) for the first 5 to 10 years after the menopause as described on page 385. In a sense, this is a 'spray shot' method as individual women lose bone in the early postmenopausal years at differing rates. It is now possible to measure the density of a woman's bones, at least those of the spine and the hip or arm, using special machines. If the woman's bone density at the time of her menopause is in the normal range, she is not at great risk of developing osteoporosis. However, it is not yet clear if she will lose bone at a low or a high rate after the menopause, so that further bone density measurements are probably needed at intervals of 2 or 3 years. If the woman's bone density, measured at the time of her menopause is low, she needs treatment at once.

Until scientists have reached a consensus about screening bone density, it is more effective for all menopausal women to consider taking oestrogen (and progestogen if she has her uterus) for 10 years after she ceases to have periods.

As well as taking hormones, the following measures will help to reduce bone loss.

- Increasing calcium intake either in foods (Table 22/1) or as calcium tablets, taken each evening, to give a total intake of about 1.5 grams of calcium daily.
- Stopping tobacco smoking.
- Taking regular exercise, choosing the form of exercise which you enjoy. Brisk walking for half an hour three times a week is as effective as any more complicated exercise programme.

The treatment of osteoporosis

The treatment of osteoporosis is much more difficult to achieve than its prevention. It has been suggested that hormone replacement treatment which prevents the development of osteoporosis may also be useful in treating the condition. But because of the lack of certainty that HRT works in established osteoporosis several other drugs are being

Table 22/1
Calcium content of average servings of common foods

Food			Calcium (mg)
Milk	250ml	(8½oz)	280
Cheese:			
Cheddar, Swiss or processed	30	(1oz)	260
Cottage	200g	(7oz)	190
Salmon (canned)	30g	(1½oz)	110
Fish	100g	(3½oz)	50
Orange	large		60
Broccoli	60g	(2oz)	60
Baked beans	100g	(3½oz)	40
Carrots	90g	(3oz)	30

investigated. The most hopeful are injections of a type of male hormone called nandrolone decanoate (Deca-Durabolin), or the use of a drug called etidronate (Didronel). Deca-Durabolin is given by injection every 3 to 4 weeks, but some women's voices become gruff and others start growing hair on their face. Didronel is given by mouth twice daily for 2 weeks and the course is repeated every 14 weeks. In the interval the woman takes at least 1500mg of calcium a day. Another drug being tested is calcitonin which is sniffed or injected.

CHAPTER 23

Growing Old Gracefully and Happily

When a woman reaches the menopause she can expect to live another 32 years, five years longer than a man, and seven years longer than she would have expected to live 100 years ago. The reasons for the increased life span of women and men today have not been fully clarified, but in part they are due to better nutrition throughout life, better health care and better social support.

By the year 2000 it has been estimated that in many Western countries, one person in six will be aged 65 or more, and women will predominate over men. This has social consequences, particularly if the person has had a hard impoverished life and has no resources beyond her pension. Such women, living alone, can be the poorest, the most deprived of all age groups. Many elderly women live a life of penury, existing in substandard, damp, dirty accommodation, often unable to afford adequate heating, and unable to purchase or to prepare nutritious food.

Growing old is inevitable, feeling old is not. In past years Western society tended to place old people into a special subordinate category. Older people were expected to behave in what society had decided was an 'appropriate manner' for an old person. It was believed that older people's feelings, their needs and their behaviours should conform to what society perceived as 'old'. If they did not conform (although most did) they were considered peculiar, eccentric or, if their sexual behaviour was not kept secret, shameless or lecherous.

Today's society is much less condemnatory and more supportive of older people, and in consequence older people can live fuller, more enjoyable, independent lives, provided that they have reasonable health, supportive relatives or friends and sufficient money for their needs.

How can a woman grow old but feel young?

There are several ways in which you can achieve this. First, remain curious about life and be or become passionate about causes. This will stimulate your brain. There is a belief that as people grow old their mental capacity diminishes. This is true for a few older people, particularly if they develop Alzheimer's disease, or if they are alcoholic or have a chronic illness, such as atherosclerosis or high blood pressure. But most older people's mental capacity remains excellent, at least until very old age. Being curious and passionate is a good way of keeping mentally alert. It has been observed that older people are more emotional, or at least show their emotions more openly, weeping more readily and being more sentimental. This has been construed as showing that older people are mentally less controlled. It could be argued, equally plausibly, that middle-aged people who do not show emotion are too tightly controlled and would be healthier if they expressed emotions more openly.

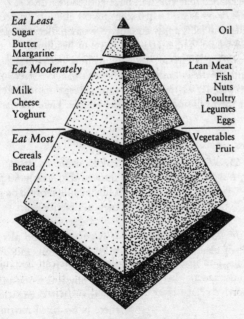

FIG. 23/1   Healthy diet pyramid.

Second, eat a healthy diet which contains fresh vegetables and fruit (providing fibre and vitamins), bread and reducing the amount of fat eaten in the form of butter, pastries, cakes and confectionery and that on meat. This does not mean that an older person should not eat cakes and the other 'goodies' from time to time, it merely means that a woman should try to eat a sensible diet, the principles of which are shown in Figure 23/1.

Third, if you smoke try to limit the cigarettes or to stop altogether.

Fourth, take regular enjoyable exercise. Walking is a wonderful way of keeping fit. It costs nothing, it gives the person the chance of seeing other people and places, and it is easy to do, even if you have a disability. It is recommended by many doctors that a woman should walk, fairly briskly, for about 20 to 30 minutes three times a week. But of course as you grow older you have to adjust this to fit in with your mobility.

Fifth, if you are obese, try and reduce your weight so that it falls into the normal range (see page 347). Obesity aggravates arthritis, increases the risk that the person will develop high blood pressure and increases the chance that you will have gallbladder disease.

In my book *Every Man*, I listed some myths about older people. These myths and the true facts apply equally to women. Because of this I have reprinted them here. The myths can have an insidious effect, reducing an older person's self esteem, and diminishing her confidence that she can contribute to the community. The myths also affect middle-aged and younger people, as they perpetuate perceptions of ageing to the detriment of their relationships to older people. Here they are.

Myth	Fact
After about 65, all old people get progressively less fit mentally and physically.	False: evidence from the USA showed that nearly 60 per cent of older people showed no physical or mental deterioration.
Old people should retire as they are incapable of meeting the demands of work.	It is true that hard physical work may prove too much; but old people are fully able to do less heavy physical work and all mental work. In occupations where there is no fixed retiring age and where people can work part-time

Myth	Fact
	if they wish, the individuals are healthier both physically and mentally than when they are forced to retire at a fixed age. Older people have less absenteeism, less injuries, and are more helpful than younger workers.
After 65, your mind degenerates and you will inevitably become senile.	You may respond slightly more slowly, and some of this is due to the way society patronizes old people – you learn to behave as it expects an old person to behave. Fewer than one person in every hundred develops senile dementia: in other words, goes mad.
Most old people live in the past, and forget the present.	Some do, many do not. 'How much of the actual failure of old people is due to society's expectation that old people are going to be forgetful, repetitious and living in the past?' asked Dr Soddy in a study of middle age.
Most old people neither want, need, nor enjoy sex.	Rubbish!
Most old people need to live in institutions, they cannot cope with living outside.	Only 5 to 10 per cent of people over 70 live in hospitals or homes: and given a proper degree of financial and social support many of them need not and would prefer not to.
Most old people are bed-ridden.	This is false. It is true that more old people are chronically ill, but fewer are more acutely ill than

Myth	Fact
	younger people. And, given help, many bed-ridden people can get up, get out, and do things. As a person grows older bed continues to be a splendid place for sleep and sex, ideal for short illness but lethal for chronic illness if the person can be induced to be mobile. An older person should not stay in bed for more than four days unless ordered to do so by a doctor.
Old people really want to opt out of having to participate in everyday matters.	They are not asked, we tell them when they get old that they need to opt out. We make them disposable objects – 'non-people'. And unhappily we forget that soon we will be old and that unless we change societal attitudes we will be eased out and made 'non-people' too.
Old people spend their time sitting, dreaming, reminiscing, and watching television – they do not want to do anything.	We have created a situation in which old people are prevented from working and are regarded as mentally and physically ineffective. We have made them feel unwanted and despised. To protect their self-respect many old people sit, dream, and watch television. If we treated them differently, they would do different things.
Old people need less food and only eat slops.	It is true that *inactive* old people need fewer calories, and if they have poor teeth cannot chew as easily. It is also true that, because

Myth	Fact
	of poverty and ignorance, many old people (and many younger people) eat the wrong kinds of foods.
Old people are usually serene, content with their lot, and grateful for what society provides.	Often old age is not a time of serenity, except in novels. Many old people are full of anxiety about their future and concern about their health. Much of this concern and anxiety is occasioned by the way younger people treat the old, some is due to the person's own perception of how old people are expected to behave.
The older a person is, the more helpless she is.	You are as old as you feel, not as old as your birth certificate states.

As the years pass inevitably a woman will grow and look old. Streaks of grey first appear in her hair and eventually all her hair becomes grey and less profuse, and later it turns white.

Her skin becomes less taut, and wrinkles (which started in middle age) increase on her face, her arms and her body. If in her youth she enjoyed lying in the sun, she is likely to have more wrinkles than a woman who avoided the sun. Wrinkles are also more likely to occur in certain families. If your mother or father had extensive wrinkles, you are likely to have extensive wrinkles.

As she grows older her teeth become looser and may have to be extracted.

As well as alterations to her physical appearance as a woman ages, three of her five senses become affected. Her hearing becomes less acute and she is no longer able to hear higher sounds clearly. If there is a lot of background noise, she may not be able to distinguish the words spoken to her from the noise. By the age of 70 about one woman in four has some degree of hearing loss. As well as ageing affecting her hearing, her

397

sense of smell diminishes, which may be beneficial or distressing depending on your life style and your viewpoint.

An older woman may find that she cannot see as well as formerly, in other words, her vision is less acute and she may require spectacles or have to change her existing glasses. Some women develop cataracts and their sight is considerably impaired. For this reason, and because glaucoma may also develop, older people would be wise to have their eyes checked at regular intervals, perhaps every 2 years. If a cataract or glaucoma is detected, it can be treated effectively. Cataracts need not cause blindness today. With modern surgical techniques, the cataract can be removed painlessly and a new lens implanted into the affected eye.

As the years pass, a woman's immune system, which helps to protect her from getting viral and other infections, becomes less effective. If she catches 'flu, for example, she may have a more severe infection and may find it harder to shake off. Minor illnesses like common colds may be more severe and lead to longer periods of restricted activity.

After the age of 70 a woman is likely to have less strength in her muscles and may find it uncomfortable to walk up stairs or for long distances. Although in all older people muscle strength diminishes, the decrease can be retarded if the person regularly takes exercise.

With increasing age, a woman's sense of balance becomes less effective and she has to take care that she does not trip and fall. A less secure sense of balance is added to by less acute vision, impaired hearing, and less mobility of the joints, making a fall more likely as a woman ages. Most falls cause no problems apart from a feeling of being stupid to have fallen, but some falls result in broken bones. This is more likely to occur if the woman has osteoporosis (see page 388), when she may sustain a broken wrist or hip if she trips and falls.

Most falls occur within the home. Because of the danger of tripping and falling a woman should check what she has in her house. If there are loose rugs on the floor she should put them away. She should avoid having small tables in unexpected places, that she might trip over. She should make sure that she has a hand rail in her shower or bath for ease of getting in and out. She needs to be particularly careful of the stairs. Stairs are often narrow and steep, and all too easy to fall down.

The physical and physiological changes of ageing are inevitable, andaffect people to differing degrees. Those who are least affected have not misused their bodies during their earlier years by smoking, by drinking

Table 23/2
Percentage of women aged 65 or older who
have a chronic disease (USA, 1978)

Arthritis	52
Hypertension	30
Hearing impairment	26
Visual impairment	23
Heart disease	19
Obesity	10
Diabetes	9
Urinary tract disease	7

heavily and by failing to take exercise and have chosen the right parents! If your parents lived to a good age, it is likely that you will live to a good age.

The changes may lead to certain health problems. Studies have shown that by the age of 70, one woman in 2 has arthritis, one woman in 3 has high blood pressure, one woman in 5 has a heart or circulation problem, one woman in 7 has urinary incontinence and one person in 12 has chronic bronchitis or some other respiratory problem (Table 23/2).

Arthritis (osteoarthritis)

By the age of 70, one woman in 2 complains of arthritis or 'rheumatism' which may be relatively painless except at certain times, or may be incapacitating. Arthritis can affect any joint in the body, but usually affects the large joints, particularly the knees and the hips. It may also affect smaller joints, particularly those of the fingers and wrists. If the arthritis affect the woman's hands, doing simple things like turning on taps, washing clothes or cooking may be a painful, slow experience. However, there are tricks which can be learnt and devices which can be purchased which reduce the pain and the incapacity.

You cannot prevent arthritis occurring but when you notice increasing stiffness of your joints (usually starting in middle age) you can take steps to prevent the disease getting very bad. You should take regular exercise, to keep the joints as mobile as possible, but avoiding any activity which puts sudden strains on joints. If you are overweight you should try to get your weight down so that your hips, knees and ankles do not have so much weight bearing on them.

399

Unfortunately arthritis is usually slowly progressive, and as you grow older the disability may increase. If a woman's hips or knees become very painful, she may consider having a replacement joint. The surgery is complicated, there is some pain for a few days (which can be relieved by drugs) but the freedom from pain and the increased mobility after surgery is welcomed by many women.

High blood pressure

As a woman grows older her blood pressure tends to rise because her arteries are less elastic and stiffer. By the age of 70 as mentioned above, one woman in three will have high blood pressure. To diagnose high blood pressure your doctor will put a cuff around your arm and raise the pressure in the cuff until the blood flow below the cuff is stopped. The doctor will then release the pressure in the cuff slowly until the blood starts to flow again and the pulse can be detected by listening through a stethoscope. This gives the height of your blood pressure when your heart is beating. The doctor continues to release the air in the cuff as he listens to your pulse until the beats cease. This measures your blood pressure when your heart is relaxed. The two measurements are recorded. If the reading exceeds 160/95 and this level or higher is found on three occasions at least three weeks apart, you have high blood pressure.

High blood pressure may be treated by changing your life style to a more relaxed one, and if you are obese by losing weight. However, doctors increasingly are prescribing treatment using diuretic drugs (which reduce the blood pressure but increase your need to pass urine), betablocker drugs or drugs which are called ACE inhibitors, both of which relax the arteries.

A reason for controlling blood pressure is that it reduces the chance that you will have a stroke and lessens the risk of a heart attack.

Dizzy spells

As well as leading to high blood pressure, the reduction of elasticity and stiffening in a woman's arteries prevent them from responding efficiently to the flow of blood through them. This may lead to a temporary reduction of blood flowing into the heart and a less efficient flow of blood from the heart. A consequence of this is that the elderly person may have a sudden fall in her blood pressure and complain of dizziness and light-headedness. She may even faint and fall, particularly when she sits up quickly. Between 10 and 20 per cent of women over the age of 70 are affected in this way.

To avoid the dizzy spells, an elderly person who has experienced them should take preventive action. She should stand up slowly, shower rather than have a bath, but if she chooses to have a bath stand rather than sit in it, avoid going outside on very hot days, and keep her house as cool as possible in hot weather.

Some elderly people become dizzy when eating meals. If this happens to you it is better to eat small meals often and add a bit more salt to the food.

Strokes and transient ischaemic attacks

Elderly people occasionally have an unexpected black out which leads to a fall, a temporary weakness in an arm or leg, a slurring of speech or a transient loss of vision. The attack only lasts a few minutes. It is called a transient cerebral ischaemic attack or a TIA, and is caused by a transient blockage of an artery supplying part of the brain. A TIA should be taken seriously and the person should visit her doctor to be checked. This is because a person who has a TIA may suffer a stroke months or a few years later.

After a stroke the person is affected much more seriously than after a TIA. Often one side of the body is partially paralyzed and the speech is badly slurred. The chance of having a stroke increases with age, and over half of strokes occur after the age of 75. After a stroke about one person dies in the first few days. Of those women who survive about one third are bedridden and need care in an institution; one third are disabled to some extent and may need help to cope with daily living and one third recover so well that they can manage their lives satisfactorily. Strokes occur more commonly in women who have high blood pressure, are overweight, have diabetes, and are smokers. If a woman has her blood pressure checked at regular intervals and takes medication if it is high; if she eats a prudent diet (see page 394) and stops smoking, her risk of a stroke is reduced considerably.

A stroke is a devastating illness for the victim and for her family. She needs a good deal of emotional and physical support. But with help and encouragement from her family and care from a rehabilitation team, considerable physical and emotional recovery is possible, but it is a slow process.

Table 23/3
Mortality from Coronary Heart Disease.
Male v Female. (England and Wales, 1987–9)

	Mortality per 100 000 in age group	
Age	Male	Female
40–44	50	8
45–49	125	20
50–55	225	45
55–59	425	110
60–65	725	250
65–69	1100	450

Heart disease

Heart disease has been discussed in the previous chapter, when it was noted that women at all ages, have fewer heart attacks than men (Table 23/3). After the menopause the difference diminishes, unless the woman takes oestrogen when the difference is maintained. It was also pointed out that the chance of having a heart attack can be reduced by changing life style, changing diet, taking exercise and ceasing to smoke. These measures are effective until the age of 70, but after that age it is not known if they will prevent a heart attack. In fact most elderly women die of a heart attack or a stroke.

Urinary incontinence

As a woman ages, many of her bodily functions become less efficient. For example, increasingly large numbers of women wet themselves, having developed urinary incontinence. Urinary incontinence can affect the woman's enjoyment of life considerably. Studies in Britain and Sweden have shown that by the age of 65, one woman in 7 wets herself once a week, and one woman in 14 wets herself each day. The same investigators found that by the age of 80, one woman in four wets herself each day. Most of these women put up with the discomfort and embarrassment and wear sanitary pads to mop up the urine. This is sad as for many of them effective treatment is now available.

There are two main types of urinary incontinence. These have been discussed on page 363. Once a diagnosis has been made the treatments recommended in that discussion may be tried, but if these fail to control the problem, operations are now available which will help the woman become dry. If a woman loses the fear that she may wet herself when she goes out, her enjoyment of life will be much improved.

Dementia

As a person grows older it is more likely that she will develop senile dementia, in other words her brain will no longer function properly. In children, brain function develops as an infant becomes a toddler and the toddler a child, and each year the child is able to do more, express more thoughts and develop more concepts. In some elderly people, it seems that the function of the brain is reversed and the brain regresses from being adult, to being like that of a child and finally to that of an infant.

By the age of 75, one person in 7 (rather more men than women), shows signs of dementia, and it is severe in one-third of them. Dementia may be caused by chronic alcoholism, by small strokes, by combinations of medications and by Alzheimer's disease, which may affect middle-aged people, but is more common among elderly people.

Dementia is characterized by a loss of initiative, decreased judgment, the inability to select appropriate words or to perform calculations, and to changes in the personality. Many older people have some of these symptoms, but not to the degree of a person who has dementia. As the years pass, dementia tends to get worse.

Dementia is not just one person's illness it affects the whole family, and it is the family which has to care for the person, as there is no effective drug treatment.

In its early stages, when only the person's memory and language abilities are diminished, the person may retain insight and develop feelings of frustration, anger and depression. The demented person can be helped by finding out which brain functions are operating best and by concentrating on them. For example, if the woman cannot remember things said to her but has a reasonable visual memory, she may feel less frustrated if written directions, pictures or signs are provided, rather than giving her verbal information, which she tends to forget.

One effective way of delaying the deterioration of brain function is to try to stimulate parts of the brain not affected by the illness, so that the affected woman obtains some enjoyment. As short term memory is most affected, affected people may be stimulated by music from an earlier period of life and by talking about old memories, or by looking at old photograph albums.

The help that the family, and more particularly the 'carer' gives to the person with dementia, is very time consuming and wearing. One author called his book about the management of Alzheimer's Disease, *The 36 Hour Day*. Carers can become very tired and frustrated. This may prevent them from being supportive, from praising the person for successes and from speaking to the demented person slowly, simply, using short sentences, and talking about specific things.

Carers also need help. One way is to persuade the demented person to spend the day in a day care centre several times a week. In the early stages of dementia such an initiative may be rejected as the person feels it demeaning, but in the middle stages of the disease it may be a help to the person and especially to her carers.

In the advanced stages of dementia, the family may find it impossible to cope and may have to put their demented relative into a nursing home. Making this decision may be very difficult and traumatic, and the main carer (who is usually a woman) may need help to overcome her feelings of guilt, depression and despair.

Medications

One of the consequences of an ageing population, such as is occurring in most Western countries, is that more resources are needed for health care. Older people are bigger consumers of health care than any other group. Older people visit their doctor more frequently, are more often referred to specialists, and are prescribed more medications than other age group.

Today's medications have enabled many older people to live more comfortable and longer lives, but have also caused social and medical problems. This is because older people, who predominantly have degenerative diseases, often of different body systems, may be referred to different specialists who prescribe different medications, and who may forget to find out what other medications have been prescribed by other doctors. The result is that some older people become walking pharmacies. An investigation in Manchester, England in 1991, found that one in four elderly patients were suffering from adverse drug reactions, half of which were attributable to inappropriate medications prescribed by a doctor.

This is causing considerable concern to doctors and at regular intervals articles appear in medical journals pointing out the damage to the elderly person's health that multiple medications may cause. For example, another study in England made in 1988 found that 2 people in every 100 over the age of 65 had been taking benzodiazipines (Valium-like drugs) for over a year. More women than men are prescribed benzodiazipines and elderly women consume a disproportionate amount of the total benzodiazipines prescribed. In many cases the drugs are given to treat depression. As well, elderly people react more strongly to the drugs than younger people. If they are prescribed in the same dose as that prescribed for a younger person, they may develop side effects such as dizziness, confusion, memory impairment, depression and dementia.

Benzodiazipines are tranquillizers and are not indicated as treatment for depression. When prescribed for anxiety, or to help the woman sleep, they should not be taken for longer than 4 weeks as they can become addictive, lose their effect and may dull the woman's mind. If a Valium-like drug is taken for more than 6 months, one woman in three will experience 'withdrawal symptoms' when the drug is stopped. These withdrawal symptoms can be severe and most distressing.

Benzodiazipines are not the only drugs which are prescribed more to older people than to younger people. As mentioned earlier, some elderly people have been found to be taking six or more medications, some of which were first prescribed months or years previously. The use of multiple drugs may cause considerable mental confusion.

For example, a woman aged 72 who was asthmatic had been treated with drugs for asthma for some years. In her sixties she developed osteoarthritis and was given drugs to relieve her pain and stiffness. When she was 70 she started being unable to sleep and was prescribed drugs to help her sleep. She was also taking drugs for 'her heart', and had episodes of wetting herself.

After she had taken the sleeping pills and all the other drugs for about three months, she became increasingly confused, disoriented and incapable of looking after herself. Her family thought that she was becoming senile and demented and that she should be cared for in a mental hospital. However, her daughter did not like the idea of her mother being in a 'loony bin' and volunteered to care for her, but said that if her mother got worse she would agree to have her seen by a psychiatrist. She took her mother into her home and asked her family doctor, in whom she had great confidence, to call. The doctor took the elderly woman's history as best she could, examined her carefully and asked to see the medications that the woman was taking. Having collected all the information, she explained to the daughter that the medications were probably causing the problems and suggested that they should be stopped, giving the daughter reasons. After some discussion the daughter agreed. Within 48 hours her mother had improved dramatically, and within a week she had recovered almost completely.

This story has been replicated many times in the past 20 years, but it still seems that many elderly people are taking too many medications for which there is no valid medical reason.

The message is clear. Older people should check with their doctor, every year or so, that the medications that they are taking are really necessary, and find out if some could be stopped and others replaced by newer medications. Doctors too have their part to play. They should review periodically the drugs prescribed to their patients and ask themselves if they are really necessary, or if some of them could be stopped.

Insomnia

As a woman grows older she may find it increasingly difficult to sleep. Her sleep may be disturbed because of emotional upset, or because she drinks excessive amounts of coffee or tea. She may catnap during the day or doze in a chair and when she goes to bed can't sleep.

Lack of sleep is not a problem in itself and will not affect your health, the important thing is to find out what has produced the insomnia and to correct it. As well as visiting your doctor and discussing the problem, you can take measures yourself which will help you sleep at night (Table 23/4).

Sexuality after the menopause

One of the more insidious myths about a woman's sexuality is that her sexual capacity and sexual desire diminish as she grows older. This is quite untrue; our bodies and minds are capable of sexuality all our lives, from birth to death, but are only capable of reproduction for a part of that time. The idea that only young people enjoy and have the desire for sex is unfair to older women whose sexuality is often enhanced. This is because the sexual drive is a learned activity and is not dependent on the sex hormones as some male sexologists believe.

Table 23/4
How to help you sleep at night

- Avoid dozing during the day
- Avoid stimulants such as tea or coffee in the late evening
- Avoid alcohol beverages in the late evening
- Alcohol is a sedative and may help you to fall asleep but you may find that you wake up early in the morning
- If you find that a glass of warm milk helps you relax, then take it
- Try to deal with any problems during the day
- Spend at least one hour before going to bed, relaxing and becoming calm
- Remember that insomnia is not a disease in itself; it is the result of something else that should be treated first. Sleeping pills taken for *short periods* help to tide you over while your doctor finds out the cause of your insomnia. But if you take them for longer periods, you will find that they only help you sleep if you increase the dose, and after a while you may find it hard to give them up. If you have been taking sleeping pills for a long time, you will need to give them up, and you must realize that you may get 'withdrawal' symptoms (particularly insomnia), which can go on for weeks.

In a US survey of sexuality at and after 'the change of life' it was found the sexual desire and sexual drive were unaltered in 60 per cent of women, 20 per cent had a reduced drive and in 20 per cent sexual desire was increased. Most women enjoy sexual intercourse well into old age, and coitus only ceases because of the death or incapacity of their partner. A few women, who have never really enjoyed sexual intercourse in their youth are not concerned, as they grow older, if coitus becomes less and less frequent. Other women may, for the first time, find a greater sexual fulfilment, either by reaching a new understanding with their partner or with a new partner.

Sexually active older women, with sympathetic partners, report a change in their attitude towards sex. In youth, sex was a rather simplistic, mechanical affair; as the woman grows older she finds that sexual activity has greater variety, a greater subtlety and a greater enjoyment. For many, sex ceases to be mainly genital and expands to include body contact, touching, and hugging, as well as sexual intercourse. Sexuality after the change of life is determined largely by the pattern established in youth; if you have had an active pleasurable sex life when young, you are more likely to have a similarly enjoyable sexual life when you are older.

A woman's sexual potential persists for longer than that of a man, so that any decline is more likely to be due to her partner's failing capacity than her ability to respond. But this can be improved if the partners are willing to try. Studies in the USA have shown that 7 out of every 10 couples investigated were sexually active after the age of 60, many continuing until their seventies or eighties.

Because women live longer than men and because of the belief that the man should initiate sex, problems do occur. In our society, older women, either single or widowed, have a smaller chance of finding a suitable sexual partner than do older men. This is aggravated by the earlier, erroneous view that an older woman should not have sexual desire. An older woman who is single or widowed should not feel guilty if she has sexual desires. These can be satisfied if she can find a man with whom she can relate.

A woman may feel unable to find a new partner, or does not wish to do so at least for a while after her husband's death, but still has a powerful sexual drive. She can still enjoy sexuality by masturbating and should feel neither shame nor guilt, nor embarrassment if she does. It is a normal, healthy activity. Studies from the USA show that older non-married women masturbate twice as frequently as married women of a similar age.

A problem of sexuality in some older women is that intercourse may become painful because the vaginal wall becomes thin and inflamed. This condition is due to a lack of oestrogen, and is easily corrected by taking oestrogen tablets or the use of a vaginal oestrogen cream.

An older woman should not feel embarrassed about showing affection, about cuddling and touching her partner, or about trying different sexual positions. In fact, it may be more than ever necessary for her to encourage her partner to take the initiative in love-making, as some men who have led active sex lives in their youth may have inhibitions about sex as they grow older.

As women live longer than men, a woman may miss the physical intimacy she experienced before her partner's death. She may accept the deprivation or it may cause her considerable emotional distress. If she forms a relationship with a man, she may have to overcome the prejudices of society; whilst if she has a close woman friend, she should not feel guilty or different if they find warmth and pleasure in intimacy, which may include fondling and clitoral stimulation.

Institutional care

Although only about 10 per cent of elderly women accept or require institutional care, the change from living in her own home or that of a relative may be traumatic to an elderly woman. Even if she takes with her some of her dearest possessions, she often has to share her room and her privacy is constantly invaded. A further problem is that some carers in institutions treat elderly inhabitants as if they have regressed mentally and are asexual. They may be segregated on the basis of sex and have restricted opportunities to meet elderly men living in the institution except in public areas. Elderly women need to be able to feel that they are able to express their need for intimacy in their own way. This may be unacceptable to the carers who are usually younger and have a different set of values and prejudices.

Some elderly women have to be placed in an institution, because of illness or destitution, but most are able to make a decision, at some stage of their life, whether to stay on in the family home, change to a smaller more easily run apartment, or go to live in a 'retirement village' or a nursing home. Whatever the decision, it is important for the elderly person's self-esteem that, if she is capable, she discusses the options with her family and, if needed, with a counsellor, and that she makes the final choice.

Most elderly women do not choose to live in a nursing home, but in some cases it may be necessary or desirable. Unfortunately the choice of nursing home may be difficult. Most provide pleasant, clean, light surroundings and the nursing staff are supportive, compassionate and devoted. In some, the residents are treated in a dehumanizing way or as delinquent children. There is little or no privacy, and the woman has no area she feels is her own. The residents are not provided with stimuli appropriate for their physical and mental health and deteriorate quickly.

Inevitably each of us will die. Death comes, when it does come, in a variety of ways. Death may be welcomed as a relief from pain or disease. But in most instances the period before death is not painful, but may be feared. Talking with an informed person may reduce the fear. In many societies, the hours before death are supported by rituals, and the dying person is involved.

In societies such as Britain, Australia and the United States, the rituals before death tend to be ignored, or death is commercialized.

After the death of a loved one, the relatives have a need to grieve. Bereavement is normal, grieving is normal, and is handled in different ways by different people. There is no right way to cope with mourning.

For the person who dies let us hope that her end is as gentle as her beginning.

Glossary

Abruptio placentae
Separation of some or most of the placenta from the uterus by bleeding.

Alveoli (pron. al-*vee*-o-li)
The plural of alveolus, which means a small cavity. The outermost parts of the duct system of the breast, where milk is secreted, are called alveoli.

Amenorrhoea (pron. a-men-or-*e*-a)
The absence of menstruation for an interval twice that (or more) of the patient's usual menstrual cycle.

Amniotic fluid
The fluid in the 'bag of waters' (or the amniotic sac) in which the fetus grows.

Amniocentesis
The procedure of introducing a narrow needle through the abdominal wall into the amniotic sac to obtain a sample of the amniotic fluid.

Analgesic
A pain-relieving drug.

Antenatal period
The period between conception and childbirth. Also called the prenatal period.

Aphrodisiac
A drug or substance which increases sexual desire.

Areola (pron. aree-*o*-la)
The brownish-coloured pigmented area which surrounds the nipple.

Bacillus

A small form of life, made up of a single cell shaped like a tiny rod, often called a germ. Germs may be harmful to man, for example the pneumococcus which causes pneumonia, and the streptococcus which causes sore throats; or they may be helpful, as the lactobacillis which lives in the vagina.

Coitus (pron. *ko*-it-us)

The act of sexual intercourse, or copulation. The verb is 'to copulate'.

Coitus interruptus

Coitus in which the penis is withdrawn from the vagina before male orgasm, and the semen is ejaculated externally to the vagina.

Conception sac

The embryo (or fetus) contained in the fluid-filled amniotic membranes is called the conception sac.

Copulate

To practise sexual intercourse.

Eclampsia

The occurrence of convulsions or fits in a pregnant woman who has other signs of pregnancy-induced hypertension.

Ejaculate

To spurt out. Applied in this context to the spurting out of semen at the time of orgasm.

Embryo (pron. *em*-bry-o)

The product of conception (or conceptus) from the day of fertilization of the egg cell (ovum) by the spermatozoon until the beginning of the 7th week. During this short period almost all of the major structures have formed.

'Eye' of the penis

The part of the end of the penis through which the urinary tube passes to reach the outside.

Fetus (pron. *fee*-tus)

The product of conception from the end of the 7th week until birth, at whatever period of the pregnancy this may be, is called a fetus.

FSH

Follicle-stimulating hormone. The substance secreted by the pituitary gland which lies beneath the brain. This hormone stimulates some of the egg follicles of the ovary to manufacture oestrogen.

Heterosexual
A person whose sexual affections are directed to a person of the other sex.

Homosexual
A noun (i.e. a person is called a homosexual) or an adjective (i.e. a homosexual act) implying that the object of a person's sexual desire is of the same sex. In slang, the male homosexual is called a fairy, a pansy, a queen or a queer, while a female homosexual is referred to as a dike or a butch. Butch is also used as an adjective to describe a female homosexual who displays outward manifestations of masculinity in behaviour or in dress.

Hormone
A substance which is released from special glands into the bloodstream and stimulates other glands or tissues into activity.

Lactation
Suckling. The period when the child is nourished from the breast. It also means the secretion or formation of milk.

Lanugo
The downy delicate hair which is found on the body of the fetus. It is replaced after birth by rather thicker hair.

Lesbian
A female homosexual.

LH
Luteinizing hormone. The second of the pituitary gonadotrophic, or ovary-stimulating, hormones. It converts the cells of the stimulated egg follicle, from which the egg has been expelled by ovulation, to produce the female sex hormone, progesterone. The cells which produce progesterone become bright yellow (for which the Latin word is '*luteus*'), hence luteinizing hormone.

Lochia
The discharge from the uterus which lasts for about 4 weeks after childbirth. For the first few days it is profuse and red, later becoming pale and scanty.

Masturbation
The mechanical stimulation, usually with the hands or finger, of the penis, the clitoris or other erogenous zones of the body leading to orgasm.

Menarche (pron. men-*ar*-kee)
The time of onset of the first menstrual period.

413

Menstrual cycle

The interval of time from the start of one menstruation (the 'period') to the next. It includes the time during which bleeding occurs and the interval between bleeding episodes.

Monilia

A fungus infection of the vagina, also called *candidosis*; and *vaginal thrush*.

Oedema (pron. *e-de*ma)

Swelling of the tissues under the skin due to retention of water in these tissues.

Oestrogen (pron. *ee*-strogen)

The female sex hormone manufactured in the ovary, and in pregnancy in the placenta. The word derives from *oestrous*, or heatmaking, because the hormone was found to be necessary to bring animals 'on heat'.

Orgasm

Intense excitement occurring at the climax of sexual intercourse culminating in involuntary jerking movement of the pelvis, a feeling of warmth, well-being and release, and followed by a feeling of relaxation. In the male it is accompanied by the ejaculation, or spurting out, of semen from the penis.

Ovum

The egg cell, which has matured and is ready to be expelled from the ovary, is called the ovum.

Partogram

A graphic display of the progress of labour.

Parturition

The process of giving birth.

Peer-group

Individuals of approximately the same age and similar social values who form groups.

Penis

The male sexual organ. Normally it lies soft and limp, but during sexual stimulation it becomes erect. Erections may occur spontaneously at night during sleep, after visual stimuli from magazines, from the sight of sexually desirable women, or during the preliminaries of love-making. Erection is not under the control of the mind.

Perineum

The area between the thighs which contains the entrance to the vagina and the other female external genitals, which comprise the vulva.

Pica
A longing to eat substances which are not foods, such as clay or coal.

Pregnancy-induced hypertension
A rise of blood pressure occurring in pregnancy, often associated with protein in the urine, is called pregnancy-induced hypertension, or pre-eclampsia. It used to be called 'toxaemia of pregnancy' which was an inexact term.

Progesterone (pron. pro-*gest*-erone)
The second main sex hormone produced by the ovaries. The hormone prepares the body, especially the uterus, for pregnancy. Progesterone is also manufactured by the placenta from its earliest days.

Progestogen
A synthetic substance which acts in the body in a way similar to the natural hormone, progesterone.

Promiscuity
A woman may be considered promiscuous if she has sexual intercourse with several casual acquaintances over a short period of time. Premarital coitus with a single partner is not promiscuity.

Prophylactic treatment
Treatment, usually with drugs, given to prevent the onset or spread of disease.

Psychosomatic disorder
A condition in which a disturbed emotion manifests itself as a disorder of one part of the body or another, and mimics disease of that part.

Puerperium
The period between childbirth and the time when the uterus has returned to its normal size, which is about 6 to 8 weeks.

Regimen
A specific course or plan of diet or drugs to maintain or improve health, or regulate the way of life.

Renal tract
See urinary tract.

Reproductive years
The years during which a woman is ovulating, or able to ovulate, and so is able to have a baby. It is the time when the female sex hormones are regularly and rhythmically produced by the ovaries.

415

Semen

The fluid ejaculated by the male at orgasm. It consists of spermatozoa, mixed with secretions from the ducts and collecting areas which link the testicles (where the spermatozoa are manufactured) and the penis (from which the semen is ejaculated).

Sexual drive

The desire to have sex. It varies in strength in different people and at different ages of the same person. Probably everyone starts with the same sexual drive but the differences found are due to inhibitions about sex produced by parental attitudes to sex and those of peer-groups.

Speculum

A small metal instrument, made like a duck's bill which a doctor introduces into a woman's vagina so that he can see her cervix.

'Toxaemia of pregnancy' (see pregnancy-induced hypertension).

Urinary tract

The kidneys, the tubes which connect the kidneys to the bladder (called the ureters), the urinary bladder, and the tube between the bladder and the vulva (called the urethra) form the renal tract.

Voiding

Emptying the urinary bladder (urinating, micturating).

Zona pellucida

The strong translucent outer membrane which surrounds the human egg, rather as the shell surrounds a hen's egg. The zona pellucida only disappears when the fertilized egg reaches the uterine cavity after spending three days in the oviduct.

Further Reading

You may wish to supplement (or confirm!) what you have read in this book with other readings. The following list may help you. Much of the material in *Everywoman* is based on that found in my textbook for medical students, doctors and nurses.

Fundamentals of Obstetrics and Gynaecology (6th edition, 1993), Mosby, London.

Chapters 3 and 4

Money, J. & Ehrhardt, A. A. (1972). *Man & Woman, Boy & Girl*, Johns Hopkins University Press, Baltimore.

Llewellyn-Jones, D. and Abraham, S. (1992). *Everygirl*, Oxford University Press, Melbourne.

Chapters 4 and 5

Abraham, S. and Llewellyn-Jones, D. (1992). *Eating Disorders – The Facts*, Oxford University Press, Oxford.

Brecher, E. (1969). *The Sex Researcher*, Little, Brown & Co., Boston.

Hite, S. (1976). *The Hite Report: a nationwide study of female sexuality*, Collier-Macmillan, London.

Llewellyn-Jones, D. (1988). *Understanding Sexuality* (2nd edition), Oxford University Press, Melbourne.

Llewellyn-Jones, D. (1992). *Getting Pregnant*, Ashwood House Medical, Melbourne.

Masters, W. & Johnson, V. (1966). *The Human Sexual Response*, Little, Brown & Co., Boston.

Chapters 8–15

Kitzinger, Sheila (1970). *The Experience of Childbirth*, Pelican, London.

Leboyer, F. (1975). *Birth Without Violence*, Wildwood House, London.

Pearce, Caroline (1976). Newsletter, Nursing Mothers of Australia Journal, 12 April.

FURTHER READING

Chapter 16

Green, C. (1989). *Babies* (2nd edition), Simon & Schuster, Sydney.

Llewellyn-Jones, D. (1983). *Breast Feeding: How to Succeed*, Faber and Faber, London.

Phillip, V. (1976). *Successful Breast Feeding*, Nursing Mothers Association, Australia.

Chapter 20

Boston Health Collective, (1984). *The NEW Our Bodies, Ourselves*, Simon & Schuster, New York and Penguin Books, UK.

Llewellyn-Jones, D. (1990). *Sexually Transmitted Diseases*, Faber and Faber, London.

Chapter 22

Llewellyn-Jones, D. and Abraham, S. (1992). *Everywoman's Middle Years*, Ashwood House Medical, Melbourne.

Index

EVERYWOMAN

Discover more about our forthcoming books through Penguin's FREE newspaper...

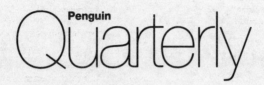

Penguin
Quarterly

It's packed with:

- exciting features

- author interviews

- previews & reviews

- books from your favourite films & TV series

- exclusive competitions & much, much more...

Write off for your free copy today to:
Dept JC
Penguin Books Ltd
FREEPOST
West Drayton
Middlesex
UB7 0BR
NO STAMP REQUIRED

READ MORE IN PENGUIN

In every corner of the world, on every subject under the sun, Penguin represents quality and variety – the very best in publishing today.

For complete information about books available from Penguin – including Puffins, Penguin Classics and Arkana – and how to order them, write to us at the appropriate address below. Please note that for copyright reasons the selection of books varies from country to country.

In the United Kingdom: Please write to *Dept. JC, Penguin Books Ltd, FREEPOST, West Drayton, Middlesex UB7 0BR*

If you have any difficulty in obtaining a title, please send your order with the correct money, plus ten per cent for postage and packaging, to *PO Box No. 11, West Drayton, Middlesex UB7 0BR*

In the United States: Please write to *Penguin USA Inc., 375 Hudson Street, New York, NY 10014*

In Canada: Please write to *Penguin Books Canada Ltd, 10 Alcorn Avenue, Suite 300, Toronto, Ontario M4V 3B2*

In Australia: Please write to *Penguin Books Australia Ltd, 487 Maroondah Highway, Ringwood, Victoria 3134*

In New Zealand: Please write to *Penguin Books (NZ) Ltd,182–190 Wairau Road, Private Bag, Takapuna, Auckland 9*

In India: Please write to *Penguin Books India Pvt Ltd, 706 Eros Apartments, 56 Nehru Place, New Delhi 110 019*

In the Netherlands: Please write to *Penguin Books Netherlands B.V., Keizersgracht 231 NL–1016 DV Amsterdam*

In Germany: Please write to *Penguin Books Deutschland GmbH, Friedrichstrasse 10–12, W–6000 Frankfurt/Main 1*

In Spain: Please write to *Penguin Books S. A., C. San Bernardo 117–6° E–28015 Madrid*

In Italy: Please write to *Penguin Italia s.r.l., Via Felice Casati 20, I–20124 Milano*

In France: Please write to *Penguin France S. A., 17 rue Lejeune, F–31000 Toulouse*

In Japan: Please write to *Penguin Books Japan, Ishikiribashi Building, 2–5–4, Suido, Tokyo 112*

In Greece: Please write to *Penguin Hellas Ltd, Dimocritou 3, GR–106 71 Athens*

In South Africa: Please write to *Longman Penguin Southern Africa (Pty) Ltd, Private Bag X08, Bertsham 2013*

READ MORE IN PENGUIN

WOMEN'S INTEREST

A History of Their Own   Bonnie S. Anderson and Judith P. Zinsser
Volumes One and Two

This is an original and path-breaking European history, the first to approach the past from the perspective of women. 'A richly textured account that leaves me overwhelmed with admiration for our fore-mothers' ability to survive with dignity' – *Los Angeles Times Book Review*

Our Bodies Ourselves   Angela Phillips and Jill Rakusen
A Health Book by and for Women

'The bible of the women's health movement' – *Guardian*. 'The most comprehensive guide we've seen for women' – *Woman's World*. 'Every woman in the country should be issued with a copy free of charge' – *Mother & Baby*

Women's Experience of Sex   Sheila Kitzinger

Sheila Kitzinger explores the subject in a way that other books rarely aspire to – she places sex in the context of life and writes about women's feelings concerning their bodies, and the many different dimensions of sexual experience, reflecting the way individual attitudes can change between adolescence and later years.

The Past Is Before Us   Sheila Rowbotham

'An extraordinary, readable distillation of what [Sheila Rowbotham] calls an "account of ideas in the women's movement in Britain" … This is a book written from the inside, but with a clarity that recognizes the need to unravel ideas without abandoning the excitements and frustrations that every political movement brings with it' – *Sunday Times*

READ MORE IN PENGUIN

WOMEN'S INTEREST

When a Woman's Body Says No to Sex Linda Valins

Vaginismus – an involuntary spasm of the vaginal muscles that prevents penetration – has been discussed so little that many women who suffer from it don't recognize their condition by its name. Linda Valins's practical and compassionate guide will liberate these women from their fears and sense of isolation and help them find the right form of therapy.

Against Our Will Susan Brownmiller
Men, Women and Rape

Against Our Will sheds a new and blinding light on the tensions that exist between men and women. It was written to give rape its history. Now, as Susan Brownmiller concludes, 'we must deny it a future'. 'Thoughtful, informative and well researched' – *New Statesman*

The Feminine Mystique Betty Friedan

First published in the sixties, *The Feminine Mystique* was a major inspiration for the Women's Movement and continues to be a powerful and illuminating analysis of the position of women in Western society.

Understanding Women Luise Eichenbaum and Susie Orbach

Understanding Women, an expanded version of *Outside In ... Inside Out*, is a radical appraisal of women's psychological development based on clinical evidence. 'An exciting and thought-provoking book' – *British Journal of Psychiatry*

Psychoanalysis and Feminism Juliet Mitchell

The author of the widely acclaimed *Woman's Estate* here reassesses Freudian psychoanalysis in an attempt to develop an understanding of the psychology of femininity and the ideological oppression of women.

READ MORE IN PENGUIN

A SELECTION OF HEALTH BOOKS

Twins, Triplets and More Elizabeth Bryan

This enlightening study of the multiple birth phenomenon covers all aspects of the subject from conception and birth to old age and death. It also offers much comfort and support as well as carefully researched information gained from meeting several thousands of children and their families.

Meditation for Everybody Louis Proto

Meditation is liberation from stress, anxiety and depression. This lucid and readable book by the author of *Self-Healing* describes a variety of meditative practices. From simple breathing exercises to more advanced techniques, there is something here to suit everybody's needs.

Endometriosis Suzie Hayman

Endometriosis is currently surrounded by many damaging myths. Suzie Hayman's pioneering book will set the record straight and provide both sufferers and their doctors with the information necessary for an improved understanding of this frequently puzzling condition.

My Child Won't Eat Nick Yapp

Written by a qualified nutritionist, this reassuring guide will provide parents with the facts, help and comfort that will put their minds at rest and allow them to feed their children with confidence.

Not On Your Own Sally Burningham
The MIND Guide to Mental Health

Cutting through the jargon and confusion surrounding the subject of mental health to provide clear explanations and useful information, *Not On Your Own* will enable those with problems – as well as their friends and relatives – to make the best use of available help or find their own ways to cope.